PHARMACOLOGY FOR DENTAL HYGIENE PRACTICE

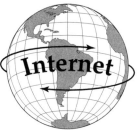

PHARMACOLOGY FOR DENTAL HYGIENE PRACTICE

Elena Bablenis Haveles, Pharm.D.

Clinical Associate Professor of Pharmacology
Old Dominion University
Norfolk, Virginia

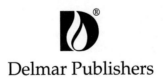

Delmar Publishers

an International Thomson Publishing company I(T)P®

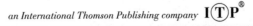

Albany • Bonn • Boston • Cincinnati • Detroit • London • Madrid
Melbourne • Mexico City • New York • Pacific Grove • Paris • San Francisco
Singapore • Tokyo • Toronto • Washington

Cover Design: Brucie Rosch

Delmar Staff

Publisher: Susan Simpfenderfer
Acquisition Editor: Kimberly A. Davies
Developmental Editor: Debra M. Flis
Project Editor: Coreen Filson

Production Coordinator: John Mickelbank
Art and Design Coordinator: Vincent S. Berger
Editorial Assistant: Donna L. Leto
Marketing Manager: Dawn Gerrain

COPYRIGHT © 1997
By Delmar Publishers, Inc.
an International Thomson Publishing Company

The ITP logo is a trademark under license.

Printed in the United States of America

For more information, contact:

Delmar Publishers
3 Columbia Circle, Box 15015
Albany, NY 12212-5015

International Thomson Publishing Europe
Berkshire House
168-173 High Holborn
WC1V7AA London,
England

Thomas Nelson Australia
102 Dodds Street
South Melbourne, 3205
Victoria, Australia

Nelson Canada
1120 Birchmount Road
Scarborough, Ontario
Canada, M1K 5G4

International Thomson Editores
Campos Eliseos 385, Piso 7
Col Polanco
11560 Mexico D F Mexico

International Thomson Publishing GmbH
Königswinterer Strasse. 418
53227 Bonn
Germany

International Thomson Publishing Asia
221 Henderson Road
#05-10 Henderson Building
Singapore 0315

International Thomson Publishing—Japan
Kyowa Building, 3F
2-2-1 Hirakawacho
Chiyoda-ku, Tokyo 102
Japan

1 2 3 4 5 6 7 8 9 10 XXX 02 01 00 99 98 97 96

Library of Congress Cataloging-in-Publication Data

Haveles, Elena Bablenis
    Pharmacology for dental hygiene practice / Elena B. Haveles.
      p.   cm.
    Includes bibliographical references and index.
    ISBN 0-8273-6602-7 (alk. paper)
    1. Dental pharmacology. 2. Clinical pharmacology. 3. Dental hygienists. I. Title
    [DNLM; 1. Pharmacology. 2. Drug therapy. 3. Prescriptions, Drug.
  4. Dental Hygienists. QV 4 H384p 1996]
  RK701.H38 1996
  615'.1'0246176—dc20
  DNLM/DCL
  for Library of Congress
                            96-17639
                              CIP

CONTENTS

PREFACE

Society has become information conscious and it is expected that the dental hygienist be knowledgeable about medications. Dental hygienists are called upon to complete medication/health histories, administer certain medications, provide basic counseling about oral hygiene, and, in some states, provide basic counseling about medications. The intent of this textbook is to provide the dental hygienist with the necessary knowledge of pharmacology to assess for medical illnesses, adverse reactions, and drug interactions that may interfere with dental treatments and oral health care. It is not intended that the dental hygienist take the place of the dentist in providing the patient with information about medications, but to work with the dentist in providing appropriate care to the patient.

My purpose is to make this a readable and clinically applicable resource in pharmacology that specifically addresses the needs of the dental hygienist. The textbook is divided into four sections: general principles of pharmacology, drugs used in dentistry, drugs that the patient is taking, and topics of general interest. Generic drug names are in bold the first time that they appear in a chapter to let the reader know their importance in the chapter. Each chapter includes dental concerns and case studies that help to strengthen clinical skills. This textbook will help meet the needs of today's dental hygienist through its emphasis on communication and clinical pharmacology.

Elena Bablenis Haveles, Pharm.D.

In memory of my mother:
Mary Georgeadys Bablenis

To my husband Paul and son Andrew:
Thank you for allowing me the time to spend countless evenings and weekends working on this project. I love you both.

To my father Harry C. Bablenis:
Thank you for all your guidance and love throughout these many years.

LIST OF FIGURES

PART I

INTRODUCTION

CHAPTER 1

General Principles of Pharmacology

Key Terms

Controlled Substance Act of 1970   Pharmacology
Federal Regulatory Agencies   Prescription
Generic Equivalence   Trade Name
Generic Name

LEARNING OBJECTIVES

After completion of this chapter and its learning activities, the student should be able to:

1. Define pharmacology.
2. List and describe the related disciplines associated with pharmacology.
3. Describe the role of the dental hygienist in pharmacology.
4. List where detailed and updated information on medications can be found.
5. Describe the different names used to identify medications and explain how they can impact counseling a patient and obtaining a medication history.
6. Define generic equivalence and how it is related to drug substitution.
7. List the different parts of the prescription.
8. Define the role of the dental hygienist in the prescription writing process.
9. List the federal regulatory agencies involved in the regulation of medications.
10. Review the Controlled Substance Act of 1970.

INTRODUCTION

In today's changing health-care environment it is important for the dental hygienist to know more than the name of a medication. Patients rely on the dental hygienist to provide them with the correct information regarding their medication and oral health care. Basic knowledge of pharmacology and its related disciplines will help the dental hygienist provide more effective care to the patient.

PHARMACOLOGY

Pharmacology is the study of drugs and their effects on living organisms. It is one of the most important disciplines of medicine and other health professions. In addition to pharmacology, the dental hygienist should know about its related disciplines, as listed and defined in Table 1-1.

THE ROLE OF THE DENTAL HYGIENIST IN PHARMACOLOGY

A sound knowledge of pharmacology is necessary for today's practicing dental hygienist. Dental hygienists may be called upon to complete medication/health histories, administer medication, or respond to a medical emergency. This section focuses on some of these areas.

Obtaining a Medication/Health History

Obtaining a medication/health history is the first step in safely treating a patient (Table 1-2). Patients may be taking any number of medications that may interact with medications used in dentistry. An understanding of their mechanism of action, adverse reactions, indications for use, and interactions can help avoid potential problems during a dental procedure. Because many drug names sound alike and many drugs look alike, it is important to determine what the patient is taking before starting any dental procedure. A detailed health/medication history allows the dental hygienist to provide the best possible care for the patient.

Medication Administration

Dental hygienists can administer several different medications in the dental office and knowledge of these agents is of great importance. Hygienists commonly apply fluoride treatments, and in some states administer local anesthetics and nitrous oxide. In some states, dental hygienists are working toward attaining solo practices and limited prescriptive authority. Both require an in-depth knowledge of pharmacology.

Table 1-1   Disciplines Related to Pharmacology

Areas of Pharmacology	*Definition*
Pharmacotherapy	The use of medications to treat different disease states
Pharmacodynamics	The study of the action of drugs on living organisms
Pharmacokinetics	The study of what the body does to the drug; the measurement of the absorption, duration of action, distribution, metabolism, and excretion of a drug from the body
Pharmacy	The practice of compounding, preparing, dispensing of drugs, and counseling of patients about their medication
Toxicology	The study of the harmful effects of drugs on living tissues

---

Table 1-2   Obtaining a Medication/Health History

---

1. **Do you take any medication for _____ ?**
   Heart
   Lungs
   Sugar
   Ulcer/Nervous Stomach
   Thoughts, Sleep, Nerves
   Arthritis (Rheumatism)
   Seizures

---

2. **What are the names of your medicines and how many times a day do you take them?**

3. **How many times a day did your doctor tell you to take your medicine?**

---

4. **Do you take any medicine that you can buy without a prescription? (for example)**
   Acetaminophen, Aspirin, Ibuprofen, Naproxen
   Antihistamines/Decongestants (Diphenhydramine, Pseudoephedrine)
   Contraceptives
   Cough and Cold Products
   Sleep Aids
   Laxatives

---

5. **Do you have any allergies to medicines?, If yes, what medicines?**

6. **What happened to you when you took the medicine?**

Appointment Scheduling

A knowledge of pharmacology is also important when scheduling a patient for an appointment. Some systemic illnesses require appointments at specific times of the day. Patients with asthma do best with morning appointments. Stress can precipitate asthma attacks, and most patients are under less stress in the morning when they have less time to think about upcoming stressful events such as dental appointments. Diabetic patients requiring oral surgery should be scheduled for morning appointments 1 to 1-1/2 hours after breakfast and their morning antidiabetic medication. This places the patient under the least amount of stress. All other appointments should be scheduled around meal times.

Information Sharing

The dental hygienist often discusses the patient's medications with the dentist, other health-care professionals, and the patient. A sound knowledge base about mechanisms of action, therapeutic uses, adverse reactions, and drug interactions will help facilitate discussions with the patient, dentist, or other health professionals. Also, the patient may ask the hygienist to explain a prescription that the dentist has just written.

Medical Emergencies

Dental hygienists help respond to emergency situations that may arise in the dental office. A knowledge of pharmacology may prevent the emergency or will help the hygienist respond appropriately should one occur.

SOURCES OF INFORMATION

There are many different medications available and it is important for the dental hygienist to know where to look for information about medication. There are many sources, including reference texts and association journals, where pertinent drug information can be found. Table 1-3 reviews several different sources of information.

DRUG NOMENCLATURE

Medications have several different names. It is important for hygienists to know these names so that they are better able to discuss them with the patient, family members, and other health professionals.

Chemical Name

The first name that a drug receives is its chemical name. The chemical name is determined by the chemical structure of the drug. If the chemical structure of the drug has not been identified, then the drug receives a code name that is a combination of letters and numbers.

Trade Name

Once a drug has been found to be useful, safe, and effective it is given its proprietary/brand or trade name. The *trade name* is the registered property of the company and is protected for 17 years under the Federal Patent Law. Trade names are usually chosen so that they can be easily remembered. The brand name is used interchangeably with the trade name.

Generic Name

The drug receives its generic name prior to marketing. The *generic name* is the official name of the drug determined by the United States Adopted Names Council. It appears on all prescription labels. Figure 1-1 provides an example of the chemical, generic, and trade names of **ibuprofen,** a popular prescription and nonprescription analgesic medication.

Trade Name vs. Generic Name Products. It is especially important for the dental hygienist to know both the trade and generic names. The 17-year patent on the more popular trade name medications has expired and other companies now manufacture and distribute *generic equivalents* of the trade products. Patients remember either the

Table 1-3   Selected Drug Information References

Reference	Brief Description
AHFS Drug Information	Updated annually with quarterly supplements by the American Society of Health System's Pharmacists. It provides detailed, unbiased information on all aspects of a medication.
Drug Facts and Comparison	Published yearly with monthly updates *Facts and Comparison*. It provides detailed information on most prescription and nonprescription drugs and is arranged by pharmacologic class.
Drug Interaction Facts	Published yearly with monthly updates *Facts and Comparison*. It provides information on reported drug interactions and rates clinical significance of those interactions.
Handbook of Nonprescription Drugs	Published every 3 years by the American Pharmaceutical Association. This textbook provides the reader with detailed information about all classes of nonprescription drugs available in the United States. It also reviews the pathophysiology of the different disease states and their treatments. This book has excellent drug monographs at the end of each chapter.
Merck Manual	Published every 5 to 6 years by Merck Research Labs. This reference book provides the reader with general information on disease states and drug therapy.
Physicians Desk Reference (PDR)	Published yearly by Medical Economics Data. This reference book lists those higher-volume drugs of pharmaceutical companies that have purchased space in the book. It is indexed by manufacturer, product name, generic name, product category, and product information. It gives a brief description of the drug including pharmacology, pharmacokinetics, indications for use, adverse reactions, drug interactions, and dosages. The information in the PDR is identical to that found in the package inserts required for each drug.
United States Pharmacopeia— Drug Information (USP DI), Vol. 1, *Drug Information for the Health Care Professional,* and Vol. 2, *Advice for the Patient*	The USP DI, volumes 1 and 2, are published yearly with monthly updates by the United States Pharmacopeial Convention. Volume 1 provides the health professional with necessary information regarding basic pharmacology and pharmacokinetics, drug interactions, adverse reactions, and dosages. Volume 2 is written in laymen's terms regarding pharmacology, pharmacokinetics, dosing, adverse reactions, and drug interactions.
Goodman and Gilman's, The Pharmacological Basis of Therapeutics	This pharmacology textbook is published every 5 years by Pergamon Press. This is the standard pharmacology textbook for pharmacy and medicine. It provides the reader with in-depth information regarding the chemistry, mechanism of action, pharmacologic effects, pharmacokinetics, adverse reactions, and therapeutic uses of drugs.

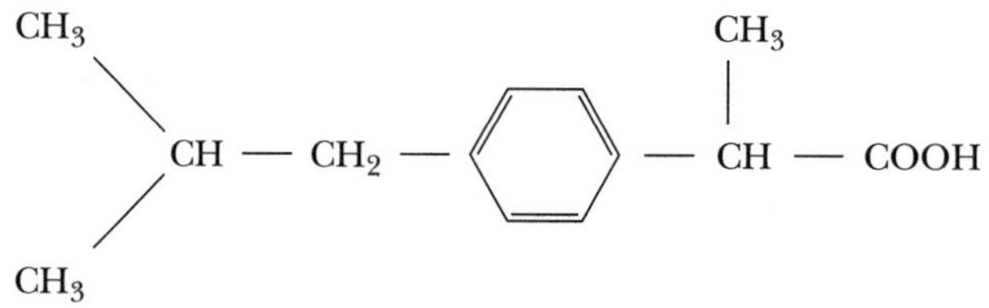

Chemical Name: (±)-2-(p-isobutylphenyl) propionic acid
Generic Name: Ibuprofen
Trade Name: Motrin®, Rufen®

Figure 1-1   *A comparison of the chemical, generic, and trade names of Ibuprofen*

trade name or generic name of their medication depending on which name appeared on the prescription label. The dental hygienist should know both the generic and trade names of medication. Patients should bring in their medications and the dental hygienist should review each prescription label and check the generic name to determine what the patient is taking.

GENERIC EQUIVALENCE

Many patients and health professionals have concerns about the effectiveness of generic medications. They want to know if the generic product is equivalent and as effective as the trade product. In 1984, Congress passed the Drug Price Competition and Patent Term Restoration Act allowing generic companies to receive expedited review from the Food and Drug Administration (FDA) without having to go through the same testing as the trade companies. Generic companies are required to prove that their product is biologically equivalent to the trade company's product, which means that the generic drug produces similar concentrations in the blood and other tissues as the trade drug. The generic drug must also enter the bloodstream at the same rate as the trade drug. The majority of generic drugs meet FDA guidelines and can be safely substituted for trade products.

PRESCRIPTION WRITING

It is important for dental hygienists to become familiar with prescription writing. Although they do not write prescriptions, they may be asked to review them with patients. Knowledge about prescription writing can help the hygienist provide a double-check for the prescriber. The double-check can help prevent delays at the pharmacy if information is missing from the prescription.

Definition of a Prescription

A *prescription* is an order for a specific medication for a specified patient at a particular time, with appropriate instructions for how the patient is to use the prescribed medication. The prescription order may be given to a pharmacist by a physician, dentist, podiatrist, physician's assistant, pharmacist, nurse practitioner, veterinarian, or any other legally recognized medical provider either as a written prescription, or a verbal or telephone order (which in certain instances may also require a written prescription as confirmation).

Composition of the Prescription

A complete prescription is composed of several parts (Figure 1-2). The name, address, and phone number of the prescriber appears at the top of the prescription. The body of the prescription is defined as follows.

Superscription. The superscription includes the name, address, age of the patient, date prescribed, and the R_x symbol, which means "take thou" in Latin. For children, the exact age and weight should be noted so the pharmacist can monitor the prescribed dose. The date prescribed is an accurate record of when the prescriber issued the prescription. The dental hygienist can review each prescription for all necessary information.

Ted E. Jones, DDS
315 Main Street
Anytown, USA 02220
(111)-222-3333

Patient Name _____   Age _____

Address _____   Date _____

R_x Amoxicillin 500 mg

Disp: #40

Sig: T cap q 6h × 10 days

Refills   0 1 2 3 4 5 prn

_____   _____

Substitution Allowed   Dispense As Written

DEA#_____

Figure 1-2 *Example of a prescription*

Inscription. The inscription contains the name, strength, dose form, and quantity of the drug prescribed.

Subscription. The subscription contains the directions to the pharmacist as to the quantity or method of preparation.

Transcription (Signature). The "Sig" means "mark thou" in Latin and is the directions for the patient. They should be written as completely and clearly as possible; use of the phrase "as directed" is discouraged since many patients may forget the instructions that the provider has given to them. Certain Latin abbreviations and phrases remain in use and are listed in Table 1-4.

The prescription is closed with the prescriber's signature, Drug Enforcement Agency (DEA) number if required, refill instructions, and instructions for either dispensing the generic product or as written by the prescriber.

Instructions to the Patient. Once the prescription has been written, the dental hygienist should review it with the patient to make sure the patient understands what medication is prescribed and how it should be taken. The dental hygienist should also review how long to take the medication, possible adverse reactions and what to do should they occur, drug interactions, and the reason for taking the medication. Well-informed patients are often more compliant with their medications. The den-

Table 1-4   Common Latin Abbreviations in Prescriptions

Abbreviation	*Interpretation*
a.	Before
a.c.	Before meals
A.D.	Right ear
A.L.	Left ear
b.i.d.	Twice a day
gtt.	Drop
h.	Hour
h.s.	Bedtime
o.u.	Each eye
o.d.	Right eye
o.s.	Left eye
p.o.	By mouth
p.c.	After meals
p.r.	By rectum
p.r.n.	As needed
q.d.	Once a day
q.i.d.	Four times a day
q.o.d.	Every other day
q 6 h	Every six hours
sl.	Sublingual
supp.	Suppository
t.i.d.	Three times a day
u.d.	As directed

tal hygienist should make sure that the prescribed medications are recorded in the patient's record.

Prescription Safety. Prescription pads should be kept in secure places. Substance abusers or others may try to steal the prescription pads for personal use or sell them. The prescriber's DEA number should be written down only when necessary—that is, if a controlled substance is prescribed or when required by a patient's prescription coverage plan.

FEDERAL REGULATORY AGENCIES

Several different *federal regulatory agencies* are involved in the production, marketing, advertising, labeling, and prescribing of medication. The FDA approves drugs for marketing in the United States after considering safety, efficacy, and physical and chemical data. The FDA also requires quality control of manufacturing facilities, determines what drugs are sold by prescription, and regulates the advertising and labeling of prescription drugs.

   The DEA is a division of the Department of Justice and administers the Controlled Substance Act of 1970. The DEA regulates the manufacturing and distribution of substances with a potential for abuse, such as opioid narcotics, benzodiazepines, and barbiturates.

DRUG LEGISLATION

Prior to 1906, there were no laws that helped regulate medications. The Food and Drug Act of 1906 helped regulate interstate commerce of drugs. This act was followed by a series of acts and amendments that helped set the standards for prescription medications. The various laws required certain medications to be sold by prescription only and to be labeled as such, and prevented the interstate commerce of drugs that were not proven safe.

   In 1914, Congress passed the Harrison Narcotic Act of 1914, which provided the federal government with control over narcotic drugs. It also mandated that all practitioners prescribing narcotics be registered with the federal government.

   In 1962, the Kefauver-Harris Bill was passed, which required manufacturers to prove the efficacy of all drugs, follow strict rules for testing, and report all adverse effects from drugs already on the market. Manufacturers were also required to list drugs by their generic names in labeling and advertising and to state adverse reactions, contraindications, and drug efficacy.

   Other amendments and acts were subsequently passed in 1965 and 1970 regulating controlled substances, for example the Drug Abuse Control Amendment of 1965 and the Controlled Substance Act of 1970.

Controlled Substance Act of 1970

The *Controlled Substance Act of 1970* set the current requirements for the prescription writing of drugs with a potential for abuse such as narcotic analgesics, antianxiety drugs, and barbiturates. It also placed medications with a potential for abuse into any one of five schedules. Table 1-5 reviews those schedules.

Table 1-5   Controlled Substance Act of 1970

Schedule	Definition	Example
Schedule I	1. High potential for abuse 2. No accepted medical use in the U.S.	Heroin, PCP
Schedule II	1. High potential for abuse 2. Substance has currently accepted use in the U.S. or currently accepted use with severe restrictions 3. Abuse may lead to severe psychological or physical dependence	Oxycodone, Morphine
Schedule III	1. Potential for abuse less than I or II 2. Currently accepted medical use in the U.S. 3. Abuse may lead to moderate or low physical dependence and high psychological dependence	Anabolic Steroids, Codeine
Schedule IV	1. Low potential for abuse relative to III 2. Current accepted medical use in the U.S. 3. Abuse may lead to limited physical or psychological dependence relative to III	Benzodiazepines, Phenobarbital
Schedule V	1. Low potential for abuse relative to IV 2. Current accepted use in the U.S. 3. Limited physical and psychological dependence relative to IV	Some codeine-containing cough syrups

The current requirements of the act are:

1. Prescriptions for a controlled substance require a DEA number.
2. Schedule II–V drugs require a prescription.
3. Schedule II prescriptions must be signed in ink, cannot be telephoned into the pharmacy (except in an emergency), and are not refillable. If a prescription is called into a pharmacy, the signed original must be delivered to the pharmacy within 72 hours of the phone call. Only an authorized practitioner with prescribing privileges may sign the prescription.
4. Certain states require duplicate or triplicate prescriptions for Schedule II drugs. The state of New York requires a triplicate prescription form for benzodiazepines, which are Schedule III drugs. With a duplicate prescription, one copy is kept in the pharmacy and the other is sent to the state board of pharmacy. With a triplicate prescription, one copy is kept in the prescriber's office, one is kept in the pharmacy, and the other is sent to the state board of pharmacy. These prescription blanks must be ordered through the state board of pharmacy.
5. Schedule III–V drugs can be telephoned into the pharmacy and can be refilled if noted on the prescription. There is a maximum on the number of refills allowed. The patient is allowed up to 5 refills over 6 months.

Summary

Today, the dental hygienist is often the first contact that the patient has in the dental office. Patients rely on hygienists to provide them with the correct information about their medications and oral health care. Patients also expect the hygienist to know all about the medications that they may be taking.

A good understanding of pharmacology and how it relates to dental hygiene is very important in today's health-care environment. There are many references (textbooks, reference books, and journals) available to help the dental hygienist learn about pharmacology. Dental hygienists should have several references in their office and should know how to use reference materials.

Medications have several different names that the hygienist needs to know. Also, many brand name medications are available as generic equivalents. Familiarity with these names will help when asking patients questions during a medication history. Medications can be chemically, biologically, and therapeutically equivalent. The dental hygienist should be familiar with these terms and their application in the practice of dental hygiene.

Though dental hygienists do not prescribe medications, they should be familiar with the process of prescription writing and the components of a prescription.

Case Study: Susan Jones

Susan Jones is new to your practice. She is 35 years old, married, and has two children. Since this is her first appointment, you must conduct the health/medication history.

1. What types of questions would you ask during a health/medication history?
2. What is the importance of the health/medication history?

During the history you learn that Mrs. Jones is a healthy individual whose only prescribed medication is the medroxyprogesterone acetate shot. She does have a family history of depression and hypertension. Upon further questioning you learn that Mrs. Jones self-treats with an occasional acetaminophen or ibuprofen.

3. Where can you look up information about medroxyprogesterone acetate?
4. What is a good reference source for over-the-counter medications?

Mrs. Jones returns for another visit and is prescribed an antibiotic for an abscess. The prescription reads as follows: Penicillin 250 mg Sig: 1 q.i.d. × 10 days. The dentist asks you to review the prescription with Mrs. Jones.

5. Please explain the prescription to Mrs. Jones.

Case Study: Jamal Taylor

Jamal Taylor is a 50-year-old male who has been coming to your practice for the past 15 years. He is married and has two daughters, one who is currently a senior in high school. His daughter is considering a career in dental hygiene and Mr. Taylor was hoping that you could answer some questions for him at the end of his appointment.

1. Why does the dental hygienist need to study pharmacology? Mr. Taylor was always under the impression that only the dentist spoke to the patient about medications.
2. Mr. Taylor required a prescription for ibuprofen 600 mg, 1 tablet three times a day, for dental pain that was a result of his procedure. You take this opportunity to explain the prescription to him and what a dental hygienist needs to know about writing prescriptions. What would you tell him about the prescription?
3. Mr. Taylor would also like to know why drugs have different names. Please explain this to Mr. Taylor.
4. Mr. Taylor would like to know where he can get information about this medication and any others that he may take. What would you tell him?

Review Questions

1. What is the role of the dental hygienist in pharmacology?
2. What are some of the different disciplines associated with pharmacology? Explain them.
3. Compare and contrast the different names that each drug is assigned.
4. What is generic equivalence and why is it a concern of health professionals and the lay public?
5. What are the different parts of the prescription? What should the dental hygienist tell the patient about the prescription?
6. What is the Controlled Substance Act of 1970?
7. What are the different schedules of the Controlled Substance Act? Explain them.
8. Why is it important to have good reference materials in your office practice?

BIBLIOGRAPHY

Bills GW, Soderberg RC: *Principles of Pharmacology for Respiratory Care.* Delmar Publishers Inc. ITP, Albany, 1994.
Cramer JA, Mattson RH, Prevey ML, Scheyer RD, Ouellette VL: How often is medication taken as prescribed? A novel assessment technique. *JAMA* 261:3272–3277, 1989.
Kessler DA, Rose JL, Temple RJ, Shapiro R, Griffin JP: Therapeutic-class wars—drug promotion in a competitive marketplace. *N Engl J Med* 331:1350–1353, 1994.
Overstreet Price K, Andel Goldwier M: Drug information resources. *Am Pharm* NS34:30–39, 1994.
Smith CM, Reynard AM: *Textbook of Pharmacology,* 1st ed. W. B. Saunders, Philadelphia, 1992.
Smith DL: Compliance packaging: A patient education tool. *Am Pharm* NS29:42–53, 1989.

CHAPTER 2

Drug Action

Key Terms

Absorption
Adverse Reaction
Allergy
Distribution
Excretion

Metabolism
Potency
Side Effect
Therapeutic Index

LEARNING OBJECTIVES

After completion of this chapter and its learning activities, the student should be able to:

1. Briefly describe a dose-response curve and its relationship to pharmacology.
2. Briefly describe the following terms and their relationship to drug dosing: potency, therapeutic index, idiosyncrasy, allergy, tolerance, therapeutic effect, side effect, toxic effect, adverse reaction.
3. Discuss the different transport mechanisms available for drug absorption.
4. Discuss the importance of lipid solubility and drug ionization in relation to drug absorption.
5. Discuss the factors that affect drug passage across biologic membranes.
6. Discuss drug distribution including plasma protein binding, tissue affinity, and blood flow.
7. Discuss drug metabolism and how it can affect drug dosing.
8. Discuss the different routes of drug excretion and what factors can influence them.
9. Discuss the different routes of drug administration including time of onset and use.
10. Discuss the different factors that can alter drug effects.

INTRODUCTION

A drug is a biologically active substance that can modify cellular function. A general understanding of drug action is important for all health professionals and will allow the dental hygienist to make informed decisions regarding possible drug interactions or adverse reactions for the dental patient. The intent of this chapter is to review some of the quantitative aspects of drug action, the different routes of drug administration, and the action of drugs in the body.

QUANTITATIVE ASPECTS OF DRUG ACTION

Dose-response curve, potency, and efficacy are terms used to measure drug response. These concepts and those used to describe both desired and undesired drug responses are reviewed in this section.

Dose-Response Curve

Whenever a drug exerts its effect on a biologic system, it is possible to measure the response to the dose of the drug given. The dose of the drug is plotted against the intensity of the effect, resulting in a dose-response curve as demonstrated in Figure 2-1.

If this curve is replotted using the log of the dose versus the response of the drug, another dose-response curve is formed that can help to determine the potency and efficacy of the drug's action (Figure 2-2).

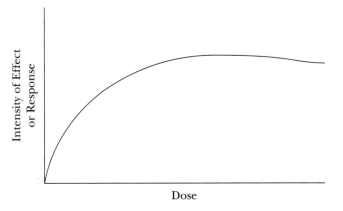

Figure 2-1   *Dose-response curve*

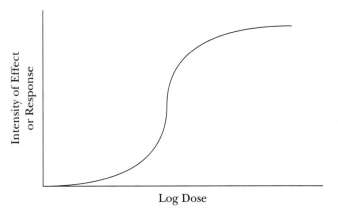

Figure 2-2   *Log dose-response curve*

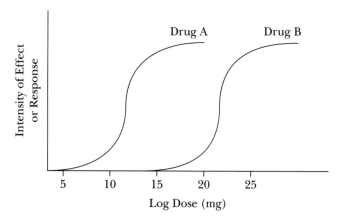

Figure 2-3   *Two different drugs of the same therapeutic class*

In both figures, dose and response increase in a corresponding fashion. Eventually, further increases in dose will not coincide with further increases in drug response. Additional increases in dose may actually lead to toxic or adverse reactions.

Potency

The *potency* of a drug is determined by the dose needed to produce the desired therapeutic effect. In Figure 2-3, drug A is more potent than drug B because a smaller dose of drug A is required to produce the desired therapeutic effect. A higher dose of drug B is required to produce an effect equal to drug A.

The potency of drugs should not be an issue as long as appropriate doses of medication are used. Less potent drugs require higher doses to produce therapeutic effects whereas more potent drugs can reach toxic levels at lower doses. Review the proper dosage of each drug before it is prescribed to the patient.

Therapeutic Index

The *therapeutic index* (TI) is a ratio of the median lethal dose (LD_{50}) to the median effective dose (ED_{50}) and can be expressed as follows:

$$TI = \frac{LD_{50}}{ED_{50}}$$

The LD_{50} is the dose of the drug required to produce death in 50% of test animals. The ED_{50} is the dose of the drug required to produced the desired clinical effect in 50% of test animals. The greater the TI, the safer the drug. Drugs with a low TI (closer to zero) require careful monitoring in order to avoid toxic reactions. An example of a drug with a low TI is **digoxin** (Lanoxin), a drug used to treat congestive heart failure.

Drug Effects

Drugs can produce both therapeutic and undesirable effects. The therapeutic effect of the drug is the intended drug effect (e.g., sleep, pain relief). *Adverse reactions* effects can be an extension of the drug's pharmacologic effect, a *side effect,* or *allergy* and are reviewed in Table 2-1.

PHARMACOKINETICS

This section discusses the pharmacokinetics of drugs, that is, what happens to the drug once it has been administered to the patient. Pharmacokinetics is collectively known as drug absorption, distribution, metabolism, and excretion (ADME).

Absorption

Once a drug has been introduced into a patient's body, it is *absorbed,* by varying degrees, into the systemic circulation. As the drug is absorbed through the complex structure of cells and tissues, it must negotiate various transport mechanisms as well as its own degree of lipid (fat) solubility and ionization.

Transport Mechanisms. Drugs are absorbed into the body with the assistance of several different transport mechanisms. The most common is passive diffusion, which is regulated by a concentration gradient. During passive diffusion (Figure 2-4), a solute or drug moves from an area of high concentration to one of lower concentration.

In some instances a drug may require assistance in crossing a biologic membrane, which can be described as carrier-assisted transport. The most important type of carrier-assisted transport is active transport. During active transport the drug crosses the membrane against a concentration of electrochemical gradient and requires an energy source.

Table 2-1   Classification of Drug Reactions

Drug Reaction	*Definition*
Therapeutic effect	Desired pharmacologic effect
Adverse reaction	Exaggerated effect on target and nontarget tissues and organs
A. Side effect	Predictable, dose-related effect that acts on nontarget organs
B. Toxic reaction	Predictable, dose-related reaction that acts on target organs
	Extension of the drug's pharmacologic effects
C. Idiosyncratic reaction	Genetically related abnormal drug response
D. Allergic reaction	Nonpredictable, non-dose-related reaction
	Immunologic response of the body toward the drug

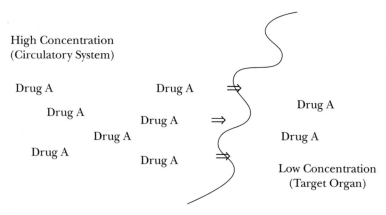

High Concentration
(Circulatory System)

Drug A   Drug A   ⇒

Drug A   Drug A

Drug A   Drug A   ⇒

Drug A   Drug A

Drug A   Drug A   ⇒

Low Concentration
(Target Organ)

Figure 2-4   *Passive diffusion*

Facilitated diffusion is another type of carrier-assisted transportation. During facilitated diffusion the drug is transported down the concentration gradient. It is more efficient and tends to occur at a greater rate than passive diffusion.

Lipid Solubility. The cell membrane is made up of significant amounts of lipid materials that can influence drug absorption. Drugs that are lipid soluble can readily pass through these membranes whereas lipid-insoluble drugs are barred passage. Examples of lipid-soluble drugs include general anesthetics and benzodiazepines.

Drug Ionization. Drugs that are water soluble or partially lipid soluble present a more complex problem in their ability to cross a biologic membrane. These drugs must be either weak acids or bases in order to be absorbed into the membrane. Weak acids and bases, when in solution, tend to be nonionized and are much more readily absorbed across biologic membranes. Absorption is difficult for drugs in their ionized state because ionized molecules are less lipid soluble and have more difficulty in crossing biologic membranes. Also, small ionized molecules are highly charged particles that have difficulty crossing membranes because of repulsion by fixed charges in the membrane channels and on the membrane surface.

As a result, the pH of tissue fluids is an important factor in the rate of drug absorption. The more neutral the drug, the better it will be absorbed. The pH of the tissue fluid will determine the ratio of the unionized to the ionized form of the drug that is present. This relationship can be best described using the Henderson–Hasselbach equation:

$$pH = pK_a + \log \frac{\text{ionized drug}}{\text{unionized drug}}$$

This equation tell us that acidic drugs are more readily absorbed in an acidic environment and basic drugs in a basic environment. For example, acidic drugs are more readily absorbed than basic drugs in the low pH of gastric fluids. Other medications, such as antacids, can raise the pH of the stomach and decrease the absorption of acidic drugs. Some basic drugs (or acidic drugs, which can be irritating to the gastrointestinal tract) are coated so that they can be absorbed in the small intestine, which is a more basic environment.

Passage across Biologic Membranes. In order for a drug to be absorbed into the body it must pass across any one of a number of biologic membranes. Biologic membranes act as barriers to drug absorption and can include the layers of cells in the gastrointestinal tract and capillaries or the plasma membrane of a cell. Figure 2-5 diagrammatically reviews one of the more commonly accepted concepts of biologic membranes and is commonly referred to as the fluid mosaic model.

The cell or biologic membrane is composed of two layers of lipid material interspersed with various sizes of protein that constantly change their position. There are also several small openings or channels that can allow for the passage of water or water-soluble molecules. Lipid soluble molecules much more readily pass across this lipid membrane.

Some membranes, such as the capillary endothelium, have larger openings that allow for the passage of small and medium-size molecules of water or water-soluble drug molecules into blood and into and through intestinal villi. Other biologic membranes have such small channels that only lipid-soluble substances are allowed to pass through, for example, the blood-brain barrier of the central nervous system.

Drug Receptors. Once a drug passes through the biologic membrane, it is carried to many different areas of the body, or site of action, to exert its therapeutic or adverse effect. In order for the drug to exert its effects, it must bind with the receptor site on the cell membrane. Drug receptors appear to consist of many large molecules that exist either on the cell membrane or within the cell itself. More than one receptor type or identical receptors can be found at the site of action. Usually, a specific drug will bind with a specific receptor in what is known as the lock and key fashion (Figure 2-6).

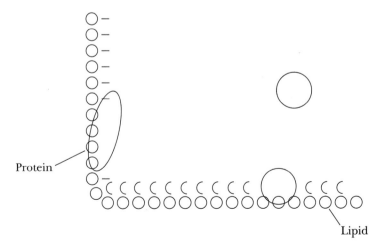

Figure 2-5 *Fluid mosaic model*

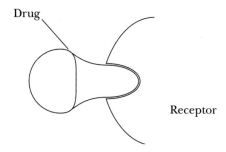

Figure 2-6 *Drug-receptor interaction*

Most drug-receptor interactions consist of weak chemical bonds and the energy formed during this interaction is very low. As a result, the bonds can be formed and broken very easily. Once a bond is broken, another drug molecule immediately binds to the receptor.

Different drugs often compete for the same receptor sites. The drug with the higher affinity for the receptor will bind to more receptors than the drug with the weaker affinity. More of the drug with the weaker affinity will be required to produce a pharmacologic response (see Figure 2-7). Drugs with a higher affinity for receptor sites are more potent than drugs with a weaker affinity.

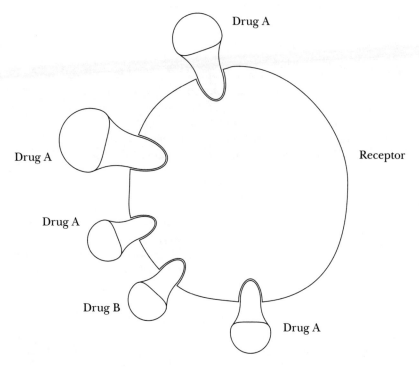

Figure 2-7 *Drug-receptor affinity*

More than one drug can bind to the same receptor and can cause an intensified drug action. These drugs are called agonists. Other drugs bind to the same receptor and no effect is produced. These drugs are referred to as antagonists.

Drug Distribution

Once a drug is absorbed, it is *distributed* throughout the body by blood. Those areas with the highest amount of blood flow have a higher concentration of drug distribution. The drug is frequently distributed to areas in which it does not immediately exert its pharmacologic effect. If all the drug were allowed to travel freely throughout the body, very little would be available for drug action; much of the drug would be metabolized and excreted from the body. This section discusses several different factors that influence drug distribution.

Protein Binding. Within plasma, there are different types of proteins that exert a chemical attraction to different drugs. These molecules are large and have a difficult time crossing biologic membranes. Once a drug binds to a protein, it cannot exert its pharmacologic effect, whereas a portion of the drug that does not bind to protein can exert its pharmacologic effect. The drug remains in constant equilibrium between the bound and unbound form and a slight change in protein binding can significantly alter drug effects. Some drugs compete for the same protein binding sites and the drug with the stronger affinity can displace the other drug, causing adverse or toxic reactions. Elderly patients and those with compromised nutritional states have low protein levels and are more at risk for toxic reactions.

Tissue Binding. Some drugs bind to other body tissues as well as protein molecules. The tissues serve as additional storage sites for the drug and cause significant clinical effects. For example, **tetracycline** antibiotics have a high affinity for developing bones and teeth of the fetus and young children. As a result, these medications are contraindicated in pregnant and nursing women and children under 8 years of age. Benzodiazepines, which are lipid soluble, tend to be stored in fat cells, which may be a problem in elderly patients who have a higher fat to muscle ratio. Lower doses should be used and any dose increases should be gradual.

Drug Metabolism

One of the first places to which a drug is distributed is the liver, which is the primary site of drug *metabolism.* Drug metabolism or biotransformation can also take place in plasma, kidneys, and other tissues. During drug metabolism the drug is altered, inactivated, changed, or prepared for elimination. Biotransformation also makes the drug more polar and water soluble and thus more readily excreted by the kidneys.

One of the most important biochemical systems available for biotransformation is the microsomal enzyme system located within the smooth endoplasmic reticulum of the liver. Of the different enzyme systems, the cytochrome P450 system is the most important. Examples of drugs metabolized by the cytochrome P450 system include **cimetidine, phenytoin,** and **phenobarbital.** Age, gender, and drugs can increase or decrease drug metabolism which can increase or decrease drug concentration in the body.

Drug Excretion

A drug can be *excreted* from the body by several different routes including the kidneys, sweat, saliva, respiratory tract, gastrointestinal tract, and breast milk in lactating mothers. The majority of drugs are excreted through the kidneys. Blood passes through the kidneys and both ionized and unionized drugs are filtered through the glomerulus of the nephron. Drugs bound to plasma proteins are reabsorbed into the body because they are too large for the pores of glomeruli. Urinary waste products and drugs metabolized into a water-soluble, ionized form are then excreted from the body. Urinary pH can be altered to enhance drug excretion from the body or drug reabsorption into the body.

ROUTES OF ADMINISTRATION

In order for a drug to produce its effect on the body it must first enter the body by any one of the routes listed in Table 2-2. The oral route is the most common route of administration and is considered the most convenient, acceptable, and safest route. In cases of overdose or toxic reactions, an antidote or gastric lavage can be given to counteract the negative drug effects. Disadvantages include slow onset of drug action; irregular drug absorption as a result of food, pathologic disease states, or other drugs, gastrointestinal upset due to the irritating effects of the drug, and patient age. Younger children, elderly patients, and even some adults have a hard time swallowing tablets and capsules.

The intravenous (IV) route of administration provides the patient with the most rapid drug response. It is used during emergency situations or for drugs that are destroyed or inactivated in the gastrointestinal (GI) tract or too poorly absorbed by the GI tract to produce an adequate drug response. It is also used for patients who are unconscious, uncooperative, or otherwise cannot take oral medication. Absorption by the IV route produces more predictable blood levels than oral dose forms. The main disadvantage to IV administration is that the drug is injected directly into the patient's bloodstream, making the reversal of toxic or overdose situations difficult.

Other routes of parenteral administration include intramuscular, subcutaneous, intraarterial, intracardiac, intrathecal, intraosseous, intraarticular, intrasynovial, and intracutaneous or intradermal. Drugs that are destroyed in the GI tract or are irritating to the skin or bloodstream are administered as intramuscular (IM) injections.

Other routes of administration include sublingual, buccal, transdermal, topical, conjunctival, aural, intraocular, oral and nasal inhalation, rectal, and vaginal. Transdermal patches are becoming more popular because of their convenience and dosing intervals. Transdermal patches are convenient because they are placed on the skin, and dosing intervals can be any time from 3 to 7 days.

FACTORS THAT AFFECT DRUG ABSORPTION

There are many different factors that can affect drug absorption. In this section we review several of these factors.

Table 2-2   Selected Routes of Administration

Route	Onset of Action	Reason for Use	Example
Oral	15 minutes to 1 hour	Patient convenience	Most all prescription and nonprescription medications
Sublingual	Minutes	Rapid response is necessary	Nitroglycerin tablets
Buccal	Minutes	Rapid response is necessary	Nitroglycerin tablets, nifedipine capsules
Inhalation			
Oral	Within 1 minute	Local effects to the lungs	Bronchodilators Ephedrine,
Nasal	Within 1 minute	Local effects to the nasal passages	beclamethasone (steroid inhalers)
Conjunctival	Minutes	Local effects to the conjunctiva	Various eye ointments
Intraocular	Minutes	Local effect to the eye	Treatment of glaucoma
Aural	Minutes	Local effect to the ear	Various over-the-counter and prescription drops
Topical	Minutes	Local or systemic effects to a portion or the whole body	Hydrocortisone cream, nitroglycerin ointment
Genitourinary			
Rectal	30 minutes	Infants or adults who are nauseous and vomiting	Acetaminophen, anti-nausea medications
Vaginal	Minutes	Local effects	Antibiotics, antifungal medications
Transdermal	Minutes	Continuous dosing over an extended period of time	Nicotine patches, estrogen patches, fentanyl patches
Parenteral			
Intravenous	Minutes	Emergency situations or for drugs that have poor oral absorption	Antibiotics, general anesthesia
Intramuscular	15–30 minutes	Drugs that are irritating in the IV form and drugs that have poor oral absorption	Opioid analgesics, antibiotics
Subcutaneous	30–45 minutes	Drugs that have poor oral absorption	Insulin, tuberculin skin test
Intradermal	Minutes	Local effects or continuous dosing over an extended period of time	Local anesthetics, progesterone implants (Norplant)

Patient Compliance

Patient compliance is important to ensure proper drug absorption. If the patient does not take the medication, it cannot be absorbed. Patients are noncompliant for any number of reasons including lack of faith in medication or the health professional, a poor understanding of their illness, and more importantly lack of money to pay for medication. Today many medications are very expensive and patients cannot afford them. It is important for the dental hygienist to question patients whenever possible as to how they will pay for medications. In some instances, prescribing a less expensive yet equally effective generic equivalent will help the patient.

Other forms of noncompliance include taking the medication incorrectly or stopping the medication midway through therapy, for example, many patients stop taking their antibiotics because they are feeling better or because the antibiotic was prescribed prophylactically. In each instance the patient is not able to achieve adequate blood levels, which can lead to further complications.

Age

The very young and the very old are more sensitive to drug effects. This may be a result of total body weight, muscle to fat ratios, size, and immature kidney and liver function in young children. Elderly patients have more body fat, less protein stores, and decreased kidney and liver function. Unfortunately, drug dosing research is not typically done in pediatric and geriatric populations, although this is beginning to change.

Sex

It is often stated that women are more susceptible to drug effects. Differences in drug response may occur because of differences in total body weight, physical size, muscle mass, and metabolic rate. Drug response may also be altered by pregnancy and breast-feeding.

Pathologic State

Many different illnesses can affect drug absorption, including liver or kidney disease, which can slow down drug metabolism and excretion, leading to toxicity. Hyperthyroidism can increase drug metabolism, which can lead to lower blood levels of medication.

Genetic Variations

Some people metabolize medications at a different rate than the general population because of genetic variations in liver microsomal enzyme systems. This fact may explain why some individuals are more susceptible to adverse reactions.

Placebo Effect

Some patients may respond to drug therapy because of their faith in the prescriber and/or the drug. Negative drug effects can also be due to placebo effects. If a patient does not have faith in his prescriber, or only focuses on the negative aspects of the drug, then he may only have adverse results with the drug.

Time of Administration

Some medications are best taken early in the morning, at bedtime, or with meals. Others, such as antibiotics, need to be taken on an empty stomach to ensure proper absorption into the body. Diuretics (water pills) are best taken in the morning in order to avoid nocturnal awakenings to urinate. Sedative-hypnotics and some opioid pain relievers are best taken at bedtime to avoid daytime sedation. Lastly, food can prevent or minimize GI irritation associated with many medications.

Other Drugs

Many patients take more than one medication for different medical or psychological illnesses. Medications can interact with each other and increase or decrease drug metabolism and excretion. The patient's medications should be carefully reviewed to ensure that the proper medications are prescribed.

Summary

A general understanding of drug action is important when prescribing and administering medications to patients. Many different factors are involved in drug absorption, distribution, metabolism, and excretion. It is important for the dental hygienist to know about them and how they can affect the dental process. The dental hygienist can perform a detailed medication/health history to help minimize drug interactions and adverse reactions. A simple assessment of the patient's age, pathologic state, and physical status will remind the prescriber and the dental hygienist that lower doses and slower dose increases are required in elderly patients. Children also require dose adjustments and dental personnel can consult any one of a number of pediatric dosage reference books. Lastly, review all medications to ensure that drug interactions can be avoided.

Case Study: Fannie Smith

Mrs. Fannie Smith is a 72-year-old who has been coming to your practice for several years. A detailed medication/health history reveals a healthy 110-pound female whose only medications are hydrochlorothiazide (water pill) 25 mg every morning for high blood pressure and an occasional ibuprofen for her rheumatism. Mrs. Smith is quite proud of the fact that she still has her own teeth. However, she is not happy with the fact that she is at your office today in order to have a cavity filled.

1. Though Mrs. Smith appears healthy and weighs 110 pounds, what are your concerns regarding drug distribution?
2. Dental practitioners do not normally request liver function and renal function tests prior to administering or prescribing medications for elderly patients. What are some methods of assessing liver and renal function in Mrs. Smith?
3. Mrs. Smith will require a local anesthetic prior to having her cavity filled. What would be the route of administration?

4. What are the advantages and disadvantages of parenteral administration?
5. Mrs. Smith takes hydrochlorothiazide and ibuprofen as oral tablets. What are the advantages and disadvantages of oral administration of drugs?
6. What factors should be taken into account when medications are given to elderly persons?
7. What would be the more appropriate time of day for Mrs. Smith to take her hydrochlorothiazide and why? How does this timing affect drug absorption?
8. How can the dental hygienist help to minimize any adverse reactions or drug interactions in Mrs. Smith?

Case Study: Joanna Hernandez

Joanna Hernandez is a 35-year-old female who presents to your office with a chief complaint of swollen and aching gums. A thorough examination reveals an infection around one of her molars, which will require antibiotic treatment. Ms. Hernandez also requests something for the pain. You then refer to Ms. Hernandez's dental record and see that she is allergic to penicillin and ibuprofen.

1. What information would you like to know regarding the allergies to penicillin and ibuprofen? Where would you find that information?
2. How would allergies affect what is prescribed for Ms. Hernandez?

Upon further questioning, you find out that Ms. Hernandez experienced breathing problems, rash, and edema the last time she took penicillin. Her primary-care provider told her that she was allergic to penicillin and that she should not take it anymore. The allergy to ibuprofen sounded more like a side effect. It made Ms. Hernandez feel nauseous and it gave her heartburn.

3. What is the difference between the therapeutic and adverse effect of a drug?
4. Compare and contrast side effects, allergic reactions, toxic reaction, and idiosyncratic reactions.
5. How could Ms. Hernandez's infection affect the absorption of a locally administered (parenteral) drug?
6. How would patient compliance affect drug absorption if Ms. Hernandez were prescribed a drug that was similar to ibuprofen?
7. What can be done to help Ms. Hernandez be more compliant with her medication?

Review Questions

1. What is a dose-response curve and what is its relationship to dosing medication?
2. What is the significance of the therapeutic index of a drug?
3. Compare and contrast the different transport mechanisms needed for drug absorption.

4. How can lipid solubility and drug ionization affect drug absorption?
5. Compare and contrast agonist and antagonist drug action.
6. What is the more common enzyme system used to metabolize drugs and what can affect it?
7. What are some of the different ways that drugs can be excreted from the body?
8. How can genetic variations affect drug absorption?

BIBLIOGRAPHY

Benet LZ, Mitchell JR, Scheiner LB: Pharmacokinetics: The dynamics of drug absorption, distribution, and elimination. In Goodman Gilman A, Rall TW, Nies AS, Taylor P (eds.), *Goodman and Gilman's The Pharmacological Basis of Therapeutics*, 8th ed. Pergamon Press, New York, 1990.

Dipalma JR, Digregorio JG: *Basic Pharmacology in Medicine*, 3rd ed. McGraw-Hill, New York, 1990.

Roth JA: Drug Metabolism. In Smith CM, Reynard AM (eds.), *Textbook of Pharmacology*, 1st ed. W. B. Saunders Company, Philadelphia, 1992.

Winter JC: Dose-effect relationships, interactions, and therapeutic index. In Smith CM, Reynard AM (eds.), *Textbook of Pharmacology*, 1st ed. W. B. Saunders Company, Philadelphia, 1992.

Winter JC: Drug absorption, distribution, and termination of action. In Smith CM, Reynard AM (eds.), *Textbook of Pharmacology*, 1st ed. W. B. Saunders Company, Philadelphia, 1992.

Winter JC: Routes of administration. In Smith CM, Reynard AM (eds.), *Textbook of Pharmacology*, 1st ed. W. B. Saunders Company, Philadelphia, 1992.

CHAPTER 3

Autonomic Pharmacology

Key Terms

Adrenergic Agonists
Autonomic Nervous System
Cholinergic
Muscarinic Receptors
Neuronal Receptors

Nicotinic Receptors
Parasympathetic Nervous System
Somatic Nervous System
Sympathetic Nervous System

LEARNING OBJECTIVES

After completion of this chapter and its learning activities, the student should be able to:

1. Describe the overall function and anatomical differences of the autonomic and somatic nervous systems.
2. Describe the term *neurotransmitter* and its relationship to autonomic pharmacology.
3. List the neurotransmitters, including site of action and receptor sites, of the somatic and the sympathetic and parasympathetic nervous systems of the autonomic nervous system.
4. Describe the overall physiologic effects and function of the sympathetic and parasympathetic nervous systems.
5. Define the terms α-adrenergic, β-adrenergic, neuronal, α-adrenergic blocker, β-adrenergic blocker, and neuronal blocker.
6. List and describe the mechanism of action, main effects, clinical use, adverse reactions, and dental concerns of α-adrenergic drugs, β-adrenergic drugs, neuronal drugs, α-adrenergic blockers, β-adrenergic blockers, and neuronal blockers.
7. Define muscarinic, nicotinic, cholinergic, anticholinergic, and anticholinesterase.
8. Describe the mechanism of action of cholinergic drugs.
9. List and describe the clinical uses, adverse reactions, and dental concerns of cholinergic drugs.
10. List and describe the clinical uses, adverse reactions, and dental concerns of anticholinergic and anticholinesterase drugs.

INTRODUCTION

A general understanding of the autonomic nervous system (ANS) is essential to understanding the pharmacology of drugs that act upon the different systems associated with the ANS. Some of the medications used by dental health professionals act upon the ANS and many of the drugs that patients are already taking exert their clinical effects on the ANS. Other drugs may not exert their clinical effects on the ANS but exert their adverse reactions on the ANS. The dental hygienist should be familiar with medications that the patient may receive as a result of a dental procedure and those that the patient is already receiving.

THE AUTONOMIC NERVOUS SYSTEM

The human body responds to moment to moment decisions regarding health, life, and disease via a cycle of internal signals that primarily involves the central nervous system (CNS). Figure 3-1 depicts the constant flow of internal and external stimuli

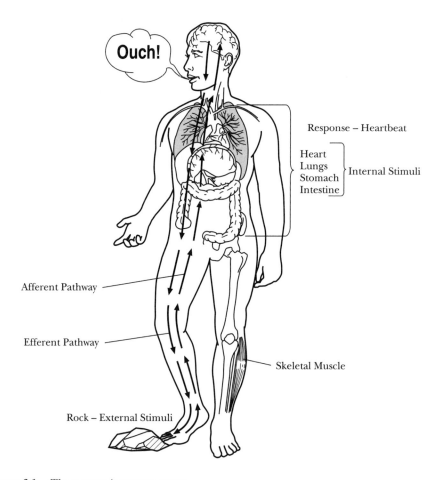

Figure 3-1   *The autonomic nervous system*

along afferent nervous pathways to the CNS. This information is processed by the brain and the appropriate response is transmitted, along efferent nervous pathways, to the *autonomic* or *somatic nervous system.*

The Somatic Nervous System

Figure 3-2 diagrammatically depicts the somatic nervous system (SNS) responsible for voluntary physiologic functions that involve skeletal muscles. The SNS originates in the CNS and extends directly to the skeletal muscle without interruption or synapse. Acetylcholine is the neurotransmitter and nicotine is the exogenous stimulating receptor subtype involved in nerve conduction.

Sympathetic and Parasympathetic Nervous System Anatomy

The autonomic nervous system is responsible for controlling involuntary physiologic functions such as breathing, heart rate, blood pressure, and digestion. The ANS also originates in the CNS and is further divided into the *sympathetic* and *parasympathetic nervous systems.* In the ANS there is an interruption in the nerve pathway between the CNS and the efferent organ. This interruption is called a synapse and is located in a ganglion (Figure 3-3).

The preganglionic neurons of the parasympathetic nervous system leave the CNS at the cranial and sacral level and the postganglionic neurons are located close to the effector organ. One preganglionic neuron usually synapses with one or two postganglionic neurons. Parasympathetic preganglionic neurons are usually longer than postganglionic neurons.

In the sympathetic nervous system the preganglionic fibers leave the spinal cord at the thoracic and upper lumbar levels and the postganglionic neurons are not close to the effector organ. One preganglionic neuron can synapse with as many as 20 to 200 postganglionic neurons. As compared to the parasympathetic nervous system, preganglionic neurons are longer than postganglionic neurons in the sympathetic nervous system and generally synapse with a single postganglionic neuron.

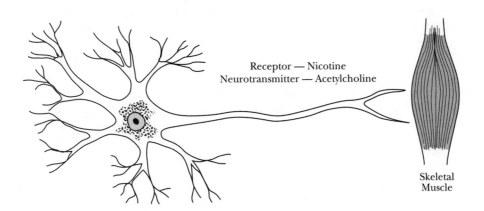

Receptor — Nicotine
Neurotransmitter — Acetylcholine

Skeletal
Muscle

Figure 3-2 *The somatic nervous system*

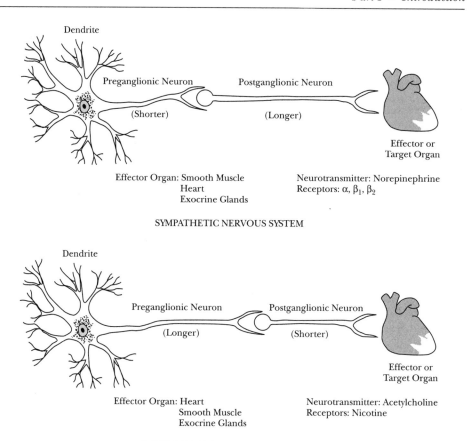

Dendrite

Preganglionic Neuron   Postganglionic Neuron

(Shorter)   (Longer)

Effector or
Target Organ

Effector Organ: Smooth Muscle   Neurotransmitter: Norepinephrine
Heart   Receptors: α, β_1, β_2
Exocrine Glands

SYMPATHETIC NERVOUS SYSTEM

Dendrite

Preganglionic Neuron   Postganglionic Neuron

(Longer)   (Shorter)

Effector or
Target Organ

Effector Organ: Heart   Neurotransmitter: Acetylcholine
Smooth Muscle   Receptors: Nicotine
Exocrine Glands

PARASYMPATHETIC NERVOUS SYSTEM

Figure 3-3 *The sympathetic and parasympathetic nervous systems*

Neurotransmitters

Once the afferent nerve pathway transmits the stimuli to the CNS, a series of events takes place to ensure that the body responds to the stimuli. An action potential is conducted over the axon of the neuron to the synaptic cleft, which is the space between the neuron and effector organ in the case of the SNS, or the preganglionic neuron and postganglionic neuron in the ANS. Neurotransmitters are released in response to the action potential and assist it in crossing the synaptic cleft and combining with postsynaptic receptors. Neurotransmitters are stored in small, membrane-bound vesicles at the end of the nerve fiber in nerve terminals. The interaction between neurotransmitters and postsynaptic receptors initiates a series of events leading to electrical signals in the postsynaptic neuron or physiologic changes in the effector organ. Table 3-1 summarizes the neurotransmitters and receptors involved in the functioning of the somatic and autonomic nervous systems.

The interaction between receptor and neurotransmitter is specific and is rapidly terminated by disposition of the neurotransmitter from the receptor. Neurotransmitter action can be terminated by enzymatic breakdown, reuptake of the neurotransmitter into the presynaptic nerve terminal, or diffusion away from the

Table 3-1 Neurotransmitters and Receptors of the Somatic and Autonomic Nervous System

Nervous System	Neuroeffector Site	Neurotransmitter at Neuroeffector Site	Neuroreceptor at Neuroeffector Site
Somatic	Skeletal muscle	Acetylcholine	Nicotinic
Autonomic			
Sympathetic	Smooth muscle, cardiac muscle, glands	Epinephrine, norepinephrine	α, β_1, β_2
Parasympathetic	Smooth muscle, cardiac muscle, glands	Acetylcholine	Nicotinic, muscarinic

Table 3-2 Effects of the Autonomic Nervous System

Organ/Tissue Site	Response to Sympathetic Nervous System	Response to Parasympathetic Nervous System
Eye	Mydriasis (dilation)	Miosis (constriction)
Heart	Increased force and rate of contraction	Decreased force and rate of contraction
Arteries	Vasoconstriction	Most are not affected
Respiratory tract	Bronchodilation	Bronchoconstriction
Urinary bladder	Relaxation	Contraction
Urinary sphincter	Constriction	Relaxation
Gastrointestinal activity	Decreased	Increased
Salivary glands	Increased secretions	Increased secretions

postsynaptic receptor. Drugs can enhance or prevent the responses of the ANS by altering the events associated with neurotransmitter action.

Physiologic Functions of the Autonomic Nervous System

Both the sympathetic and parasympathetic nervous system innervate most body organs and usually have opposite effects. The actions of the sympathetic nervous system are generalized and widespread and are often referred to as "flight or fright" responses. The sympathetic nervous system is more dominant in times of stress, increased activity, or emergency situations. Actions of the parasympathetic nervous system are more discrete and generalized and are referred to as vegetative responses, dominating when the body is at rest. The response of a specific tissue is equal to the sum of the excitatory and inhibitory responses to the stimuli. Table 3-2 summarizes the responses of the neuroeffector sites to the ANS.

THE SYMPATHETIC NERVOUS SYSTEM

The major neurotransmitters of the sympathetic nervous system, norepinephrine (NE) and epinephrine (EPI), help the body respond to stress and belong to the chemical class of compounds called catecholamines. Both are synthesized in the

Table 3-3   Adrenergic Receptors, Site of Action, and Response

Receptor	Site of Action	Response
α	Eye (iris)	Mydriasis
	Arteries	Vasoconstriction (NE and EPI)
β_1	Heart	Increased force and rate of contraction (EPI and NE)
β_2	Eye (ciliary muscle)	Relaxation for distant vision
	Lungs	Bronchodilation (EPI)
	Skeletal smooth muscle	Contraction
	Uterus	Relaxation

neuronal tissues and stored in synaptic vesicles. Norepinephrine is released from nerve endings in response to stress, and EPI is released from the adrenal medulla in response to stress and both are distributed throughout the body via the bloodstream.

The effects of NE are not immediately terminated upon connection with the appropriate receptor, causing a wait period for the effects of NE to dissipate. Norepinephrine action is terminated primarily by reuptake into the presynaptic nerve terminals. Enzymatic breakdown occurs by either monoamine oxidase (MAO) (within the neuron) or catechol-*O*-methlytransferase (COMT) (extraneuronal tissue). Norepinephrine response can also be altered by adrenergic agonists and antagonists. Once the impulse reaches the nerve ending, adrenergic drugs exert their effects by (1) directly stimulating the receptor, (2) releasing endogenous NE, which produces a response (indirect action), or (3) a combination of direct and indirect actions.

Sympathetic or Adrenergic Receptors

Once the neurotransmitter is released, it can bind to any one of the following receptors: α, β_1, β_2. Table 3-3 reviews the three receptors, site of action, and effects produced by the binding of NE and EPI to them. The stimulation of α receptors results in smooth muscle excitation or contraction, stimulation of β_1 receptors results in smooth muscle excitation, and stimulation of β_2 receptors results in smooth muscle relaxation.

Adrenergic drugs can affect NE transmission at presynaptic nerve endings by one of several mechanisms. They include creating false neurotransmitters, blocking the reuptake of NE, depleting NE from presynaptic storage vesicles, increasing the release of NE from nerve endings, and decreasing the release of NE from nerve endings. These drugs are referred to as either adrenergic agonists or blockers.

ADRENERGIC AGONISTS

Adrenergic agonists play an important role in the treatment of many different illnesses. This next section reviews the pharmacology, adverse reactions, clinical uses, and specific adrenergic agonists.

Pharmacology of Adrenergic Agonists

Table 3-4 reviews the pharmacologic action of adrenergic agonists and their receptor activity. **Epinephrine** stimulates both α and β_1 and β_2 receptors, **norepinephrine** stimulates α and β_1 receptors, **phenylephrine** stimulates primarily α receptors, **isoproterenol** primarily stimulates β_1 receptors, and **albuterol** and other adrenergic bronchodilators primarily stimulate β_2 receptors.

Adverse Reactions

The adverse reactions associated with adrenergic agonists are usually an extension of the drugs' pharmacologic effects. Adverse reactions include CNS excitation, anxiety, tremors, and tachycardia. Other cardiac adverse reactions include arrhythmias and increased blood pressure. Caution should be used when these drugs are given to patients with hypertension, angina, or hyperthyroidism. Uncontrolled hyperthyroidism is a contraindication for epinephrine use.

Clinical Use

The clinical uses of α- and β-adrenergic agonists are many and are reviewed in Table 3-5. The next section reviews some of the more commonly used α- and β-adrenergic agonists.

Epinephrine. **Epinephrine** stimulates both α and β receptors with a stronger affinity for β_1 and β_2 receptors and is primarily used to treat acute asthma attacks and anaphylaxis. It is also added to local anesthetics as a vasoconstrictor to reduce bleeding,

---

Table 3-4   Pharmacologic Actions of Adrenergic Agonists

Central Nervous System
  Excitation, alertness
  Anxiety, apprehension, restlessness, tremors (at higher doses)

Cardiovascular System
  Heart—increase the force and rate of contraction; increase in blood pressure
  Vessels—Vasoconstriction of smooth muscle (α), which increases total peripheral resistance; vasodilation of skeletal muscle (β), which decreases total peripheral resistance
  Blood pressure—increase in blood pressure

Eye
  Decrease in intraocular pressure

Respiratory System
  Bronchial relaxation

Metabolic Effects
  Increased glycogenolysis, decreased insulin release

Salivary Glands
  Decrease saliva flow

Table 3-5   Clinical Uses of Adrenergic Agonists

Central Nervous System Stimulation
   Treatment of attention deficit hyperactivity disorder, obesity, depression
   resistant to traditional therapies, narcolepsy

Cardiovascular
   Treatment of shock, hypotension, cardiac arrest

Vasoconstriction
   Prolong the action of local anesthetics and reduce systemic toxicity; hemostasis;
   nasal decongestant

Respiratory System
   Treatment of asthma and anaphylactic reactions

---

prolong the duration of action of local anesthetics, and reduce the incidence of local anesthetic systemic adverse reactions. Cardiac uses include treatment of hypotension and use as a stimulant to increase cardiac output and heart rate.

Epinephrine is administered as either intravenous or subcutaneous injections and is stored in amber-colored vials. The vials should be stored in a dark place because light can cause epinephrine to deteriorate. Any type of discoloration should be indicative of contaminated or inactive epinephrine and should be discarded.

Levonordefrin (Neo-Cobefrin). **Levonordefrin**, a derivative of norepinephrine, is a vasoconstrictor that is added to local anesthetic solutions. It is an α agonist which is considered to have less CNS and cardiac stimulation and excitation than epinephrine, although more medication is required to produce a level of vasoconstriction similar to epinephrine.

Phenylephrine. **Phenylephrine** is an α agonist that causes vasoconstriction of the nasal passages and is the active ingredient in many over-the-counter (OTC) nose drops or sprays. It provides symptomatic relief by reducing swelling of nasal passages. However, repeated use can lead to rebound congestion. Patients experience increased swelling of nasal passages and have difficulty breathing well before the next scheduled dose of medication. Treatment with oral, systemic decongestants can help to alleviate this problem.

Phenylephrine produces vasoconstriction in cutaneous vessels, which increases total peripheral resistance and increases blood pressure. It is also used to dilate pupils.

Ephedrine. **Ephedrine** is an α, β_1, and β_2 agonist and has several different uses. Ephedrine is used to treat low blood pressure due to hypotension and shock and to improve blood flow to vital organs.

Dipivefrin (Propine). **Dipivefrin** is used to treat chronic open-angle glaucoma and has both α- and β-agonist activity. Its α-agonist effects include mydriasis and β effects include increased production and increased outflow of aqueous humor. It is metabolized to epinephrine and may result in fewer side effects than epinephrine.

Phenylpropanolamine. **Phenylpropanolamine** has both α and β activity and is the active ingredient in many OTC diet aids and cold products. It is similar to ephedrine and has slight CNS properties that are similar to **amphetamines.** It is a safe medication when used appropriately.

Amphetamine and Amphetamine-like Drugs. Amphetamine, **phentermine** (Fastin), **phendimetrazine** (Plegine), **diethylpropion** (Tenuate), and **fenfluramine** (Pondimin) are prescription drugs used to treat obesity and are used as diet aids for those who are not obese.

    Methylphenidate (Ritalin), **dextroamphetamine** (Dexedrine), and **pimoline** (Cylert) are used to treat attention deficit hyperactivity disorder (ADHD) in children and in adults. These medications help to increase attention span and reduce impulsive behavior.

Isoproterenol (Isuprel). **Isoproterenol** has pure β effects and is closely related to NE and EPI. It is a bronchodilator that is used to treat asthma. However, it has significant β_1 effects that cause cardiac stimulation.

Beta$_2$ Agonists. These medications include **albuterol** (Proventil, Ventolin), **metaproterenol** (Alupent), and **terbutaline** (Brethine) and are used to treat acute and chronic asthma. These drugs and others are discussed in further detail in Chapter 15.

Dental Concerns

Both epinephrine and levonordefrin are vasoconstrictors that are added to local anesthetics. These medications can cause tachycardia with a subsequent increase in blood pressure. A detailed medication/health history will reveal patients with hypertension and whether or not it is being adequately controlled with medication, diet, exercise, or a combination of the three. The patient's blood pressure should also be taken prior to administering the vasoconstrictor. In most instances, the patient with controlled hypertension can receive the local anesthetic with a vasoconstrictor. This subject is discussed in further detail in Chapter 4.

    Both epinephrine and levonordefrin can cause CNS excitation and tremors, which may be exaggerated in a patient with existing CNS problems or with hyperthyroidism. Both can be minimized or avoided with detailed medication/health histories and a lower dose of the vasoconstrictor.

    Many patients self-treat with OTC medications and often neglect to inform their dental or medical health-care provider. The active ingredients of OTC products have both α and β activity and may interact with vasoconstrictors that are added to local anesthetics. Both may lead to an increase in blood pressure and symptoms of anxiety and nervousness. Carefully question your patient about OTC use of medications and the time of the last dose of an oral OTC medication. Those OTC medications of concern include oral decongestants and diet aids.

    Oral β-adrenergic agonists have the ability to cause tachycardia and increase blood pressure. The dental hygienist or dentist should measure the patient's blood pressure and ask specific questions about the patient's medications and health. This will help to avoid drug interactions with a vasoconstrictor.

Adrenergic Antagonists

Adrenergic antagonists or blockers may block all adrenergic receptors, may block a combination of receptors, or may block only α, β_1, or β_2 receptors. This next section reviews some of the more commonly used agents.

Phenoxybenzamine (Dibenzyline). **Phenoxybenzamine** blocks α receptors, which reduces sympathetic tone in blood vessels and causes a decrease in total peripheral resistance. It is used to treat vascular spasms due to peripheral vascular disease (Raynaud's disease) and for the diagnosis and management of pheochromocytoma. Adverse reactions include orthostatic hypotension, reflex tachycardia, profound drop in blood pressure, and miosis.

Tolazoline (Priscoline) and Phentolamine (Regitine). Both medications are α blockers used to treat Raynaud's disease. They have a shorter duration of action and are less potent than phenoxybenzamine. Adverse reactions include hypertension, cardiac stimulation, and increased gastric acid secretion.

Prazosin (Minipress), Terazosin (Hytrin), Doxazosin (Cardura). These medications block α receptors in the vasculature without producing tachycardia. They are used to treat hypertension and are discussed further in Chapter 13. They are also used to treat Raynaud's disease and benign prostatic hypertrophy.

Propranolol (Inderal). **Propranolol** is the prototype for the class of drugs known as β blockers and is discussed in detail in Chapter 13. It is a nonselective β-blocking agent used to treat hypertension, angina, cardiac arrhythmias, myocardial infarction, open-angle glaucoma, essential tremors, and for the prophylactic treatment of migraine headaches. It is also used to treat anxiety due to public speaking and stage fright.

Propranolol blocks β_2 receptors in the lungs and can precipitate an asthma attack. It should be avoided in patients with asthma or chronic obstructive pulmonary disease. It also lowers cardiac output and heart rate and should be avoided in people with congestive heart failure, hypotension, and bradycardia. Other adverse reactions include hypoglycemia and sedation.

Labetalol (Normodyne, Trandate). **Labetalol** blocks both α and β receptors and is used to treat hypertension. It lowers blood pressure without reflex tachycardia.

Dental Concerns. Drugs used to treat Raynaud's disease and hypertension have the ability to cause reflex increases in heart rate and blood pressure. Measure the patient's blood pressure and obtain a detailed medication/health history in order to avoid or minimize drug interactions or adverse reactions.

Medications such as propranolol can cross the blood-brain barrier and cause sedation and other CNS effects. Caution should be used if an opioid analgesic or antianxiety agent is prescribed. Someone should drive the patient to and from the appointment and the patient should avoid working with or operating heavy machinery, or anything that requires thought or concentration.

Adrenergic Neuronal Agonists and Antagonists

These medications affect the release of NE from presynaptic nerve endings. They also decrease adrenergic activity and influence α- and β-receptor activity. This section briefly reviews these centrally acting drugs.

Reserpine (Serapsil). **Reserpine** prevents the storage of NE in presynaptic vesicles, thus depleting NE stores and leaving little NE available for use. Use of this drug was initially curtailed because of its CNS and other adverse reaction profiles. It is used to treat mild hypertension. Adverse reactions include CNS sedation, GI discomfort, nasal congestion, and exacerbation of peptic ulcer disease.

Guanethidine (Ismelin). **Guanethidine** blocks the release of NE from presynaptic nerve terminals and is used to treat moderate to severe hypertension. Adverse reactions include postural hypotension, bradycardia, impotence, orthostatic hypotension, and aggravation of asthma.

Methyldopa (Aldomet). **Methyldopa** causes activation of the receptor site and works on presynaptic and postsynaptic nerve endings. It also stimulates α_2 receptors and is used to treat hypertension. Adverse reactions include sedation and GI discomfort.

Clonidine (Catapres). **Clonidine** reduces sympathetic tone and works directly in the brain. It is used to treat hypertension and adverse reactions include sedation and GI discomfort.

Dental Concerns. Neuronal agonists and antagonists are used to treat hypertension. As with the use of α and β blockers, the patient's blood pressure should be taken and a detailed medication/health history should be obtained to avoid or minimize drug interactions or adverse reactions. Patients should be slowly raised to a sitting position after being in the dental chair and should be instructed to rise slowly from the chair. Many of these medications can cause orthostatic hypotension, which could be precipitated by rising too quickly.

These medications are centrally acting agents, that is, they can cause CNS adverse reactions including sedation and confusion. Caution should be used if an opioid analgesic or an antianxiety agent is prescribed because both cause CNS sedation and confusion. The patient should have someone drive her to and from her appointment and should avoid driving, working with heavy machinery, or anything that requires thought or concentration.

THE PARASYMPATHETIC NERVOUS SYSTEM

The major neurotransmitter of the parasympathetic nervous system is acetylcholine (ACh) and it helps the body respond to quiet, nonstressful situations. Acetylcholine is synthesized, stored, and released from cholinergic neurons in the preganglionic and postganglionic nerves of the parasympathetic nervous system and the preganglionic nerves of the sympathetic nervous system. Other cholinergic receptors are located in the sympathetic postganglionic fibers in sweat glands, skeletal muscles, and the motor neurons of the somatic nervous system.

Table 3-6   Cholinergic Receptors, Site of Action, and Response

Receptor	Site of Action	Response
Muscarinic	Eye (iris, ciliary)	Miosis, contraction for near vision
	Heart	Decreased heart rate
	Lungs	Bronchoconstriction
	Uterus	Contraction
	Urinary bladder	Contraction
	Lacrimal, bronchial, nasopharyngeal	Increased secretions
	GI tract	Increased motility
Nicotinic	All autonomic ganglia	Stimulation of postganglionic neuron
	Skeletal muscle	Contraction

Once the action potential reaches the cholinergic nerve ending, ACh is released and initiates a response in postsynaptic tissue. Small doses of ACh produce effects in the neuroeffector junction of the parasympathetic nervous system and the postganglionic neuroeffector junctions of sweat glands and skeletal muscle blood vessels. Larger doses of ACh produce effects in the ganglionic synapses of both the parasympathetic and sympathetic nervous systems and myoneural junctions of the somatic nervous system. Acetylcholine release, under normal circumstances, is fast and is measured in microseconds. Its actions are terminated by hydrolysis by acetylcholinesterase which yields the inactive compounds choline and acetic acid.

Parasympathetic or Cholinergic Receptors

Once ACh is released, it can bind to either *muscarinic* or *nicotinic receptors*. Small doses of ACh bind to muscarinic receptors and duplicate the effects of the chemical substance muscarine. Larger doses bind to nicotinic receptors and duplicate the effects of nicotine, a chemical substance found in cigarettes. The amount of neurotransmitter released, size of the synaptic cleft, and postganglionic site determine which receptor site is activated. Table 3-6 reviews the two receptors, site of action, and effects produced by the binding of ACh to them.

CHOLINERGIC (PARASYMPATHOMIMETIC) AGONISTS

Cholinergic agonists are used to diagnosis and treat different illnesses. This section reviews the pharmacology, adverse reactions, contraindications, clinical uses, dental concerns, and specific cholinergic agonists.

Pharmacology of Cholinergic Agonists

Table 3-7 reviews the pharmacologic action of cholinergic agonists and their receptor activity. Cholinergic agonists can be classified as direct (choline ester) or indirect (anticholinesterase) acting depending on mechanism of action. Direct-acting agonists have activity on the parasympathetic nervous system, have a long duration of action, and are more selective of receptor sites. Indirect-acting agonists inhibit the enzyme acetylcholinesterase, which allows for a higher concentration of ACh.

Table 3-7 Pharmacologic Actions of Cholinergic Drugs

Cardiovascular System
  Direct Effect
    Decreased force and rate of contraction
    Decreased cardiac output
    Smooth muscle relaxation of vessels
  Indirect Effect
    Increase in heart rate and cardiac output

Gastrointestinal System
  Excitation of smooth muscles, which leads to salivation, lacrimation, urination,
    increased stomach acid production and diarrhea

Eye
  Accommodation for near vision
  Miosis
  Decreases in intraocular pressure

Adverse Reactions

The adverse reactions associated with cholinergic agonists are usually an extension of the drugs' pharmacologic effects. Adverse reactions include salivation, lacrimation, urination, and defecation. Other adverse reactions include confusion at higher doses and neuromuscular paralysis at very high doses.

Overdose of cholinesterase inhibitors can be treated with a combination of **pralidoxime** and **atropine.** Pralidoxime regenerates receptor sites bound by acetylcholinesterase inhibitors and atropine blocks muscarinic receptor sites.

Contraindications

Contraindications to cholinergic agonists are a result of the drugs' pharmacologic effects and adverse reactions. These include bronchial asthma, hyperthyroidism, mechanical obstruction of the gastrointestinal or urinary tract, severe cardiac disease, myasthenia gravis (treated with **neostigmine**), and peptic ulcer disease.

Clinical Use

The clinical uses of cholinergic agonists are reviewed in Table 3-8. This next section reviews some of the more commonly used cholinergic agonists.

Table 3-8 Clinical Uses of Cholinergic Drugs

Eye
  Treatment of glaucoma and myasthenia gravis

Genitourinary
  Treatment of urinary retention

Other
  Treatment of xerostomia; treatment of tricyclic antidepressant and
  anticholinergic overdose

Choline Esters

This group of medications stimulates muscarinic receptors. Some of the more commonly used medications are as follows.

Acetylcholine. **Acetylcholine** is an endogenous neurotransmitter with no significant clinical use because of its short duration of action and rapid breakdown by acetylcholinesterase. It is only used occasionally on the eye for its miotic effect.

Methacholine (Provocholine). **Methacholine** is a synthetic choline ester that is less affected by acetylcholinesterase than ACh and has a much longer duration of action than ACh. It is used as a diagnostic test for bronchial airway hyperactivity and to stimulate muscarinic receptors in the sphincter muscles of the iris, causing miosis.

Bethanechol (Urecholine). **Bethanechol** is similar to methacholine and possesses fewer nicotinic and muscarinic properties. It is available orally and is used to treat urinary retention following general anesthesia.

Carbachol (Miostat). **Carbachol** is not inactivated by either acetylcholinesterase or plasma cholinesterase and has a long duration of action. It has more nicotinic action than methacholine and is less affected by atropine. It is used for localized treatment of glaucoma.

Pilocarpine (Adsorbocarpine). **Pilocarpine** is a naturally occurring alkaloid that stimulates muscarinic receptors. It is used topically to treat glaucoma and orally for the treatment of xerostomia.

Anticholinesterase Drugs

This group of medications inhibits the effects of acetylcholinesterase at receptor sites throughout the CNS and the peripheral nervous system. Some of the more commonly used medications are reviewed here.

Edrophonium (Tensilon). **Edrophonium** binds directly with acetylcholinesterase, resulting in a short-term, reversible blockade of acetylcholinesterase. Its main use is for the diagnosis of myasthenia gravis. Other uses include treatment of certain types of tachycardia and as an antidote for curare poisoning.

Neostigmine (Prostigmin). **Neostigmine** does not cross the blood-brain barrier and reversibly inhibits peripherally located cholinesterase. It also has a stronger affinity for nicotinic receptors. It is used to treat myasthenia gravis.

Pyridostigmine (Mestinon). **Pyridostigmine** drug is similar to neostigmine and is also used to treat myasthenia gravis.

Physostigmine (Eserine). **Physostigmine** is lipid soluble and readily crosses the blood-brain barrier. It is used to treat overdoses due to anticholinergic or tricyclic antidepressant ingestion.

Irreversible Organophosphates. Included in this group are the agricultural insecticides **malathion** and **parathion** and the "nerve" gases used in chemical warfare: **sarin** and **tabun.**

Dental Concerns

The majority of these medications are used by anesthesiologists or ophthalmologists and are usually given as eyedrops or intravenously. Those medications available in oral dose forms can cause increased salivation and some may cause hypotension and bradycardia. Patients should use good oral hygiene to help with the effects of increased salivation. The dental hygienist should raise a patient into the sitting position slowly and have the patient rise slowly from the dental chair in order to help minimize the hypotensive effects of these medications.

CHOLINERGIC ANTAGONISTS

Cholinergic antagonists have many different medical and dental uses. This next section reviews the pharmacology, adverse reactions, contraindications, clinical uses, dental concerns, and specific anticholinergic drugs.

Pharmacology of Cholinergic Antagonists

Cholinergic antagonists or anticholinergic drugs block muscarinic receptors throughout the body and nicotinic receptors at sufficiently high doses. Anticholinergic drugs block the effects of ACh on smooth muscle, glandular tissue, and the heart. Table 3-9 reviews the pharmacologic action of some of the more commonly used anticholinergic drugs.

Adverse Reactions

The adverse reactions associated with anticholinergic drugs are usually an extension of the drugs' pharmacologic effects. Adverse reactions include xerostomia (dry mouth), blurred vision, constipation, and urinary retention. CNS adverse reactions

---

Table 3-9   Pharmacologic Effects of Anticholinergic Drugs

Central Nervous System Effects
　Low doses—sedation
　High doses—stimulation (psychosis)

Cardiovascular System Effects
　Low doses—bradycardia
　High doses—tachycardia

Eye
　Increase in intraocular pressure, cycloplegia, mydriasis

Smooth Muscle
　Relaxation of the respiratory and gastrointestinal smooth muscle

Exocrine Glands
　Reduction of secretions in the respiratory, gastrointestinal, and genitourinary tracts

---

include mental confusion, excitation, delirium, and hallucinations. Other adverse reactions include photophobia, tachycardia, fever, and hot, dry flushed skin, which is caused by a lack of sweating. High fever and dry mouth are treated symptomatically. Convulsions and respiratory depression can also occur.

Contraindications

Anticholinergic drug use is contraindicated for patients with glaucoma, prostatic hypertrophy, constipation, urinary retention, or cardiovascular disease. Anticholinergic drugs can cause an increase in intraocular pressure in patients with narrow-angle glaucoma, thereby precipitating an attack.

These drugs cause urinary retention and constipation and could aggravate existing conditions. They can also cause further urinary problems in men with prostatic hypertrophy who already have a problem urinating.

Lastly, anticholinergic drugs can block the vagus nerve and cause tachycardia. Patients with cardiovascular disease should avoid using these drugs.

Clinical Uses

The clinical uses of anticholinergic drugs are many and are reviewed in Table 3-10. Some of the more commonly used anticholinergic drugs are reviewed here.

Atropine (Atripison). **Atropine** is the prototype for this class of medications and is used for a number of clinical situations. It mainly blocks muscarinic receptors at low doses and blocks nicotinic receptors at much higher doses. It is used as a preanesthetic agent to decrease salivary flow and respiratory secretions, as an agent to increase heart rate, and to dilate pupils.

Scopolamine. **Scopolamine** is closely related to atropine and has a more obvious depressant effect on the CNS. It has been used as a preanesthetic for both its drying abilities and CNS sedative effects. It is primarily used as an anti–motion sickness agent.

Table 3-10   Clinical Uses of Anticholinergic Drugs

Preoperative Medication
   Inhibit salivary and bronchial secretions—produce dry field
   Block the vagal slowing of the heart by general anesthetics

Gastrointestinal Disorders
   Decreases GI motility—treatment of gastric ulcers, GI hypermotility

Eye Examinations
   Cycloplegia—relaxes the lense
   Mydriasis—full visualization of the retina

Central Nervous System
   Treatment of motion sickness, sleep aid, treatment of Parkinson's disease,
      treatment of Parkinson-like symptoms from antipsychotic drugs

---

Methantheline (Banthine). **Methantheline** is a synthetic atropine substitute that is widely used as an antisialagogue in prosthodontics and orthodontics. It reduces salivary flow for a brief and more reasonable period of time than atropine. It does block ganglionic activity and can cause hypotension.

Dicyclomine (Bentyl) and Propantheline (Pro-Banthine). **Dicyclomine** and **propantheline** have a strong affinity for muscarinic receptors in the gastrointestinal tract. They are used to reduce gastrointestinal motility.

Benztropine mesylate (Cogentin), Trihexyphenidyl hydrochloride (Artane), Biperiden (Akineton), and Procyclidine (Kemadrin). These medications block muscarinic receptors and have been used as first-line therapy in the treatment of Parkinson's disease. They are also used to treat the extrapyramidal adverse reactions associated with antipsychotic drug therapy.

Dental Concerns

The primary dental concern associated with anticholinergic drugs is xerostomia. Xerostomia or dry mouth is one of the leading causes of noncompliance in patients taking these medications. The dental hygienist plays an important role in teaching patients ways to minimize xerostomia. Xerostomia can be minimized or alleviated with meticulous oral hygiene including brushing and flossing. Patients should also drink plenty of water and keep a glass of water by their bedside at night. Patients should avoid both prescription and nonprescription mouth rinses that contain alcohol. Alcohol can exacerbate dry mouth. Drinks containing caffeine can actually intensify xerostomia and should be avoided. Juices may seem like a natural alternative; however, they consist of natural sugar, which can place the patient at risk for dental caries. Patients can chew sugarless gum or suck on tart, sugarless candy to help minimize dry mouth. There are artificial saliva substitutes available for patients with severe xerostomia.

Anticholinergic medications can also cause tachycardia, which can increase blood pressure. A patient's blood pressure should be taken prior to any dental procedure or administration of a medication that can cause tachycardia.

Sedation is another adverse reaction associated with anticholinergic medications. Caution should be used if an opioid analgesic or an antianxiety agent is prescribed because both cause CNS sedation and confusion. The patient should have someone drive him to and from his appointment and avoid working with or operating heavy machinery, or anything that requires thought or concentration.

Summary

Epinephrine, norepinephrine, and acetylcholine are three neurotransmitters that help the body respond to both internal and external stimuli. These neurotransmitters bind to receptors that help to produce a response to stimuli. Medications are available that either mimic or block the effects of these neurotransmitters.

Medications such as epinephrine (stimulates α and β receptors), which mimic the effects of the sympathetic nervous system, can increase heart rate and blood pressure, cause vasoconstriction, and dilate bronchial smooth muscle. Albuterol is a β agonist that relaxes bronchial smooth muscles. Propranolol blocks sympathetic receptors (β_1 and β_2), decreases heart rate and blood pressure, and causes bronchial smooth muscle constriction. Prazocin, which blocks α receptors, is also used to lower blood pressure.

Pilocarpine mimics the effects of the parasympathetic nervous system. It is used to treat glaucoma and urinary retention or other gastrointestinal motility problems. Pilocarpine relaxes GI smooth muscle and reduces intraocular pressure. Drugs that block the effects of the parasympathetic nervous system include benztropine mesylate, atropine, and scopolamine. These drugs can increase heart rate and intraocular pressure and cause dry mouth, blurred vision, urinary retention, and constipation. Lastly, neuronal agonists and antagonists are used to treat hypertension. These drugs work by affecting epinephrine and norepinephrine release and by influencing α and β activity.

Medications that affect the sympathetic and parasympathetic nervous systems are taken by many patients. Patients may self-medicate with OTC products, take medications prescribed by a health-care provider, or have health conditions that could be aggravated by medications used in dentistry. The dental hygienist can play an important role in helping to minimize adverse drug reactions (e.g., dry mouth) or interactions (e.g., with epinephrine). A detailed medication/health history and an understanding of the pharmacology of autonomic drugs can allow the dental hygienist to effectively counsel the patient about possible adverse reactions and drug interactions.

Case Study: Rolanda Elliot

Rolanda Elliot is a 46-year-old patient with a 5-year history of hypertension and asthma. A detailed medication/health history reveals that she is taking propranolol to treat her hypertension and using an albuterol inhaler to treat her asthma. She has been coming to your practice for 10 years and is meticulous about her oral hygiene. Unfortunately, she must have a cavity filled. Both her blood pressure and asthma are under control, which will allow the dentist to use a local anesthetic with epinephrine (vasoconstrictor).

1. What are the contraindications to epinephrine therapy?
2. What are some ways to minimize or avoid adverse drug reactions or drug interactions with epinephrine?
3. What is propranolol? Include mechanism of action and clinical use.
4. What are some of the adverse reactions associated with propranolol?
5. Are there any dental concerns associated with propranolol? If so, what are they and what should Mrs. Elliot be told about them?
6. What is albuterol? Include mechanism of action and clinical use.
7. What are some of the adverse reactions associated with albuterol?

8. Are there any dental concerns associated with albuterol? If so, what are they and what should Mrs. Elliot be told about them?

Case Study: Harry Karteris

Harry Karteris is a 68-year-old man who has been coming to this dental practice for 40 years. He was diagnosed with Parkinson's disease about 3 years ago. Mr. Karteris's only medications include benztropine mesylate and acetaminophen for general aches and pains. Unfortunately, he has begun to have problems with his teeth since starting benztropine mesylate.

1. What is benztropine mesylate and what are some of its clinical uses?
2. What are some of the contraindications to medications like benztropine mesylate?
3. What are some of the adverse reactions associated with benztropine mesylate?
4. What should Mr. Karteris be told about the dental adverse reactions associated with his medication?
5. What drugs prescribed in a dental office would interact with benztropine mesylate?
6. What should Mr. Karteris be told if one of these interacting medications (i.e., sedating drug) must be prescribed for him?

Review Questions

1. Compare and contrast the functions of the somatic and autonomic nervous systems.
2. Compare and contrast the functions of the sympathetic and parasympathetic nervous systems.
3. What is a neurotransmitter? How is it activated and deactivated?
4. What are the major neurotransmitters and receptors of the sympathetic nervous system?
5. What are the pharmacologic effects of adrenergic drugs on the eye, bronchioles, and salivary glands?
6. What are the clinical uses and adverse reactions of α-adrenergic blocking drugs?
7. What are the major neurotransmitters and receptors of neuronal agonists and antagonists?
8. What is the major neurotransmitter and the receptors of the parasympathetic nervous system?
9. What is the difference between choline esters and acetylcholinesterase inhibitors?
10. What are the pharmacologic and clinical uses of choline esters and acetylcholinesterase inhibitors?

BIBLIOGRAPHY

Appelt GD: Weight control products. In *The Handbook of Nonprescription Drugs,* 10th ed. American Pharmaceutical Association, Washington, D.C.,1993.

Brown OM: Adrenergic drugs. In Smith CM, Reynard AM (eds.), *Textbook of Pharmacology,* 1st ed. W. B. Saunders Company, Philadelphia, 1992.

Bryant BG, Cormier JF: Cold and allergy products. In *The Handbook of Nonprescription Drugs,* 10th ed. American Pharmaceutical Association, Washington, D.C., 1993.

Lefkowitz RJ, Hoffman BB, Taylor P: Neurohumoral transmission: The autonomic and somatic motor nervous system. In Goodman Gilman A, Rall TW, Nies AS, Taylor P (eds.) *Goodman and Gilman's The Pharmacological Basis of Therapeutics,* 8th ed. Pergamon Press, New York, 1990.

McIsaac RJ: Principles of neuroeffector systems. In Smith CM, Reynard AM (eds.), *Textbook of Pharmacology,* 1st ed. W. B. Saunders Company, Philadelphia, 1992.

McIsaac RJ: Cholinomimetic drugs. In Smith CM, Reynard AM (eds.), *Textbook of Pharmacology,* 1st ed. W. B. Saunders Company, Philadelphia, 1992.

McIsaac RJ: Cholinomimetic drugs–cholinesterase inhibitors. In Smith CM, Reynard AM (eds.), *Textbook of Pharmacology,* 1st ed. W. B. Saunders Company, Philadelphia, 1992.

McIsaac RJ: Antimuscarinic drugs. In Smith CM, Reynard AM (eds.), *Textbook of Pharmacology,* 1st ed. W. B. Saunders Company, Philadelphia, 1992.

PART II

MEDICATIONS USED
IN DENTISTRY

CHAPTER 4

Local Anesthetics

Key Terms

Additives
Amides
Esters
Ionization

Local Anesthetic
PABA
Vasoconstrictor

LEARNING OBJECTIVES

After completion of this chapter and its learning activities, the student should be able to:

1. Describe the general characteristics of local anesthetics.
2. List the classifications of local anesthetics.
3. Describe the site, mechanism of action, and ionization factors of local anesthetics.
4. Describe the pharmacology and pharmacokinetics of local anesthetics.
5. List the amide local anesthetics and discuss their advantages and disadvantages.
6. List the ester local anesthetics and discuss their advantages and disadvantages.
7. Describe the adverse effects associated with local anesthetics.
8. List the additives found in local anesthetics.
9. Discuss the rationale for adding a vasoconstrictor to a local anesthetic. (Include the mechanism of action of vasoconstrictors.)
10. Describe the relationship between vasoconstrictors and cardiovascular disease.

INTRODUCTION

Local anesthetics are drugs that produce a loss of sensation in a localized area of the body. The primary dental use of local anesthetics is the prevention and alleviation of pain. Many local anesthetics are used in today's dental practice and in some states dental hygienists administer them. Therefore, it is necessary for the dental hygienist to have a clear understanding of local anesthetic agents.

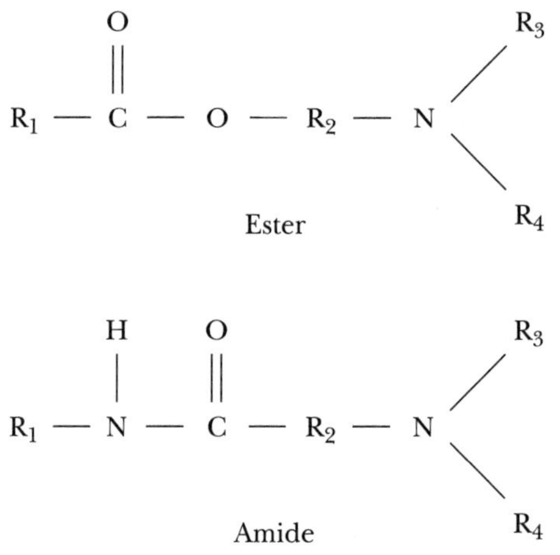

Figure 4-1   *Chemical structure of local anesthetics*

CLASSIFICATION AND STRUCTURE OF LOCAL ANESTHETICS

Local anesthetics are derived from *p*-aminobenzoic acid *(PABA)* and are divided into two groups: *esters* and *amides*. The structure of the local anesthetic is composed of an aromatic nucleus (R_1), linkage (ester or amine followed by an aliphatic chain, (R_2)), and an amino group. The aromatic nucleus is lipophilic and the amino group is hydrophilic (Figure 4-1).

SITE OF ACTION

The site of action of local anesthetics is the nerve membrane, which is responsible for conducting the nerve action potential. This area has been localized to be near the internal surface of the nerve membrane as opposed to the external surface.

MECHANISM OF ACTION

Local anesthetics reduce the transient increase in sodium flow into the nerve membrane. Activation of the action potential by painful stimuli results in an inward flow of sodium and an outward flow of potassium. Once the local anesthetic binds to the nerve membrane, the permeability to sodium is reduced. The water-soluble charged form of the local anesthetic binds to the calcium ion receptor site. The receptor channel is blocked and sodium conduction decreases. In turn, the rate of depolarization is decreased, nerve conduction is prevented, and the potential pain threshold is blocked.

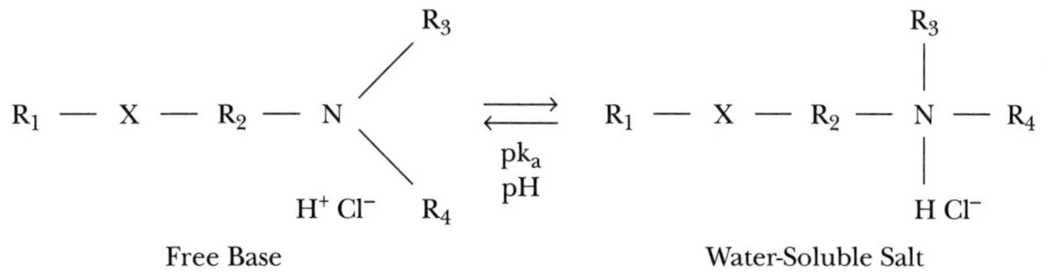

Figure 4-2 *Free base and water-soluble salt form of local anesthetics*

Table 4-1 Characteristics of the Free Base and Hydrochloride Salt Forms of Local Anesthetics

Free Base	*Hydrochloride Salt*
Lipophilic	Hydrophilic
Unstable	Stable
Basic	Acidic
Uncharged, unionized	Charged, ionized
Viscous liquids	Crystalline solids
Amorphous solids	

IONIZATION FACTORS

Local anesthetics are weak bases that occur in equilibrium between the lipid-soluble (lipophilic) free base and the water-soluble (hydrophilic) hydrochloride salt (Figure 4-2). Table 4-1 provides an overview of the characteristics of the lipophilic free base and water-soluble hydrochloride salt forms of local anesthetics. The proportion of the free base and the hydrochloride salt is determined by the pK_a of the local anesthetic and the pH of the surrounding tissue environment. The dental carpule has a pH less than 7.4, which allows for more drug to be in the ionized form and increases drug solubility. This also increases the stability of the local anesthetic in the carpule. Injection into surrounding tissue with a pH of 7.4 allows more drug to be available in the free-base, unionized form, which provides for greater tissue penetration. Inflammation and abscesses may lower tissue pH, causing less anesthetic to be absorbed, thereby slowing the onset of action and reducing potency.

PHARMACOLOGY

Local anesthetics work by reversibly blocking peripheral nerve conduction of small unmyelinated fibers and then large myelinated fibers. A loss of nerve function results, occurring in the following order: autonomic, cold, warmth, pain, touch, pressure, vibration, proprioception, and motor response. There is a variation to this order in some patients. Nerve function returns in the reverse order.

Arrhythmias and seizures are associated with abnormal or excessive excitability of nerve membranes. Local anesthetics, such as **lidocaine,** block cardiac sodium channels and depress abnormal pacemaker activity, cardiac excitability, and conduction, thereby stopping the arrhythmia. Intravenous lidocaine has also been successful in interrupting status epilepticus.

PHARMACOKINETICS

The pharmacokinetics of local anesthetics play an important role in rate of onset, duration, and intensity of action of local anesthesia. All are either directly or indirectly related to amount and concentration of drug, site of application, and procedure. This section reviews the pharmacokinetics of local anesthetics.

Absorption

The rate of absorption of local anesthetics is dependent on tissue vascularity and route of administration. Factors that affect vascularity include degree of inflammation present and the vasodilating properties of the local anesthetic. Vasodilatory activity increases blood flow to the site of injection, which increases systemic absorption and decreases the duration of action. Warmth and massage increase vasodilatory activity whereas cold temperatures decrease vasodilatory activity. Absorption is also determined by the degree of ionization of the local anesthetic.

Distribution

Once the local anesthetic has been absorbed, it is distributed throughout the body. Protein binding allows for the free-base form of the drug to bind to nerve fiber receptor sites more tightly, allowing for more potent anesthesia and a longer duration of action.

Metabolism

Ester local anesthetics are hydrolyzed in the plasma by pseudocholinesterase. An example of an ester local anesthetic is **procaine,** which is metabolized to PABA and causes allergic reactions in many people. Amide local anesthetics are metabolized by the liver except for **prilocaine,** which is metabolized by the lungs. Amide local anesthetics may not be suitable for patients with liver disease or heart failure. If they are used, the dose should be reduced significantly.

Elderly patients and those with liver failure may not be able to metabolize local anesthetics as quickly as a healthy 40-year-old patient. Higher concentrations and prolonged duration of action of the local anesthetic may result. Also, other drugs may increase the metabolism of local anesthetics, leading to lower concentrations and decreased duration of action.

Excretion

Both amide and ester local anesthetics and their by-products are excreted by the kidneys. Amides appear in the urine as the parent compound and in higher concentrations than esters. The dose of local anesthetics should be appropriately adjusted for a person with renal disease or the elderly because they may not be able to excrete the local anesthetic as quickly, thereby leading to higher concentrations and a prolonged duration of action.

TYPES OF LOCAL ANESTHETICS

Table 4-2 reviews local anesthetics available for dental use. On average, local anesthetics have an onset of action of 5 to 7 minutes and a duration of action of 1 to 3 hours and can be extended with the addition of a vasoconstrictor.

Amides

The five amide local anesthetics, **bupivacaine, etidocaine, lidocaine, mepivacaine,** and **prilocaine,** are more commonly used in dentistry. They appear to have a lower

Table 4-2   Local Anesthetics Commonly Used in Dentistry

Local Anesthetic Agent	Vasoconstrictor	Maximum Safe Dose Local Anesthetic	Maximum Safe Dose Vasoconstrictor	
			Healthy Patients	*Cardiac Patients*
Amides				
Lidocaine 2%	None	20–300 mg		
Lidocaine 2%	Epinephrine 1:50,000	20–100 mg, not to exceed 500 mg	0.2 mg	0.04 mg
Lidocaine 2%	Epinephrine 1:100,000	20–100 mg, not to exceed 500 mg	0.2 mg	0.04 mg
Lidocaine 2%	Epinephrine 1:200,000	20–100 mg, not to exceed 500 mg	0.2 mg	0.04 mg
Prilocaine 4% (Citanest)	Epinephrine 1:200,000	40–80 mg, not to exceed 400 mg	0.2 mg	0.04 mg
Mepivacaine 3% (Carbocaine)	None	54–270 mg, not to exceed 300 mg		
Mepivacaine 2% (Carbocaine)	Neo-Cobefrin 1:20,000	36–180 mg, not to exceed 400 mg	1 mg	0.2 mg
Bupivacaine 0.5% (Marcaine)	Epinephrine 1:200,000	9–90 mg	0.2 mg	0.04 mg
Etidocaine 1.5% (Duranest)	Epinephrine 1:200,000	150–300 mg, not to exceed 400 mg	0.2 mg	0.04 mg
Esters				
Propoxycaine 0.4% with procaine 2% (Ravocaine)	Neo-Cobefrin 1:20,000	7.2–36 mg	0.2 mg	0.04 mg
Procaine 2% (Novocain)	Levophed 1:30,000	36–180 mg not to exceed 400 mg	0.34 mg	0.14 mg

Reprinted with permission from *Dental Hygienist News,* Vol. 7, No. 2 (Spring 1994), through an educational grant from Procter and Gamble.

incidence of hypersensitivity reactions, a longer shelf life, a greater degree of anesthesia, and a duration of action suitable for most dental procedures.

Bupivacaine. **Bupivacaine** is ideal for dental procedures requiring more than 90 minutes of anesthesia or when postoperative pain is anticipated. It is similar to lidocaine and mepivacaine, although it has a slower onset of action but a more prolonged duration of action. Bupivacaine has a Food and Drug Administration (FDA) pregnancy category rating of C and the lowest possible dose should only be used after all other options have been explored.

Etidocaine. **Etidocaine** is also ideal for dental procedures requiring more than 90 minutes of anesthesia or when postoperative pain is anticipated. It is similar to lidocaine and mepivacaine yet it has a fast onset and prolonged duration of action.

Lidocaine. **Lidocaine** with a vasoconstrictor is well suited for dental procedures requiring 30–90 minutes of anesthesia. It has a rapid onset of action and spreads quickly throughout the affected tissue. Lidocaine has an FDA pregnancy rating category of B and is considered the drug of choice for a pregnant woman if a local anesthetic is required.

Mepivacaine. **Mepivacaine** with a vasoconstrictor is ideal for dental procedures requiring 30–90 minutes of anesthesia. It also has a rapid onset of action and produces less vasodilation than lidocaine. It is available as a 2% solution with the vasoconstrictor **levonordefrin.** Mepivacaine, without a vasoconstrictor, is suitable for dental procedures that require no more than 30 minutes of anesthesia. Mepivacaine has an FDA pregnancy category rating of C and the lowest possible dose should only be used after all other options have been explored.

Prilocaine. **Prilocaine** with a vasoconstrictor will provide anesthesia for up to 90 minutes. It appears to be less potent and toxic than lidocaine and has a slightly longer duration of action than lidocaine. Prilocaine has an FDA pregnancy rating of category B.

Esters

Ester local anesthetics are more likely to produce hypersensitivity reactions and should only be used in those patients with allergic reactions to amide local anesthetics. This section reviews the more commonly used ester local anesthetics.

Procaine. **Procaine** is only available in combination with **propoxycaine.** It has a slow onset and a toxicity and potency half that of lidocaine. It produces marked vasodilation and has a short duration of action. It should be used for dental procedures that require 30–60 minutes of anesthesia.

Propoxycaine. **Propoxycaine** with a vasoconstrictor is suitable for dental procedures requiring 30–60 minutes of anesthesia. It has a rapid onset and a relatively long duration of action.

ADVERSE REACTIONS

Local anesthetics have a relatively low incidence of adverse reactions and those factors that influence adverse reactions are reviewed in Table 4-3. Children, the elderly, and those with pathologic factors are more likely to suffer an adverse drug reaction.

The two main systems affected by adverse reactions are the central nervous system (CNS) and the cardiovascular (CV) system. CNS adverse reactions include restlessness, tremors, and convulsions followed by CNS depression, respiratory and CV depression, and coma. Some patients may experience sedation with lidocaine. Cardiovascular adverse reactions include myocardial depression and cardiac arrest with peripheral vasodilation.

Several cases of methemoglobinemia have been reported with prilocaine. Large doses of prilocaine are metabolized to orthotoluidine and toxic doses can result in cyanosis of the lips and mucous membranes, respiratory depression, and circulatory distress. It can be reversed with methylene blue. Prilocaine should be avoided in patients with chronic obstructive lung disease, asthma, and other oxygenation problems.

Local adverse reactions may be a result of physical injury caused by injection technique or rate of administration. Allergic reactions are more common with ester local anesthetics with no cross-sensitivity reactions to amide local anesthetics.

Table 4-3   Factors that Affect Local Anesthetic Toxicity

Patient Factors	*Description*
Age	
Under 6 years	Underdeveloped absorption, metabolism, excretion
Over 65 years	Decreased absorption, metabolism, excretion
Body Weight	
Thin	Increased systemic concentration of local anesthetic
Muscular	Decreased systemic concentration of local anesthetic
Obese	Increased systemic concentration of local anesthetic
Pathologic Factors	
Liver disease	Decreased metabolism of local anesthetic
Heart failure	Decreased transportation to the liver for breakdown
Pulmonary disease	Decreased metabolism of prilocaine
Renal disease	Decreased excretion of local anesthetic
Drug Factors	
Vasoactivity	Local anesthetics increase vascularity at the site of injection
Dose	Increasing the dose increases blood levels
Route of administration	Intravascular routes rapidly increase blood levels
Rate of injection	Rapid injections increase the rate of absorption at the site of injection, thereby increasing blood levels
Vascularity	The more vascular the site, the more rapid the absorption of the local anesthetic at the site of injection
Vasoconstrictor	Decreases systemic absorption of the local anesthetic at the site of injection

Reprinted with permission from *Dental Hygienist News*, Vol. 7, No. 2 (Spring 1994), through an educational grant from Procter and Gamble.

DENTAL CONCERNS

Dental hygienists should counsel all patients about the potential adverse reactions associated with local anesthetics. Patients should be advised to let the dental hygienist or dentist know if they are feeling anxious, nervous, or if they are having heart palpitations. Most of these problems can be avoided by lowering the dose of the local anesthetic or switching to another local anesthetic.

Lidocaine may cause sedation and patients should be advised of this. They should have someone drive them to and from the dental procedure. Patients should use caution if an opioid analgesic or antianxiety agent is prescribed because of the potential for increased sedation and drowsiness. If this is the case, patients should be advised to avoid working with heavy equipment or machinery, driving, or doing anything that requires thought or concentration.

Patients should also refrain from eating or drinking very hot or cold foods or drinks. The local anesthetic will make it difficult to detect temperature changes and patients may burn themselves with hot food.

ADDITIVES

Local anesthetic solutions are composed of the local anesthetic and additives, and may contain a vasoconstrictor. The *additives* are **methylparaben, sodium bisulfite, sodium bicarbonate, carbon dioxide salt, other sodium salts,** and **Dextran.**

Methylparaben. In the past, methylparaben was used in multidose vials to provide antibacterial activity. It has been removed from multidose vials because of its high incidence of allergic reaction.

Sodium Bisulfite and Sodium Metabisulfite. Both are antioxidants that help to prolong the shelf life of the local anesthetic. Caution should be used with bisulfites because many people are allergic to them. Particular caution should be exercised with asthmatic patients who are very sensitive to sulfites. Observe the patient for wheezing and shortness of breath.

Other Additives. Other additives include salts of carbon dioxide, sodium chloride, sodium hydroxide, or Dextran, which have a higher pH, allowing for a faster onset of action and more profound effect.

VASOCONSTRICTORS

Vasoconstrictors are important additions to local anesthetic solutions and **epinephrine** and levonordefrin are the vasoconstrictors of choice in the United States. The duration of action of most local anesthetics is 30 minutes to 3 hours and may be extended by adding a vasoconstrictor. Table 4-2, page 35, reviews the concentrations of vasoconstrictors added to the more commonly used local anesthetics. A vasoconstrictor should be used with a concentration that allows for adequate depth, duration, and safety.

Mechanism of Action

The local α effects of vasoconstrictors cause blood vessels to constrict, which decreases the amount of blood flow to the site of injection, in turn, decreasing systemic absorption of the local anesthetic. A higher concentration of the local anesthetic remains locally, leading to a prolonged duration of action. Blood vessel constriction also results in hemostasis, which improves visibility at the surgical site.

Vasoconstrictors and Cardiovascular Disease

In the past, it was felt that vasoconstrictors should not be given to patients with cardiovascular disease because of the systemic effects of the vasoconstrictor. Systemic effects include cardiac excitability, which results in increased heart rate, force of contraction, and stroke volume, which can elevate blood pressure. Patients with controlled cardiovascular disease do not have a noticeable increase in heart rate and blood pressure when given a vasoconstrictor. All patients can release endogenous levels of epinephrine in excess of a vasoconstrictor if a local anesthetic is given without a vasoconstrictor. This is due to the patient's normal physiologic response to the injection and the pending procedure.

Cardiovascular patients with controlled hypertension or angina can receive local anesthetics with epinephrine. The local anesthetic with a vasoconstrictor should be administered in the lowest possible dose using techniques that minimize systemic absorption. Table 4-2, page 35, reviews the maximum allowable doses of a vasoconstrictor for healthy adults and cardiovascular patients and these doses should not be exceeded.

Patients with uncontrolled hypertension, hyperthyroidism, unstable angina, controlled arrhythmias, and those who have had a myocardial infarction or cerebrovascular accident within the past 6 months should delay elective dental procedures. Caution should be used if a vasoconstrictor is administered to these patients. Vasoconstrictors are contraindicated in patients with uncontrolled arrhythmias, pheochromocytoma, and uncontrolled hyperthyroidism.

Dental Concerns

A detailed medication/health history will determine whether or not a patient is taking medication for hypertension or angina or has had recent cardiovascular or cerebrovascular problems. The dental hygienist, dentist, or dental assistant should check the patient's blood pressure and then the dentist should make the decision about whether or not to use a vasoconstrictor with the local anesthetic. Often, the dentist may make this decision after consulting with the patient's physician.

Adverse Reactions

Adverse reactions include such central nervous effects as patient anxiety, apprehension, and nervousness. These can be minimized by having a calm staff member remain with the patient or by administering a lower dose of vasoconstrictor.

Table 4-4   Drug Interactions with Vasoconstrictors

Interacting Drug Group	Examples	Outcome
Tricyclic antidepressants	Amitriptyline	Increased pressor effects of epinephrine, arrhythmias
Monoamine oxidase inhibitors	Phenelzine	Serious potentiation of epinephrine—hypertensive crisis
Phenothiazines	Haloperidol	Increased risk for hypotension
β Blockers	Propranolol	Hypertension and reflex increase in vagal tone resulting in bradycardia
Antidiabetic agents	Insulin, chlorpropamide	Increase in blood sugar
Antihypertensives	Guanethidine	Increased effects of epinephrine, development of severe hypertension
Antimanics	Lithium	Decreases the efficacy of epinephrine
Cocaine abuse	Cocaine	Stimulates the release of norepinephrine, increased sympathetic activity, which can lead to ischemia, arrhythmias, angina, and myocardial infarction
Anticonvulsants	Phenytoin	Decreased efficacy of epinephrine

Reprinted with permission from *Dental Hygienist News,* Vol. 7, No. 2 (Spring 1994), through an educational grant from Procter and Gamble.

Drug Interactions

Table 4-4 reviews some of the more common drug interactions with vasoconstrictors. They are not absolute contraindications to using a vasoconstrictor, but great caution should be exercised when a patient is taking these medications. Assess the general health of the patient and monitor her for any signs of a drug interaction. Also, use the least concentrated solution of a vasoconstrictor that will allow for anesthesia over a sufficient period of time. Lastly, the local anesthetic and vasoconstrictor should be injected slowly with frequent aspiration to minimize systemic absorption and accidental intravascular injection.

TOPICAL LOCAL ANESTHETICS

Several local anesthetics are commercially available in topical dose forms and are rapidly absorbed when applied to the mucous membranes. In order to avoid adverse reactions to both the patient and hygienist, one should know both the relative toxicity and concentration of the drug used. One should limit the area of application and use the smallest volume of the least toxic topical local anesthetic.

The commonly used topical local anesthetics in dentistry are **benzocaine, lidocaine,** and **tetracaine.**

Benzocaine. **Benzocaine,** an ester of PABA, is the most commonly used topical local anesthetic. Dental staff should wear gloves when administering it because it can cause contact dermatitis. It is also available in many over-the-counter products for teething, sunburn, hemorrhoids, and insect bites.

Lidocaine. **Lidocaine** 2–5% is available as the hydrochloride salt or the base. The base is not very water soluble; the hydrochloride salt is water soluble, causing greater tissue penetration and the potential for systemic adverse reactions. Viscous lidocaine 2% is available as an oral rinse.

Tetracaine. **Tetracaine** is an ester of PABA and has a slow onset and long duration of action. It is rapidly absorbed from the mucosal surface and has a high toxicity rate. It is available as a 2% solution and no more than 20 mg should be used at any one time.

DENTAL CONCERNS

Topical local anesthetics can be absorbed into the mucous membranes of the oral cavity very quickly and can cause adverse reactions. The dental hygienist should know the concentration of the drug being used and should use the smallest volume and lowest concentration of the least toxic local anesthetic. The dental hygienist should also limit the area of application in order to reduce the risk of further systemic absorption and adverse reactions.

The dental hygienist should instruct the patients not to swallow topical local anesthetics. These medications are numbing and may interfere with swallowing and gag reflexes. Patients should be instructed to avoid very hot or very cold foods and drinks because they may not be able to sense temperature changes with a tongue that has been numbed by a topical local anesthetic.

Summary

Local anesthetics are important in providing the patient with "painless" dentistry. On average, local anesthetics have a duration of action of 1 to 3 hours and can be extended with the addition of a vasoconstrictor. Many different factors affect the ability of the body to absorb the local anesthetic. They include drugs such as epinephrine that decrease the amount of drug absorbed into the systemic circulation of the body and create a dry field. The rate of injection, patient age, infection, and heat or cold applied to the area of injection all affect the amount of drug that is absorbed. Local anesthetics have a relatively low adverse reaction profile and the more common adverse reactions involve the central nervous and cardiovascular systems. Several drug interactions have been reported with vasoconstrictors. These interactions can cause increased heart rate and blood pressure and can also affect cardiac rhythm. Local anesthetics with vasoconstrictors can be used in patients with controlled cardiovascular disease. Several local anesthetics are available in topical dose forms. Be familiar with the relative toxicity and concentration of the drug used to avoid adverse reactions.

Case Study: Louisa Mendoza

Louisa Mendoza is a 32-year-old woman who is a long-time patient of your practice. Since this is a scheduled maintenance visit, you review her medication/health history. She tells you that she gave birth to her daughter, whom she is nursing. Mrs. Mendoza is here today to have the cavity filled that was found during her last trimester of pregnancy. The cavity was not filled at that time because Mrs. Mendoza was uncomfortable in the dental chair as she was near term.

1. What other questions would you ask during the medication/health history?
2. Which local anesthetic could be used and why?
3. Should the local anesthetic be used with or without a vasoconstrictor? Why or why not?
4. What should Mrs. Mendoza be told about the local anesthetic that was chosen?
5. What are the adverse reactions associated with vasoconstrictor use? How can they be minimized?
6. What are the systemic and local adverse reactions associated with local anesthetics?
7. Mrs. Mendoza has concerns about the local anesthetic and its effect on her infant (local anesthetics cross into breast milk as they do across the placenta). What should she be told about local anesthetics and nursing?

Case Study: Frank Castinelli

Frank Castinelli is 55 years old, slightly overweight, and has been coming to your practice for close to 10 years. He has a somewhat stressful job that takes up quite a bit of his time. His medications include nitroglycerin sublingual tablets for angina, ibuprofen for aches and pains, and antacids for heartburn. Mr. Castinelli comes in today for a scheduled oral health maintenance visit and tells you that he suffered a heart attack 3 months ago. He is in good spirits and seems to be recovering from his heart attack. His only new medication is an aspirin tablet each day to prevent further heart attacks. Unfortunately, you note two cavities during your oral examination and cleaning of Mr. Castinelli.

1. Would you and the dentist recommend that Mr. Castinelli have his cavities filled within the next 2 weeks? Why or why not?
2. When should Mr. Castinelli have his cavities filled?
3. Would a local anesthetic with a vasoconstrictor be appropriate in this patient?
4. What is the relationship between vasoconstrictors and cardiovascular disease?
5. If Mr. Castinelli were to have his cavities filled in 6 to 8 months, what should be recommended and why?
6. What should Mr. Castinelli be told about his new health status (post–heart attack) and vasoconstrictors?

Review Questions

1. What is the mechanism of action of local anesthetics?
2. What are the ionization factors of local anesthetics and how do they impact on drug absorption into the surrounding tissue?
3. What factors can affect the rate of absorption of local anesthetics?
4. What factors can affect the metabolism of local anesthetics?
5. Which local anesthetic would be appropriate for a dental procedure requiring 30 to 60 minutes of anesthesia?
6. List three additives found in local anesthetics. Why are they added to the local anesthetic?
7. Why are vasoconstrictors added to local anesthetics?
8. What are some of the drug interactions associated with vasoconstrictors?

BIBLIOGRAPHY

Adriani J., Zepernick R: Clinical effectiveness of drugs used for topical anesthesia. *JAMA* 188:711, 1964.
Ayoub ST, Coleman AE: A review of local anesthetics. *Gen Dentistry* 40:285–287, 289–290, 1992.
Bablenis Haveles E: Local anesthetics: A review. *Dental Hygienist News* 7:3–7, 1994.
Cassidy JP, Phero JC, Grau WH: Epinephrine: Systemic effects and varying concentrations in local anesthetics. *Anesth Prog* 33:289–295, 1986.
Covino BG: Pharmacokinetics of intravenous regional anesthetics. *Regional Anesthesia,* Jan–March, 5–8, 1979.
Goulet JP, Perusse R, Turcotte JY: Contraindications to vasoconstrictors in dentistry: Part III. *Oral Surg Oral Med Oral Pathol* 74:692–697, 1992.
McEvoy, G.K., ed: Local anesthetics. *American Hospital Formulary Service.* ASHP, Bethesda, Maryland, 1995, pp. 1946–1959.
Ritchie JM, Greene NM: Local anesthetics. In Goodman A, Rall TW, Nies AS, Taylor P (eds.), *Goodman and Gilman's The Pharmacological Basis of Therapeutics,* 8th ed. Pergamon Press, New York, 1990, pp. 311–331.
Young ER, MacKenzie TA: The pharmacology of local anesthetics—a review of the literature. *J Can Dent Assoc* 58:34–42, 1992.

CHAPTER 5

General Anesthetics

Key Terms

Anesthesia
Conscious Sedation
Dissociative Anesthesia
General Anesthetics
Induction

Inhalation Anesthetics
Minimal Alveolar Concentration
Nitrous Oxide
Volatile Anesthetics

LEARNING OBJECTIVES

After completion of this chapter and its learning activities, the student should be able to:

1. Define anesthesia.
2. Demonstrate a general knowledge of the mechanism of action of general anesthetics.
3. Describe the stages and planes of anesthesia.
4. Describe the physical factors that regulate the rate of onset and recovery of anesthesia.
5. Discuss the adverse reactions associated with general anesthetics.
6. Discuss the pharmacologic and pharmacokinetic actions of nitrous oxide, including time course of action, organ system effects, drug interactions, dental concerns, and adverse reactions.
7. Discuss the volatile anesthetics, including pharmacology, pharmacokinetics, drug interactions, dental concerns, and adverse reactions.
8. Discuss the use of ultrashort-acting barbiturates in the induction phase of anesthesia. Include pharmacology, pharmacokinetics, drug interactions, dental concerns, and adverse reactions.
9. Define the term *conscious sedation* and its relationship to anesthesia. Include drug pharmacology, pharmacokinetics, drug interactions, dental concerns, and adverse reactions.
10. Define the term *dissociative anesthesia*. Include drug pharmacology, pharmacokinetics, drug interactions, dental concerns, and adverse reactions.

INTRODUCTION

Anesthesia is the combination of reversible unconsciousness and the absence of response to painful stimuli. It is produced by a group of chemical substances *(general anesthetics)* that are potent central nervous system (CNS) depressants. Patients experience unconsciousness, analgesia, immobility (thus permitting surgery), and amnesia upon recovery. Because the patient has lost consciousness and the ability to respond to and remember major changes in sensory input, it is mandatory for the health professional to provide constant monitoring and evaluation of the patient.

Most of the general anesthetics used today have only been recently introduced into medicine. The administration techniques used provide a balanced combination of drugs that help to minimize adverse reactions and take into account the preanesthetic and postanesthetic needs of the patient. Health professionals working with general anesthetics have special training in pharmacology and administration techniques.

General anesthetics are usually administered in hospital operating rooms, which have the equipment and trained personnel necessary to monitor the patient and, if necessary, resuscitate the patient. General anesthetics have been safely used by oral and maxillofacial surgeons for many years. General dentists have used nitrous oxide for its antianxiety effects as opposed to its anesthetic effects, and other general anesthetics are being used for conscious sedation in general dental practices. The dental hygienist should have a general knowledge of the pharmacology of these drugs as well as adverse reactions and drug interactions.

MECHANISM OF ACTION

The many theories and explanations surrounding the mechanism of action of general anesthetics involve the functional interactions among the varying intervening levels of neuronal organization of the person receiving the drug. These medications depress the CNS and affect memory, sensation, and volitional movements. Cardiovascular and respiratory function are only depressed when lethal levels of a general anesthetic are administered.

STAGES AND PLANES OF ANESTHESIA

The stages and planes of anesthesia were initially developed by Guedel to describe the levels and progression of anesthesia produced by ether. Although this information is somewhat outdated, it has proven to be conceptually and clinically useful in learning about anesthetics (Marshall and Longnecker, 1990). Table 5-1 reviews the stages and planes of anesthesia.

Induction from stage 1 through stage 2 can be uncomfortable for some patients because emesis and incontinence may occur. This can be minimized by providing the patient with a smooth and rapid induction through stages 1 and 2 into stage 3 by administering an ultra-short-acting barbiturate.

Stage 3 is divided into four planes differentiated on the basis of eye movements, depth of respiration, and muscle relaxation. Decreased skeletal muscle tone, dilated pupils, tachycardia, and hypotension are indicative of stage 3, plane 3. Plane 4 is

Table 5-1   Stages and Planes of Anesthesia

Stage and Plane	*Patient Response*
Stage 1—Analgesia	1. Patient is responsive 2. Reduced sensation to pain 3. Can still respond to commands 4. Reflexes are present 5. Regular respiration 6. Some amnesia 7. Loss of consciousness (end of stage)
Stage 2—Delirium or Excitement	1. Unconsciousness 2. Amnesia 3. Involuntary movement and excitement 4. Irregular respiration 5. Increased muscle tone 6. Sympathetic stimulation—tachycardia, mydriasis, hypertension
Stage 3—Surgical Anesthesia	1. Return to regular respiration, muscle relaxation, and normal heart and pulse rates 2. Divided into four planes
Stage IV—Respiratory or Medullary Paralysis	1. Cessation of respiration 2. Subsequent circulatory failure 3. Respiration must be artificially maintained

characterized by intercostal muscle paralysis, absence of all reflexes, and extreme muscle flaccidity. Patients can progress to stage 4 with cessation of all respiration.

A more recent approach to explaining the different levels of anesthesia is reviewed next. Flagg proposed that the levels of anesthesia be redefined as induction, maintenance, and recovery.

Induction

The induction phase of anesthesia includes all preoperative medications, adjunctive medications to anesthesia, and the anesthetics required for anesthesia. This phase takes place prior to the actual operation or procedure.

Maintenance

This phase begins when the patient has reached an anesthetic level deep enough to allow the surgical procedure to begin. It continues until the procedure has been completed.

Recovery

This phase begins as the surgical procedure is completed and continues throughout the postoperative period until the patient is fully responsive.

FACTORS REGULATING ONSET AND RECOVERY OF ANESTHESIA

The onset of anesthesia is regulated by the respiration rate, depth, respiratory minute volume, alveolar membrane-blood translocation, cardiac output and functional perfusion, partial pressure of the anesthetic in the inspired mixture, and solubility of the general anesthetic in blood and tissues. Induction can be hastened by having the patient rapidly breathe high concentrations of the general anesthetic. Concentration and rate of delivery can be decreased to maintenance levels once the desired depth of anesthesia has been reached.

The solubility of the general anesthetic in blood and tissues is measured as the blood:gas partition coefficient. Low solubility is indicative of rapid onset and recovery whereas highly soluble drugs have a slower rate of onset and recovery.

The term *minimal alveolar concentration* (MAC) is used to measure and compare the relative potency of general anesthetic agents. General anesthetics with MACs greater than 1 are less potent than general anesthetics with an MAC less than 1. General anesthetics (volatile anesthetics) with low MACs are used in combination with **nitrous oxide** (MAC of 100) to reduce the concentration of each and improve MAC values.

Factors that regulate the rate of recovery from anesthesia include those involved in the rate of onset, solubility in adipose (fat) tissue, and the circulatory perfusion of tissues, especially adipose for potent, highly lipid-soluble general anesthetics.

ADVERSE REACTIONS

The adverse reactions associated with general anesthetics are often a result of lethal doses. At high enough doses general anesthetics can produce arrhythmias, increased (stage 2) or decreased blood pressure, and cardiac arrest. Respiratory adverse reactions include respiratory depression (stage 3) and respiratory arrest (stage 4). Other adverse reactions include headache, fatigue, irritability, and nausea and vomiting.

Health professionals, in particular operating room personnel, are at risk for developing hepatoxicity as a result of repeated exposure to general anesthetics. Both female health professionals and spouses or significant others of male health professionals who work with general anesthetics may experience a higher rate of fetal abnormalities and spontaneous abortions. Lastly, explosions have been associated with **cyclopropane** and **ether.**

DRUG INTERACTIONS

Essentially, all drugs that cause CNS depression cause additive CNS depressant effects with general anesthetics. Drugs that cause CNS depression or sedation include opioid analgesics, barbiturates, benzodiazepines, **chloral hydrate,** antipsychotics, antidepressants, other anesthetics, antihistamines, and alcohol. The patient should be questioned about his use of these medications, including the time of the last dose of the CNS depressant medication. The dose of the anesthetic may have to be lowered in order to avoid serious adverse reactions. On the other hand, patients receiving amphetamine and amphetamine-like drugs may require a higher dose of the general anesthetic.

DENTAL CONCERNS

Sedation and amnesia are an accepted and desired state of general anesthetic drugs. Patients should be reminded of this and should have someone drive them to and from their dental appointment. They should also avoid operating or working with heavy machinery and anything else that requires concentration for at least several hours after their dental appointment.

The dental hygienist should question patients about their medication use in order to avoid any interactions with general anesthetic drugs. Medication/health histories of patients should be reviewed in order to avoid or minimize adverse reactions.

INHALATION ANESTHETICS

Inhalation anesthetics can be categorized as gases at standard temperature and atmospheric pressure and volatile liquids. This section reviews the more commonly used gases and volatile liquids and briefly discusses some of the older drugs.

Nitrous Oxide

Nitrous oxide (N_2O) is a colorless gas with little or no odor. It has little potency and is used in clinical outpatient dentistry as an inhaled sedative. It produces intoxication, analgesia, and amnesia in most patients and does *not* produce complete unconsciousness or complete general anesthesia in concentrations used in dentistry. Nitrous oxide in combination with oxygen (N_2O-O_2) allows the patient to remain conscious with his reflexes intact and provides relief from anxiety when administered properly.

Nitrous oxide is administered with oxygen by varying the concentration of nitrous oxide to titrate the patient to the desired level of sedation. The gas mixture is administered using a gas machine with accurately calibrated flow meters that control the volume flow and percentage of nitrous oxide and oxygen. One hundred percent oxygen is administered for the first 2–3 minutes and nitrous oxide is then added in 5–10% increments until the desired state of sedation is attained, usually within 3–5 minutes. Table 5-2 reviews the percent of nitrous oxide in oxygen and patient response. The average patient requires 35% of nitrous oxide in oxygen with a range of 10–50%.

Once the procedure is terminated, the patient should receive 100% oxygen for at least 5 minutes. The effects of nitrous oxide wear off rapidly as it is removed from the tissues. If the breathing mask is removed too quickly (without oxygen recovery), the patient breathes room air and can develop hypoxia. Hypoxia is a result of the rapid outward flow of nitrous oxide, oxygen, and carbon dioxide. Patients may complain of headache, which can be treated with 100% oxygen administration.

The advantages to nitrous oxide–oxygen administration include rapid onset and recovery, easy administration, close control of the patient, acceptability for children, and a more calm dental team. The proper depth of sedation can be easily controlled with nitrous oxide. Patient response to questions is a good indication of the level of sedation. Patients may demonstrate slow, slurred speech, appear sleepy yet open their eyes if asked to do so, and can maintain an open-mouth position during the procedure. Patients are also relaxed, cooperative, and may experience feelings of euphoria, hence the term "laughing gas." The patient's time frame is also distorted by

Table 5-2   Patient Response to Nitrous Oxide–Oxygen Mixtures

Nitrous Oxide Concentration	*Patient Response*
10–20%	Body warmth
	Tingling of hands and feet
20–30%	Circumoral numbness
	Numbness of thighs
20–40%	Numbness of tongue
	Numbness of hands and feet
	Droning sounds present
	Hearing distinct but distant
	Dissociation begins and reaches peak
	Mild sleepiness
	Some analgesia
	Euphoria
	Feeling of heaviness or lightness of body
30–50%	Sweating
	Nausea
	Amnesia
	Increased sleepiness
40–60%	Dreaming, laughing, giddiness
	Further increased sleepiness, tending toward unconsciousness
	Increased nausea and possible vomiting
Greater than 50%	Unconsciousness and light general anesthesia

Adapted from Bennett CR: *Conscious-Sedation in Dental Practice.* Mosby, St. Louis, 1974. Used with permission.

nitrous oxide so that the patient assumes that the procedure was much shorter than it actually was. This may be due to the amnestic qualities of nitrous oxide.

Nitrous oxide is advantageous in managing apprehensive children and adults, although it cannot be used in patients who are hysterical or uncontrollable. Calm patients allow for the dental team to remain calm and relaxed during the dental procedure.

Pharmacology

Nitrous Oxide. **Nitrous oxide** produces predictable, dose-related effects on the CNS resulting in sedation, analgesia, and amnesia.

Pharmacokinetics. The onset of effects of nitrous oxide are rapid due to its rapid absorption from pulmonary alveoli into the circulatory system. Nitrous oxide has low solubility in blood and tissues, which allows for the equilibrium between the inhaled nitrous oxide–oxygen mixture in body tissues to be reached within minutes.

Adverse Reactions. The adverse reactions most commonly occurring with nitrous oxide have been the result of misuse or faulty installation of equipment. Nitrous oxide cylinders are blue and oxygen cylinders are green to avoid confusion and both are "pin coded" to avoid inadvertent mixing of cylinders and lines. Inhalation administration equipment is now equipped with a fail-safe system that shuts down the nitrous oxide if the oxygen runs out and also limits the amount of nitrous oxide that can be released.

Other adverse reactions include nausea and vomiting. The dental hygienist should advise the patient to eat a light meal prior to the appointment and avoid eating a large meal within 3 hours of the appointment.

Contraindications. Although nitrous oxide is safe and easy to use, it is contraindicated in several patient populations. Patients with any type of respiratory obstruction, including a stuffy nose, should not receive nitrous oxide since the patient needs clear nasal passages to breathe in the mixture and for gaseous exchange. Other respiratory diseases, such as asthma, must be carefully evaluated.

Patients with chronic obstructive pulmonary disease, particularly emphysema, have respirations that are driven by a lack of oxygen and not by elevated carbon dioxide levels. These patients would have great difficulty if they received more oxygen than they normally breathe.

One of the effects of nitrous oxide is euphoria, which could be exacerbated in patients with mental illness or other types of emotional instability. Also, young children and emotionally unstable adults can often become uncooperative in a dental office. This type of behavior would make it difficult for them to inhale nitrous oxide and achieve any type of conscious sedation.

Indirect evidence has indicated that female dental personnel with chronic exposure to nitrous oxide or pregnant women who receive nitrous oxide may have a higher incidence of miscarriage or spontaneous abortion than those who are not exposed. Also, women who were exposed to greater than 5 hours per week of nitrous oxide were less fertile than unexposed women.

This issue is of particular concern to all female dental personnel and patients who are pregnant or of childbearing potential. The female dental hygienist should be aware of the level of nitrous oxide present in her place of practice. Machines are available to monitor the levels of nitrous oxide in the office and scavenger systems can retrieve much of the expired gas and turnover of room air can be increased.

Drug Interactions. The most serious drug interactions occur with drugs known to produce CNS depression and sedation. The combination of a CNS depressant with nitrous oxide can lead to a state of general anesthesia. If nitrous oxide is combined with other methods of sedation, the general dental staff must be trained and prepared for the resulting general anesthetic state.

Nitrous Oxide Abuse. Unfortunately, the euphoric feelings of nitrous oxide make it a drug of abuse by both the patient and dental personnel. Chronic exposure to nitrous oxide can lead to peripheral neuropathy, which is a numbness and paresthesia of the hands and legs, and continued abuse can lead to more serious neurological problems. Other signs of chronic abuse are liver and kidney problems.

Dental Concerns. A detailed medication/health history will reveal patients with emotional/psychiatric problems as well as medications for depression, bipolar disorder, schizophrenia, other psychosis, anxiety, and other emotional disorders.

Some patients may have fanciful dreams that seem real to them upon discontinuation of the nitrous oxide. A female staff member should be present when a female patient receives nitrous oxide in the presence of a male dentist, dental hygienist, or dental assistant. This should help to avoid problems such as unfounded accusations.

Volatile Anesthetics

Volatile anesthetics are liquids that evaporate easily upon exposure to room temperature and are classified chemically as halogenated hydrocarbons because they contain fluorine, chlorine, or bromine in their structure. This section reviews the more commonly used volatile anesthetics.

Halothane (Fluothane). **Halothane** is a potent anesthetic with an MAC of 0.75 that is nonflammable, nonexplosive, and has a distinct fruity odor. It provides for smooth rapid induction of anesthesia with little laryngeal and bronchial spasm. Muscle relaxation is not complete and patients may require **d-tubocurarine,** a peripheral neuromuscular-blocking drug. Recovery is largely due to exhalation of the anesthetic from the lungs (80%).

Halothane dosage must be carefully titrated to avoid respiratory depression. Halothane also causes cardiovascular depression and presents as bradycardia and hypotension and can also cause arrhythmias. Other adverse reactions include uterine smooth muscle relaxation and depressed renal function.

There is little evidence to support the theory that halothane causes liver damage. However, there have been reports of postanesthetic hepatitis attributed to halothane. Repeated exposure to halothane or any other halogenated hydrocarbon may increase the likelihood of an occurrence or recurrence. As a result, halothane or any of the other halogenated hydrocarbons should not be used in patients with a history of postanesthetic hepatitis due to halothane.

Enflurane (Ethrane). **Enflurane** is a colorless, nonflammable liquid with a sweet odor with an MAC of 1.68 that is lowered to 0.57 when combined with nitrous oxide. Its low MAC allows for both rapid induction of and recovery from anesthesia. Skeletal muscle relaxation occurs to a greater extent with enflurane than halothane. Enflurane also causes respiratory depression, depression of myocardial contractility, and low blood pressure. Arrhythmias are less likely to occur with enflurane than halothane. Adverse reactions include seizure activity, hypotension, and a transient decrease in kidney function.

Isoflurane (Forane). **Isoflurane** is a potent agent with a pungent smell and is the most commonly used general anesthetic. Its low tissue solubility allows for rapid *induction* and recovery from anesthesia. Isoflurane's pungent smell may make it difficult for some patients to have a smooth induction period. This can be minimized by giving the patient an intravenous barbiturate as the induction to anesthesia.

Isoflurane also produces respiratory depression, hypotension, and smooth muscle relaxation. It does not sensitize the heart to epinephrine and it does not produce seizure-like activity. The most serious adverse reaction is respiratory acidosis with deeper levels of anesthesia.

INTRAVENOUS GENERAL ANESTHETICS

Intravenous general anesthetics include barbiturates, benzodiazepines, and opioid analgesics and provide the patient with *conscious sedation,* which will allow for short-lasting surgical procedures. The patient is calm, sedated, and has both analgesia and amnesia and has the ability to answer questions and respond to his environment. These medications are also used as induction agents in combination with inhaled anesthetics.

Barbiturates

Thiopental sodium (Pentothal), **methohexital sodium** (Brevital), and **thiamylal sodium** (Surital) are ultra-short-acting barbiturates that are used to induce sleep and anesthesia. These medications have an onset of action of 30–40 seconds when given intravenously and the rapid onset of sedation and sleep is the direct result of translocation of the drug from the blood to the brain. Its short duration of action is attributed to its redistribution from the brain to areas of low perfusion such as adipose (fat) tissue. Repeated dosing can lead to storage in adipose tissue, which will prolong recovery time. Patients with more adipose tissue, whether overweight or elderly, will have longer recovery times and may be at a higher risk for CNS adverse reactions.

These medications are not analgesics and should not be used as the sole anesthetic agent. They should be given with local anesthetic or as part of balanced anesthesia.

Complications of ultra-short-acting barbiturates include laryngospasm, bronchospasm, and some patients may experience hiccups, increased muscle activity, and delirium upon recovery. Other adverse reactions of barbiturates are discussed in Chapter 20.

Intravenous, ultra-short-acting barbiturates are irritating to the skin and intraarterial area. Extravascular (on the skin) exposure can result in tissue tenderness or even tissue necrosis or sloughing. Intraarterial injection can cause arteriospasm with ischemia of the arm and fingers and severe pain.

Dental Concerns. Patients should be carefully examined prior to any injection for suitable veins for administration of the ultra-short-acting barbiturates; these drugs are contraindicated in patients without suitable veins. Other contraindications to ultra-short-acting barbiturates include status asthmaticus, porphyria, and known sensitivity to the medications. This information can be obtained from a detailed medication/health history. Patients with asthma, liver disease, renal disease, cardiovascular disease, or who are elderly require dose reduction and should be carefully monitored for potential adverse reactions.

Benzodiazepines

Benzodiazepines have been an integral part of conscious sedation and preanesthesia because of their excellent antianxiety and amnestic properties. Patients are calm, relaxed, yet able to respond to simple commands. **Diazepam** (Valium) and **midazolam** (Versed) are the two benzodiazepines used for conscious sedation and as preanesthetics. Midazolam is less irritating on intravenous administration than diazepam, though it is sometimes more difficult to manage than diazepam. There is a significant lag between administration of dose and CNS effects, which could lead to drug overdose. Also, midazolam appears to have significant respiratory depressant effects and can cause respiratory depression and cardiac arrest. This can be avoided or minimized by carefully titrating the dose based on the individual patient and carefully monitoring the patient's vital signs. The benzodiazepines are an integral part of reducing patient anxiety and are further discussed in Chapter 9.

Ketamine (Ketalar). **Ketamine** is chemically related to phencyclidine (PCP) and produces an anesthetic situation where the patient, though not asleep, fails to respond to her environment. The patient does not respond to painful stimuli and does not remember the procedure (amnesia), yet respiratory and cardiac behaviors and functions remain intact. Pharyngeal and laryngeal reflexes also remain intact and muscle tone is sustained with small and nonpurposeful movements. The term *dissociative anesthesia* refers to the fact that there is a dissociation between the patient's response and her environment.

The main disadvantage to ketamine is its ability to cause hallucinations, delirium, confusion, irrational behavior, or bizarre dreams, which may make it uncomfortable for many patients. This seems to occur more frequently in the elderly, children, and those with a history of substance abuse. Ketamine is contraindicated in these patients as well as those with cerebrovascular disease, hypertension, and known drug hypersensitivity. Ketamine can cause excessive salivation and an anticholinergic drug may be required to create a dry field. Detailed medication/health histories will help to determine whether or not a patient should receive ketamine.

Opioid Analgesics

Opioid analgesics have been used as part of balanced anesthesia to provide the patient with analgesia during surgery and postsurgery as well as a preanesthetic medication. **Fentanyl** (Sublimaze), **alfentanil** (Alfenta), and **sufentanil** (Sufenta) are the more commonly used opioid analgesics because they are rapid acting and short lasting. The major disadvantage of these medications is respiratory depression. They do not significantly alter cardiovascular function or peripheral vascular resistance. Opioid analgesics are further discussed in Chapter 8.

Droperidol Plus Fentanyl (Innovar). **Droperidol** is an antipsychotic drug and **fentanyl** is a potent opioid analgesic. They have been combined to produce a wakeful anesthetic state. Droperidol produces significant sedation and catatonia and fentanyl provides potent analgesia. The return to consciousness is rapid though the effects of droperidol are long lasting.

The adverse reactions associated with these medications are the same as for other antipsychotics and opioid analgesics and are further discussed in Chapters 8 and 21. This combination of drugs should be used with caution in patients with Parkinson's disease and pulmonary insufficiency. A boardlike chest, which requires ventilatory assistance, has occurred in some patients.

Summary

General anesthetic drugs are an important part of "painless" dentistry. Several different classes of drugs are used to minimize adverse reactions and take into account the patient's preanesthetic and postanesthetic needs. General anesthetics are thought to work by depressing the CNS and affect memory, sensation, and volitional movements. The onset of anesthesia is regulated by the patient's respiratory rate, depth, respiratory minute volume, alveolar membrane-blood translocation, cardiac output and functional perfusion, partial pressure of the anesthetic in the inspired solution, and the solubility of the general anesthetic in blood and tissues. General anesthetic adverse reactions include headache, fatigue, irritability, nausea, and vomiting. Cardiac and respiratory adverse reactions occur at high doses. Drugs that cause CNS depression cause additive CNS depressant effects with general anesthetics.

General anesthetics include inhalation anesthetics that are broken down into gases and volatile liquids. Nitrous oxide is the most common gas that is used as an inhaled sedative to provide the patient with conscious sedation. Volatile general anesthetics include halothane, enflurane, and isoflurane. They are often used in combination with intravenous general anesthetics for a balanced anesthetic effect. Intravenous general anesthetics include the barbiturates, benzodiazepines, ketamine, opioid analgesics, and droperidol plus fentanyl.

The dental hygienist plays an important role in determining the patient's health and medication status through detailed medication/health histories. A general knowledge of these medications will help to prevent or minimize adverse reactions, drug interactions, and contraindications and provide the patient with a positive dental experience.

Case Study: Shalanda Riviera

Shalanda Riviera is a 21-year-old college student who comes to the university dental clinic for a scheduled oral examination. Unfortunately, Ms. Riviera needs to have a tooth extracted, which will require an appointment with the oral surgeon. Ms. Riviera has never had a tooth extracted and is concerned about the procedure. Since the oral surgeon is in the same office suite as the dental clinic, he requests that you conduct the medication/health history for Ms. Riviera.

1. What questions would you ask during the medication/health history?
2. Ms. Riviera's only medications include occasional over-the-counter ibuprofen and acetaminophen and cough and cold products. She is currently taking a combination decongestant/antihistamine for a head cold. Would this interfere with a general anesthetic?
3. Which volatile general anesthetic could be used and why?
4. Compare and contrast the volatile general anesthetic drugs.
5. What should Ms. Riviera be told about the volatile general anesthetic that was chosen?
6. Would an opioid analgesic be necessary? Please explain your answer.

Case Study: Tiesha Wilkins

Tiesha Wilkins is a 23-year-old newly licensed dental hygienist who has recently started working with the local dental practice. She is engaged and will be married in 6
months. Ms. Wilkins has some general concerns regarding the use of general anesthetics in this office practice. These concerns are of importance because Ms. Wilkins
and her fiancé would like to start a family someday.

1. What are some of Ms. Wilkins's concerns?
2. Nitrous oxide is a general anesthetic with several contraindications. How do
   they relate to Ms. Wilkins?
3. What can be done to help prevent these problems in Ms. Wilkins and other
   dental personnel?
4. Miscarriage can also happen with volatile anesthetic drugs. Who is at risk and
   what can be done to prevent or minimize it?
5. Should Ms. Wilkins inform patients about the risk of miscarriage?

Review Questions

1. What is the general mechanism of action of general anesthetics?
2. Compare and contrast the stages of anesthesia as described by Guedel and
   Flagg.
3. What are the factors regulating the onset and recovery of anesthesia?
4. What are the adverse reactions associated with all general anesthetics?
5. What are the dental concerns of all general anesthetics?
6. What is conscious sedation and what drugs are used to achieve this state?
7. What is dissociative anesthesia and what is used to achieve it?
8. What is Innovar and what is its role in balanced anesthesia?

BIBLIOGRAPHY

Bennett CR: *Conscious-Sedation in Dental Practice.* Mosby, St. Louis, 1974.
England A, Jones RM: Inhaled anaesthetic agents: From halothane to the present day. *Br J Hosp Med* 48:254–257, 1992.
Jaffe JH, Martin WR: Opioid analgesics and antagonists. In Goodman Gilman A, Rall TW, Nies AS, Taylor P (eds.), *Goodman and Gilman's The Pharmacological Basis of Therapeutics,* 8th ed. Pergamon Press, New York, 1990.
Jastak JT: Nitrous oxide in dental practice. *Int Anesthesiol Clin* 27:92–97, 1989.
Mandel ID: Occupational risks in dentistry: Comfort and concerns. *J Am Dent Assoc* 124:40–49,1993.
Marshall BE, Longnecker DE: General anesthetics. In Goodman Gilman A, Rall TW, Nies AS, Taylor P (eds.), *Goodman and Gilman's The Pharmacological Basis of Therapeutics,* 8th ed. Pergamon Press, New York, 1990.

Rall TW: Hypnotics and sedatives: Ethanol. In Smith CM, Reynard AM (eds.), *Textbook of Pharmacology,* 1st ed. W. B. Saunders, Philadelphia, 1992.

Roizen MF: Anesthesiology. *JAMA* 263:2625–2627, 1990.

Ryder W, Wright PA: Dental sedation. A review. *Br Dent J* 165:207–216, 1988.

Smith CM: General anesthesia and general anesthetics. In Smith CM, Reynard AM (eds.), *Textbook of Pharmacology,* 1st ed. W. B. Saunders, Philadelphia, 1992.

CHAPTER 6

Antimicrobial Medications

Key Terms

Antagonism
Antibacterial
Antibiotic
Antifungal
Antiinfective
Antimicrobial
Antiviral
Bactericidal

Bacteriostatic
Infection
Minimum Inhibitory Concentration
Resistance
Spectrum
Superinfection
Synergism

LEARNING OBJECTIVES

After completion of this chapter and its learning activities, the student should be able to:

1. Define antiinfective, antifungal, antiviral, antibiotic, bactericidal, bacteriostatic, infection, resistance, and spectrum.
2. Discuss the general mechanism of action of antibiotics and the factors that influence antibiotic effectiveness.
3. Describe the role of antiinfective drugs in dentistry.
4. List and describe the β-lactam antibiotics including mechanism of action, spectrum, resistance, adverse reactions, drug interactions, clinical use, and dental concerns.
5. List and describe the macrolide antibiotics including mechanism of action, spectrum, adverse reactions, drug interactions, clinical use, and dental concerns.
6. List and describe the tetracyclines, clindamycin, metronidazole, vancomycin, and aminoglycosides including mechanism of action, pharmacokinetics, spectrum, adverse reactions, drug interactions, clinical use, and dental concerns.
7. List and describe the different topical antibiotics and their role in dentistry.
8. List and describe the reasons for prophylaxing a patient prior to a dental procedure. Include antibiotics used and their doses.
9. List and describe the different antifungal drugs including pharmacokinetics, spectrum, adverse reactions, drug interactions, clinical use, and dental concerns.
10. List and describe the antiviral drugs used in dentistry including mechanism of action, spectrum, adverse reactions, clinical use, and dental concerns.

INTRODUCTION

Antimicrobial drugs play an important role in dentistry and medicine and are among the more commonly prescribed drugs today. Bacteria have been implicated in the cause of dental caries, periodontal disease, and localized or systemic infections. Though dental caries are best treated by good oral hygiene and fluoride, antibiotics may be of benefit in periodontal disease and are effective for systemic dental infections. Antibiotics are also used as prophylaxis for certain at-risk patients and are discussed later in this chapter. Though not common, fungal and viral infections are also treated in the dental office.

Antimicrobial therapy has become quite extensive and dental hygienists should become familiar with the different antimicrobial drugs used in dentistry. The intent is to present an overview of the more commonly used antibiotics in dentistry. This chapter covers some general definitions and concepts as well as the mechanism of action, spectrum, pharmacokinetics, adverse reactions, drug interactions, and dental uses of the more commonly prescribed antibiotics.

DEFINITIONS

This section reviews the definitions of terms used to describe antimicrobial therapy.

Antagonism: bactericidal rate for two drugs is less than that of either drug alone.

Antibacterial: any substance that destroys or suppresses the growth or multiplication of bacteria.

Antibiotic: any drug that is produced by other microorganisms to kill or inhibit the growth or multiplication of bacteria. Antibiotics are made from living organisms and antibacterials are synthetic and created in laboratories.

Antifungal: any drug that destroys or suppresses the growth or multiplication of fungi.

Antiinfective: any drug that acts against or destroys infections.

Antimicrobial: any substance that inhibits the growth of or kills a microorganism. The terms antimicrobial, antiinfective, antibacterial, and antibiotic are used interchangeably without regard to definition.

Antiviral: any drug that destroys or suppresses the growth or multiplication of viruses.

Bactericidal: an antibiotic that kills bacteria.

Bacteriostatic: an antibiotic that suppresses the growth or multiplication of bacteria.

Infection: the invasion of the body by pathogenic organisms and the body's response to that organism. Factors that can determine the likelihood of an infection are the virulence of the organism, number of organisms present, and resistance of the host (person).

Minimum Inhibitory Concentration (MIC): lowest concentration needed to inhibit viable growth of an organism after 18–24 hours of incubation.

Resistance: occurs when organism growth is not killed or suppressed by antimicrobial drugs. This can occur naturally if the organism has always been resistant to the drug or it can be acquired. Acquired resistance may be the result of previous exposure to the drug due to spontaneous mutation or by transfer of genetic material from one organism to another. The second strain becomes resistant to the antibiotic without prior exposure.

Spectrum: range of activity of a drug. Antimicrobials with a broad spectrum act against a wide variety of organisms including gram-positive, gram-negative, and some bacteria. Narrow-spectrum antimicrobials act against either gram-positive or gram-negative organisms.

Superinfection: infection caused by the overgrowth of bacteria different from the causative infection. Antimicrobials disturb the normal flora and allow for the emergence of different organisms that are resistant to or unaffected by the antimicrobial.

Synergism: the combination of two antimicrobials is more bactericidal than either drug used alone.

GENERAL MECHANISMS OF ACTION OF ANTIBIOTICS

Antibiotics exert their bactericidal or bacteriostatic effects on three general sites and by four general mechanisms of action on the offending microorganism. The sites of action are the cell wall, cytoplasm, and cytoplasmic membrane. Figure 6-1 reviews the sites of action as well as the general mechanisms of action of different antibiotics. Table 6-1 classifies antibiotics as bactericidal, bacteriostatic, or both. The penicillins are bactericidal and the classic inhibitors of cell wall synthesis.

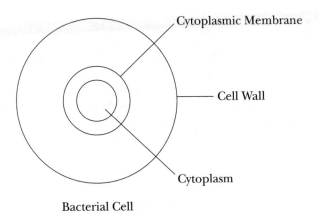

Site	Mechanism of Action
Cell wall	Inhibition of synthesis
Cytoplasmic membrane	Interference with protective function and permeability

Figure 6-1 *Antimicrobial sites and mechanism of action*

Table 6-1   Classification of Antibiotic Activity

Bactericidal Activity	Bacteriostatic Activity	Bactericidal/Bacteriostatic Activity
Aminoglycosides	Tetracyclines	Clindamycin
Bacitracin	Macrolides	Macrolides
β-lactams		
Metronidazole		
Neomycin		
Polymyxin		
Vancomycin		

Tetracycline and macrolide antibiotics are bacteriostatic and work by interfering with the microorganism's ability to synthesize proteins in the cytoplasm. This group can be further subdivided into antibiotics that bind to the 50S (erythromycin) and 30S (tetracycline) ribosomal subunit. Both **clindamycin** and the macrolides are bactericidal at higher concentrations.

Lastly, antifungals and polymixins interfere with the protective function and permeability of the cytoplasmic membrane of the microorganism.

FACTORS INFLUENCING EFFECTIVE ANTIBIOTIC THERAPY

There are many factors that influence the outcome of antibiotic therapy. First and foremost is the spectrum of the prescribed antibiotic. Ideally, the antibiotic with the most narrow spectrum should be used to reduce the incidence of superinfection and bacterial resistance. Broader-spectrum antibiotics have antimicrobial action against both gram-positive and gram-negative organisms and truly put the patient at risk for the emergence of bacterial resistance. The dental practitioner should use the antibiotic to which the microorganism is sensitive. This will help to avoid inhibiting or killing any more of the patient's normal flora than necessary.

Pharmacokinetic factors such as dose, route of administration, dosing frequency, and drug absorption, distribution, and metabolism also affect antibiotic effectiveness.

The characteristics of the infecting organism affect antibiotic outcome. Older infections require higher antibiotic doses and longer periods of therapy. These infections may also require broader-spectrum antibiotics because of the possibility of antibacterial resistance.

The patient's physical health and other drugs may interfere with the antibiotic's therapeutic effects. Some diseases, for example, cancer and diabetes, may make the patient more susceptible to bacterial, viral, or fungal infections. Some drugs, such as the corticosteroids, mask the symptoms of infection and a more potent antibiotic may be necessary. Detailed medication/health histories and a review of the literature can help the dental practitioner decide the best course of action.

DENTAL CONCERNS

The dental hygienist can help improve a patient's outcome with antibiotics by making sure that the patient knows how to take his medication. Carefully explain to the patient the drug name, dose, and how to take the medicine. Remind the patient that it is important for him to take the full course of antibiotic therapy. Many patients stop taking their antibiotics because they feel better or they feel that the infection has completely healed. This may cause the infection to develop strength and the patient may require additional antibiotic therapy.

Other patients may not understand the rationale for prophylactic therapy and may not take their medication or may take it incorrectly. Carefully explain to patients the rationale for prophylactic therapy and have them repeat it back to you. Answer all questions to the best of your ability or with the aid of the dentist.

ANTIBIOTIC TOXICITY

The adverse reactions of antibiotics can be categorized as hypersensitivity (allergic) reactions, direct toxic effects on human tissue and cells (side effects), and indirect toxic effects due to the antibiotic's ability to promote the overgrowth of bacteria not susceptible to it. The direct and indirect toxic effects are related to the dose administered and duration of drug exposure. Hypersensitivity reactions are not dose or drug exposure dependent.

Hypersensitivity reactions to antibiotics usually require a prior exposure with a 7–10-day period for the body to develop drug-specific antibodies. The next exposure to the antibiotic results in an antigen-antibody response that can provoke the typical symptoms of an allergic response. The allergic response ranges from a mild rash with itching to severe anaphylaxis.

Some patients have an allergic response to **penicillin** the first time they take the drug. The penicillins are sensitizing drugs in that first exposure leads to the production of antibodies necessary for an antigen-antibody response. This may set the patient up for a serious reaction upon subsequent exposure to penicillin.

Antibiotics can cause an indirect adverse reaction known as a superinfection. This is an overgrowth of nonsusceptible organisms that can produce their own infection, usually caused by other bacteria or fungi.

Dental Concerns

Some patients may not take any of the penicillin-like antibiotics for fear of having an allergic reaction. A detailed medication/health history will help determine if a patient has had an allergic reaction to a medication. Many patients confuse allergic reactions with side effects, so it is important to find out what the patient's symptoms are. Patients who have had a mild reaction to penicillin can receive a cephalosporin antibiotic. However, those with anaphylactic reactions should avoid any penicillin-type medication.

Once the prescription is written, the dental practitioner should review the signs and symptoms of an allergic reaction with the patient. Patients should also be instructed as to what to do if an allergic reaction should occur. This may range from stopping the medication to calling the dental or medical health-care provider or going directly to an emergency-care facility.

ANTIBIOTIC DRUG INTERACTIONS

Antibiotics have been known to decrease the effectiveness of oral contraceptives. Antibiotics reduce the flora in the intestinal tract, which decreases the amount of bacteria necessary to hydrolyze conjugated estrogen. Less estrogen is reabsorbed and more is excreted through the intestines. Signs of this interaction include breakthrough bleeding and there have been several reports of pregnancy.

Other drug interactions include oral anticoagulants. Antibiotics, such as tetracycline, change the environment that normal gastrointestinal flora require to survive and reduce the number of bacteria present that make vitamin K. Vitamin K is a natural clotting factor, and when its levels are reduced, anticoagulant effects are increased. Erythromycin may inhibit the enzymes that metabolize warfarin, resulting in increased warfarin levels. This can increase prothrombin time, which will lead to increased bleeding or even hemorrhage. Patients receiving anticoagulant therapy should be carefully monitored if they also require antibiotic treatment.

Dental Concerns

Although the interaction between oral contraceptives and antibiotics is rare, it should be discussed with female patients taking oral contraceptives who require antibiotic therapy. All female patients of childbearing years should be questioned about oral contraceptive use. It is necessary to know whether or not your patient is taking an oral contraceptive because a backup method of contraception may be necessary while taking the antibiotic. It is important for the dental practitioner to document this conversation in the patient's dental record.

ANTIBIOTICS IN DENTISTRY

The development of many new antibiotics has occurred since the 1980s, and this chapter focuses on antibiotics used in dentistry. Antibiotics are used to treat acute oral infections and are used as prophylaxis against bacterial endocarditis. Table 6-2 reviews the therapeutic and prophylactic need for antibiotic use in dentistry. The next sections review the different antibiotics including mechanism of action, adverse reactions, drug interactions, and dental concerns.

BETA-LACTAM ANTIBIOTICS

The β-lactam antibiotics include the penicillins, cephalosporins, carbapenems, and monobactams and are reviewed in Table 6-3. All four classes have a four-member β-lactam ring as part of their chemical structure (Figure 6-2) that is responsible for its antibacterial activity. The β-lactams differ by various substitutions made at the letter R.

Mechanism of Action

Beta-lactam antibiotics are bactericidal and inhibit bacterial cell wall synthesis. The inhibition of cell wall synthesis causes autolytic enzymes to be activated, which causes bacterial cell wall lysis. The β-lactam antibiotics interfere with peptidoglycans, which are substances found in bacterial cell walls.

Table 6-2 Antibiotic Use in Dentistry

Indication	Drug(s) of Choice	Alternatives
Periodontal Disease		
Acute necrotizing ulcerative gingigivitis	Penicillin VK, amoxicillin	Metronidazole, tetracycline
Abscess (periodontitis)	Penicillin VK	Tetracycline, clindamycin (refractory periodontitis)
Adult periodontitis	Not usually treated with antibiotics	
Localized juvenile periodontitis	Doxycycline, tetracycline	Amoxicillin and metronidazole or Augmentin
Oral Infections		
Abscesses, cellulitis, and other soft tissue infections	Penicillin VK, amoxicillin	Tetracycline, cephalosporin
Osteomyelitis	Penicillin VK, amoxicillin	Cephalosporin, clindamycin
Mixed infections insensitive to penicillin	Amoxicillin, metronidazole, clindamycin	Cephalosporins, tetracycline, sulfonamides
Prophylaxis for Bacterial Endocarditis		
Rheumatic heart disease, and heart valve prosthesis	Amoxicillin	Erythromycin
*Impaired Host Defense Mechanism		
Diabetes mellitus Drugs—corticosteroids, anticancer	Penicillin VK, Amoxicillin	Erythromycin, Tetracyclines

*Not all-inclusive.

Resistance

One of the major problems with antibiotic use today is resistance. Some bacteria produce the β-lactamase enzyme, which cleaves the carbon-nitrogen bond in the β-lactam ring and destroys antibacterial activity. β-lactam antibiotics have been developed that are effective against β-lactamase-producing bacteria. A discussion regarding the different types of β-lactam antibiotics follows.

THE PENICILLINS

The mold *Penicillium notatum* and its related species are responsible for producing the naturally occurring penicillins of which only penicillin G (benzyl penicillin) is still used today. All other penicillins are semisynthetic and are made by modifications to the R side chain (see Figure 6-2).

Table 6-3   The Beta-Lactams

Generic Name	Trade Name	Routes of Administration
Natural Penicillins		
Penicillin G	Pentids	Oral, IM, IV
Penicillin G procaine	Crysticillin	IM
Penicillin G benzathine	Bicillin L-A	IM
Penicillin V	Pen Vee K, V-Cillin K	Oral
Penicillinase Resistant		
Methicillin	Staphcillin	IM, IV
Nafcillin	Unipen, Nafcil	Oral, IM, IV
Oxacillin	Prostaphlin, Bactocil	Oral, IM, IV
Cloxacillin	Tegopen, Cloxapen	Oral
Dicloxacillin	Dynapen, Dycill	Oral
Amino Penicillins		
Ampicillin	Polycillin, Omnipen	Oral, IM, IV
Amoxicillin	Amoxil	Oral
Extended Spectrum		
Carbenicillin	Geocillin, Geopen	Oral, IM, IV
Ticarcillin	Ticar	IM, IV
Mezlocillin	Mezlin	IM, IV
Piperacillin	Piperacil	IM, IV
Carbapenem		
Imipenem	Primaxin	IM, IV
Monobactam		
Aztreonam	Azactam	IM, IV

IV = intravenous, IM = intramuscular.

Source: McEvoy GK, ed., Anti-infectives. In *AHFS Drug Information 95*. American Society of Hospital Pharmacists, Bethesda, MD, 1995.

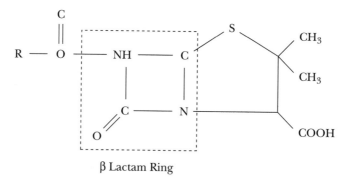

β Lactam Ring

Figure 6-2   *The β-lactam ring with the penicillins as an example*

Pharmacokinetics

Penicillins can be administered either orally or parenterally. Oral absorption is dependent on the type of penicillin given and can range from 0% to greater than 90% absorption. Penicillin G is unstable in the acid environment of the stomach and is administered parenterally whereas penicillin V is acid stable. The oral dose form offers the convenience of self-administration by the patient and less likelihood of a severe anaphylactic reaction. The disadvantages to oral penicillins are less predictable blood levels and the inactivation of some oral penicillins by gastric acid. The patient should take her medication 1 hour before meals or 2 hours after meals.

The penicillins are widely distributed throughout the body including tissue, saliva, kidneys, the placenta, and breast milk. Oral penicillins poorly distribute to the cerebrospinal fluid, bone, and abscesses. Penicillins are metabolized in the liver and excreted through the kidneys.

Spectrum of Activity

Penicillin G and penicillin V have a narrow spectrum of activity and are effective against gram-positive cocci such as *Staphylococcus aureus, S. pneumonia, Streptococcus pyogenes,* and *S. viridans;* and gram-negative cocci such as *Neisseria gonorrhea* and *N. meningitides.* Penicillin is also effective against *Actinomyces, Peptococcus, Peptostreptococcus, Bacteroides, Corynebacterum,* and *Clostridum* species, which are causative pathogens of periodontal disease.

Adverse Reactions

The major adverse reaction of the penicillins is the high incidence of allergic reaction. Table 6-4 summarizes the types of allergic reactions associated with the penicillins. Allergic reactions can range from a mild delayed reaction or rash to acute anaphylaxis. There is a high incidence of cross-allergenicity between all penicillins, which means that if a person is allergic to penicillin, he will be allergic to amoxicillin.

Large intravenous doses of penicillin can cause seizures and large doses of penicillin G have been associated with renal damage. Signs and symptoms of renal damage include fever, eosinophilia, rash, albuminuria, and an increase in blood urea nitrogen (BUN) levels. Penicillin has also been known to cause hemolytic anemia and bone marrow depression. Parenteral penicillin is irritating to the skin and can cause sterile abscesses if given intramuscularly or thrombophlebitis if given intravenously.

Gastrointestinal adverse reactions include nausea with or without vomiting. Patients often confuse gastrointestinal complaints with allergic reactions. It is important for the dental hygienist or dentist to carefully question the patient about his "reaction" to penicillin. An upset stomach or nausea does not indicate that the patient has had an allergic reaction to penicillin and the patient should be able to take amoxicillin or a cephalosporin. True allergic reactions may make a switch to either one of these antibiotics impossible.

Specific Penicillins

The following discussion includes examples, clinical use, and general information on specific penicillins.

Table 6-4   Types of Allergic Reactions Associated with Penicillin

Allergy and Hypersensitivity

Rash
1. Mild and self-limiting
2. Occurs in 80% to 90% of all penicillin allergic reactions
3. Can occasionally be severe

Anaphylaxis (Type I—IgE mediated response)
1. Characterized by bronchoconstriction, shock, and urticaria
2. Occurs within a half-hour of taking the penicillin
3. Death can result if treatment with the immediate administration of epinephrine is not given

Cytotoxic Response (Type II—IgG or IgM mediated response)
1. Hemolytic anemia

Delayed Serum Sickness (Type III—IgG mediated response)
1. Fever, skin rash, and eosinophilia
2. Can be as severe as arthritis, purpura, lymphadenopathy, splenomegaly, mental status changes, abnormal EKG, and edema
3. 6 days to develop
4. Can occur during therapy or up to 2 weeks after discontinuation of therapy

Oral Lesions-Delayed Reaction (Type IV—T-lymphocyte response)

1. Severe stomatitis, furred tongue, black tongue, acute glossitis, cheilosis

Other
1. Interstitial nephritis

Penicillin G. **Penicillin G** is the prototype penicillin and is available as sodium, potassium, procaine, or benzathine salt. The potassium salt is available as the intravenous dose form and gives the most rapid and highest blood levels. The benzathine salt is given intramuscularly and its blood levels are much lower than the potassium salt but are more sustainable. The sodium salt of penicillin should be avoided in patients who are on a salt-restricted diet, for example, those with cardiovascular disease. Potassium salts should be avoided in patients with renal disease.

Penicillin V. **Penicillin V** is acid stable and is given orally. It produces blood levels comparable to penicillin G. It is used to treat and prevent dental infections.

Penicillinase-Resistant Penicillins. These penicillins include **methicillin, nafcillin, oxacillin, cloxacillin,** and **dicloxacillin.** They are used to treat penicillinase-producing staphylococci. They are also effective against streptococcus organisms A, B, C, and G and pneumococci. They tend to have more gastrointestinal adverse reactions, bone marrow depression, and abnormal renal and hepatic function than other penicillins. Patients who are allergic to penicillin are allergic to penicillinase-resistant penicillins.

Amino Penicillins. Amino penicillins or broad-spectrum antibiotics include **ampicillin** and **amoxicillin.** They cover the same organisms as penicillin but also cover such gram-negative cocci as *Hemophilus influenzae, Escherichia coli, Proteus mirablis, Salmonella,* and *Shigella.*

Amoxicillin is the drug of choice for the prophylaxis of rheumatic heart disease because it is better tolerated and is better absorbed than the other penicillins. Both medications are also used to treat middle-ear infections, upper respiratory tract infections, urinary tract infections, and strep throat.

Ampicillin has more gastrointestinal irritation than amoxicillin and must be taken on an empty stomach. Amoxicillin is better tolerated and can be taken on an empty stomach or with food. Both can cause allergic reactions.

Extended-Spectrum Penicillins. This group of drugs includes **carbenicillin, ticarcillin, mezlocillin, azlocillin,** and **piperacillin.** These medications are effective against both gram-positive and gram-negative organisms with special activity against *Pseudomonas aeruginosa* and some strains of *Proteus.* These medications are only available intravenously.

Beta-Lactamase Inhibitors. Bacteria produce β-lactamase, which is instrumental in the development of bacterial resistance to antibiotics. Two β-lactamase inhibitors, clavulanic acid and sulbactam, have been developed to prevent resistance. They have no bacterial activity and are only present to inhibit β-lactamase and increase spectrum coverage. Clavulanic acid is combined with amoxicillin (Augmentin) and with ticarcillin (Timentin) and sulbactam is combined with ampicillin (Unasyn). Unasyn and Timentin are available for parenteral use and Augmentin is available as the oral dose form. The most common adverse reaction is gastrointestinal upset.

These medications are used to treat upper respiratory tract infections, strep throat, pneumonia, and any other bacterial infection treated by other penicillins. Augmentin has some use in the management of certain periodontal diseases.

CEPHALOSPORINS

The chemical structure and mechanism of action of cephalosporins are very similar to penicillin except that cephalosporins are more resistant to β-lactamase. They are active against a wide variety of gram-positive organisms, gram-negative organisms, *Salmonella,* and *Klebsiella.* There are more than 20 different cephalosporin antibiotics and they are available orally (Table 6-5), intravenously, and intramuscularly. Cephalosporins with poor oral absorption are administered parenterally.

Cephalosporin antibiotics are categorized into one of three generations. First-generation cephalosporins cover gram-positive and a few gram-negative organisms; second-generation cephalosporins cover gram-positive organisms, some gram-negative organisms, and anaerobes; third-generation cephalosporins are effective against gram-positive organisms, many gram-negative organisms, and anaerobes.

Cephalosporin antibiotics have a low incidence of adverse reactions and are usually well tolerated. Adverse reactions include such gastrointestinal complaints as diarrhea, nausea, vomiting, and abdominal pain. They can be minimized or avoided by taking the antibiotics with food or milk. Other adverse reactions include local reactions at the site of intramuscular or intravenous injections, hemostasis, disulfi-

Table 6-5   Cephalosporin Antibiotics

Generic Name	Trade Name	Routes of Administration
First Generation		
Cephalexin	Keflex	Oral
Cephadrine	Velosef	Oral
Cefadroxil	Duricef	Oral
Second Generation		
Cefaclor	Ceclor	Oral
Cefuroxime	Ceftin, Kefurox, Zinacef	Oral, IV, IM
Cefprozil	Cefzil	Oral
Cefpodoxomine	Van Tin	Oral
Loracarbef	Lorabid	Oral
Third Generation		
Cefixime	Suprax	Oral

IV = intravenous, IM = intramuscular.

Source: McEvoy GK, ed., Anti-infectives. In *AHFS Drug Information 95*. American Society of Hospital Pharmacists, Bethesda, MD, 1995.

ram-like reactions, superinfection, and allergic reactions. Approximately 10% of patients allergic to penicillin will have cross-sensitivity allergic responses to cephalosporin antibiotics. However, patients with histories of penicillin allergies may receive cephalosporin antibiotics.

Cephalosporin antibiotics are indicated for the treatment of a variety of community and hospital acquired infections. Dental use is limited to treatment of infections that are resistant or ineffective against more narrow-spectrum antibiotics or if the patient cannot tolerate penicillin antibiotics.

CARBAPENEM

Carbapenem is similar to penicillin but has marked resistance to β-lactamase. It is a broad-spectrum antibiotic, it is effective against more than 90% of all clinically significant bacteria, and it is combined with cilastatin to prevent renal metabolism. The drug is not effective orally and must be given parenterally. The main clinical use of the drug is in the treatment of hospital-acquired infections. Adverse reactions include pain at the site of injection, allergies, nausea, vomiting, superinfection, diarrhea, and some blood disorders.

AZTREONAM

This antibiotic is a synthetic and is effective against facultative aerobic gram-negative bacteria. It is less toxic than aminoglycosides but has the potential to cause penicillin-resistant gram-positive superinfections. It is only available parenterally and is used to treat hospital-acquired infections.

MACROLIDE ANTIBIOTICS

The macrolide antibiotics include **erythromycin, azithromycin, dirithromycin,** and **clarithromycin** (Table 6-6).

Mechanism of Action

These medications are bacteriostatic and interfere with protein synthesis at the 50S subunit of the 70S ribosome.

Spectrum of Activity

All four macrolides are effective against most gram-positive and gram-negative organisms including *Mycoplasma pneumoniae, Moraxella, Bordetella, Campylobacter, Neisseria,* and *Legionella.* They are also effective against *Chlamydia trachomatis, Treponema pallidum,* and *Entamoeba histolytica.* Erythromycin is ineffective against anaerobes including those implicated in dental infections. They include *Bacteroides, Peptococcus,* and *Peptostreptococcus* species. Both azithromycin and clarithromycin are effective against some anaerobic bacteria.

Pharmacokinetics

Erythromycin is broken down by the acidic contents of gastric fluid and, as a result, is formulated with a protective coating. Food can reduce the absorption of erythromycin and azithromycin and both should be taken 1 hour before meals or 2 hours after meals.

Table 6-6 Macrolide Antibiotics*

Generic Name	Trade Name	Routes of Administration
Erythromycin	E-Mycin	Oral
	ERYC	Oral
	Ery-Tab	Oral
	PCE Dispertab	Oral
Erythromycin estolate	Ilosone	Oral
Erythromycin ethylsuccinate	E.E.S.	Oral
	EryPed	Oral
Erythromycin lactobionate	Same as generic	IM, IV
Erythromycin stearate	Erythrocyin	Oral
Dirithromycin	Dynabac	Oral
Clarithromycin	Biaxin	Oral
Azithromycin	Zithromax	Oral

*Not all-inclusive of erythromycin base antibiotics.

IM = intramuscular, IV = intravenous.

Source: McEvoy GK, ed., Anti-infectives. In *AHFS Drug Information 95*. American Society of Hospital Pharmacists, Bethesda, MD, 1995; Hussar DA, New therapeutic agents marketed in second half of 1995. *Pharmacy Today* 2:7, 1996.

Both can cause gastrointestinal upset and patients can be advised to take them with food or milk if this should occur. Antacids can reduce azithromycin absorption, which means that the patient should not take them with azithromycin. Erythromycin is distributed to most body tissues, excreted in the bile, partially reabsorbed through enterohepatic circulation, and excreted in the urine and feces. Clarithromycin is not affected by food absorption and can be taken without regard to meals.

Adverse Reactions

Gastrointestinal upset is the most frequent adverse reaction associated with erythromycin use and is the most common cause of patient noncompliance. Problems include stomatitis, abdominal cramps, nausea, vomiting, and diarrhea. Gastrointestinal upset occurs less frequently with azithromycin and clarithromycin, though there have been reports of an abnormal, metallic taste associated with clarithromycin. Cholestatic jaundice has been reported with the estolate and ethylsuccinate forms of erythromycin. Symptoms include nausea, vomiting, abdominal cramps, jaundice, and elevated liver enzymes. Patients with a history of hepatitis should receive the erythromycin base or stearate form.

Drug Interactions

Erythromycin can increase the blood levels of theophylline, digoxin, triazolam, warfarin, carbamazepine, and cyclosporin. Clarithromycin inhibits the cytochrome P450 system and may increase the blood levels of theophylline and carbamazepine. Patients and their physicians should be notified of this if erythromycin or clarithromycin must be prescribed. The doses of these medications may have to be lowered during the course of erythromycin therapy. There have also been reports of death due to cardiac abnormalities when erythromycin was given to patients taking terfenadine. As a result, the use of erythromycin with terfenadine or astemizole is contraindicated.

Clinical Use

Currently, erythromycin is the only antibiotic used for prophylaxis and it is only used for patients who are allergic to or cannot tolerate penicillin. Clarithromycin and azithromycin are not currently used in dentistry and any use will await the results of clinical trials. All four antibiotics are used to treat upper and lower respiratory tract infections and skin infections caused by suspectible organisms.

TETRACYCLINE ANTIBIOTICS

Tetracycline antibiotics are broad-spectrum antibiotics that affect a wide range of bacteria and are reviewed in Table 6-7.

Mechanism of Action

The tetracyclines are bacteriostatic and interfere with the synthesis of bacterial protein by binding to the 30S subunit at the bacterial ribosome.

Table 6-7   Tetracycline Antibiotics

Generic Name	Trade Name	Routes of Administration
Tetracycline	Achromycin V, Sumycin	Oral
Doxycycline	Vibramycin, Doryx	Oral
Minocycline	Minocin	Oral

Source: McEvoy GK, ed., Anti-infectives. In *AHFS Drug Information 95*. American Society of Hospital Pharmacists, Bethesda, MD, 1995.

Spectrum of Activity

Tetracyclines provide coverage against gram-positive and gram-negative aerobic and anaerobic bacteria. Some examples include *Rickettsia,* spirochetes, some protozoa, *Chlamydia,* and *Mycoplasma.*

PHARMACOKINETICS

Tetracycline antibiotics are rapidly absorbed after oral administration and are distributed throughout the body. They are secreted in saliva and in breast milk of lactating mothers and cross the placenta. They concentrate in the liver and are excreted into the intestines by bile. Tetracyclines are also stored in the dentin and enamel of unerupted teeth and are concentrated in gingival crevicular fluid.

Doxycycline is excreted in the feces, tetracycline is eliminated unchanged by glomerular filtration, and minocycline is metabolized in the liver and excreted unchanged in urine. Doxycycline and minocycline can be given to patients with renal dysfunction.

Adverse Reactions

The adverse reactions associated with tetracycline antibiotics are many but occur infrequently. The most common adverse reaction associated with tetracycline antibiotics is gastrointestinal upset. Gastrointestinal adverse reactions include nausea, vomiting, diarrhea, gastroenteritis, glossitis, stomatitis, xerostomia, and superinfection due to candida. These adverse reactions are almost all a result of changes in oral, gastric, and enteric flora. Some patients have developed a yellowish brown discoloration of the tongue.

Tetracyclines are most noted for their effects on teeth and bones. They can cause a permanent discoloration of teeth and enamel hypoplasia if given during the time of enamel calcification. They should not be used during pregnancy or the first 8 or 9 years of life. If tetracycline is given during this time, it can cause a permanent staining that begins as a yellow fluorescence and progresses with time to a brown color. Large doses of tetracyclines have also decreased the growth rate of bones in the fetus and infants.

Other adverse reactions include hepatoxicity, renal toxicity, hematologic effects, and superinfection. Minocycline has been associated with lightheadedness and dizziness. Patients should be careful about doing anything that requires thought or concentration including driving a car or operating heavy machinery when taking minocycline. Minocycline has also been reported to cause a blue-black discoloration of the tongue.

Tetracycline use has been associated with photosensitivity. Patients taking tetracycline should generously apply a sunscreen lotion with a skin protection factor (SPF) of at least 15 prior to any sun exposure. This may help to avoid or minimize sunburn.

The overall allergenicity of tetracyclines is low. If a person is allergic to one tetracycline, he will be allergic to others.

Drug Interactions

Calcium, magnesium, iron, and aluminum all decrease the intestinal absorption of tetracycline by chelating with it. Dairy products, antacids, and mineral supplements should not be taken for at least 2 hours after ingesting tetracycline. Patients can take dairy products with doxycycline and minocycline but they should avoid antacids and mineral supplements.

Tetracycline can enhance the effects of sulfonylureas, digoxin, lithium, warfarin, furosemide, and theophylline. Doses of these medications should be adjusted accordingly if tetracycline is added to the patient's list of medications. The barbiturates and phenytoin have the ability to increase tetracycline metabolism because of stimulation of hepatic microsomal enzymes. As with other antibiotics, tetracyclines may reduce the effectiveness of oral contraceptives. Female patients should use a backup method of contraception if they are taking oral contraceptives and a tetracycline antibiotic is prescribed.

Clinical Use

The tetracyclines are used to treat a wide variety of medical illnesses including acne, pulmonary infections, and traveler's diarrhea.

Tetracycline antibiotics concentrate in gingival crevicular fluid greater than serum and are used to treat certain periodontal conditions when conventional methods have failed. Oral tetracycline antibiotics are dosed as follows: tetracycline hydrochloride, four times a day; doxycycline, once or twice a day; and minocycline is dosed twice a day. Recently, the Food and Drug Administration approved the use of a new tetracycline delivery system that allows practitioners to place the antibiotic directly into the periodontal pocket (site of infection). This product is called Actisite and is made up of a monofilament of ethylene/vinyl acetate that contains 12.7 mg of tetracycline. It releases medication continuously for 10 days after which the fiber is removed. It is indicated for adjunct treatment of periodontitis in conjunction with good oral hygiene, scaling, and root planing.

Tetracycline antibiotics are also used as prophylaxis against infective endocarditis in patients who are penicillin resistant to *A actinomycetemcomitans*. In these situations a full course of tetracycline should be given several weeks before dental treatment and amoxicillin or erythromycin should be given as per the guidelines of the American Heart Association.

CLINDAMYCIN

Clindamycin is a synthetic derivative of lincomycin and is an alternative to treating penicillin-1 and erythromycin-susceptible infections. It is bacteriostatic and an inhibitor of protein synthesis and is primarily effective against gram-positive organisms and the anaerobe *Bacteroides*.

Pharmacokinetics

Clindamycin can be administered orally, topically, or parenterally. Oral clindamycin is well absorbed and its absorption is not affected by food. Clindamycin is distributed throughout the body, including bone and placenta. It does not distribute to cerebrospinal fluid. The majority of the drug is excreted as the inactive metabolite in the urine and feces.

Spectrum of Activity

Clindamycin is effective against such gram-positive organisms as *Streptococcus pyogenes*, *S. viridans*, *Pneumococcus*, and *S. aureus*. It is also effective against several anaerobes including *Bacteroides melaninogenicus*, *Fusobacterium* species, *Peptostreptococcus*, *Peptococcus*, and *Actinomyces israelii*. Its gram-positive activity is similar to erythromycin and cross-sensitivity has been noted.

Adverse Reactions

The more common adverse reactions associated with clindamycin are gastrointestinal, including diarrhea, nausea, vomiting, abdominal cramps, and antibiotic-associated colitis. Antibiotic-associated pseudomembranous colitis is characterized by severe, persistent, bloody diarrhea and is caused by the toxin *Clostridium difficile*. It is treated by the discontinuation of the offending antibiotic, oral vancomycin or cholestyramine, and fluid and electrolyte replacement. It may occur during treatment or several weeks after therapy has stopped.

Other adverse reactions include superinfection, neutropenia, thrombocytopenia, agranulocytosis, and abnormal liver and renal function tests. Allergies have been reported and oral manifestations include glossitis and stomatitis.

Clinical Use

Clindamycin is used to treat oral infections caused by *Bacteroides* species and to treat some staphylococcus infections. It is also used to treat acne.

METRONIDAZOLE

Metronidazole is a synthetic nitroimidazole with bactericidal action that penetrates all bacterial cells. It is well absorbed after oral administration with peak levels occurring 1 to 2 hours after ingestion. It is somewhat concentrated in gingival crevicular fluid and distributes to cerebrospinal fluid, saliva, breast milk, and crosses the placenta. It is effective against *T. vaginalis*, *Bacteroides*, *Treponema*, *Peptococcus*, and *Peptostreptococcus* species to name a few.

Adverse Reactions

The most common adverse reactions are gastrointestinal and include nausea, anorexia, diarrhea, and vomiting. Abdominal cramping and epigastric distress have also been reported. Oral adverse reactions include glossitis, black, furred tongue, dry mouth, and an unpleasant metallic taste. Central nervous system (CNS) effects include headache, dizziness, vertigo, and ataxia. Other CNS adverse effects include confusion, depression, weakness, and insomnia. Other adverse reactions include renal toxicity and a transient neutropenia.

Drug Interactions

Metronidazole in combination with alcohol can produce a disulfiram-like reaction that is characterized by nausea, abdominal pain, flushing, headache, and vomiting. All sources of alcohol, including cough and cold products, mouthwashes, and food, should be avoided during and for several days after metronidazole therapy. In some instances, perfumes, aftershave lotions, and other alcohol-containing skin-care products can cause this reaction. The scent of these products can cause nausea, flushing, and headache in patients taking metronidazole.

Clinical Use

Metronidazole is used to treat several different sexually transmitted diseases and serious anaerobic infections of the abdomen, skeleton, and female genital tract. Dental use includes the treatment of periodontal infections.

VANCOMYCIN

Vancomycin is bactericidal and its mechanism of action is the inhibition of cell wall synthesis. It has a narrow therapeutic spectrum and is effective against penicillinase-resistant penicillin, staphylococci, and streptococci. It has minimal gastrointestinal absorption, causes irritation when administered intramuscularly, and is only administered intravenously. Large doses or prolonged use can lead to ototoxicity and nephrotoxicity.

It is used for the prophylaxis of bacterial endocarditis for patients with prosthetic heart valves who are allergic to penicillin or who cannot take anything by mouth. It must be given by intravenous infusion over a 1-hour period.

AMINOGLYCOSIDES

Aminoglycoside antibiotics include **neomycin, streptomycin, kanamycin, gentamicin, tobramycin, amikacin,** and **netilmicin.** Only gentamicin is used in dentistry.

Mechanism of Action

These drugs are bactericidal and work by inhibiting protein synthesis and appear to act directly on the 30S subunit of the ribosome. These drugs are poorly absorbed after oral administration and are only administered intravenously or intramuscularly and plasma blood levels must be monitored. They are effective against most gram-negative bacilli.

Adverse Reactions

Adverse reactions include ototoxicity, nephrotoxicity, and neuromuscular blockade. These medications are toxic to the eighth cranial nerve and can cause auditory or vestibular symptoms. Patients may have difficulty maintaining balance or may have hearing loss that could be permanent.

Clinical Use

These medications are used for the treatment of serious infections that require hospitalization. Gentamicin is combined with ampicillin in dentistry for prophylaxis in patients with prosthetic heart valves who cannot take oral medications.

TOPICAL ANTIBIOTICS

There are occasions when the use of topical antibiotics are warranted. If one is used, the dental hygienist should be aware of the fact that topical antibiotics only have superficial action and their effectiveness is only limited to the superficial organism. Topical antibiotics can cause severe local reactions and sensitization may occur more frequently when they are applied to the skin and/or mucous membranes. The drugs are highly concentrated when applied topically, which may allow some of the drug to be absorbed into the systemic circulation. Several oral antibiotics are available in topical dose forms and patients should not use both dose forms simultaneously. This may lead to an increased incidence of adverse drug reactions.

Neomycin, Polymyxin, Bacitracin

This combination is available commercially as Neosporin and is effective against gram-positive and gram-negative organisms. **Neomycin** is an aminoglycoside with bactericidal activity; **polymyxin** and **bacitracin** are both bactericidal polypeptide antibiotics. All three inhibit cell wall synthesis.

Mupirocin

Mupirocin (Bactoban) is a topical antibacterial that inhibits protein synthesis of the bacterial cell wall. It is active against certain *Streptococcus* and *Staphylococcus* species and is effective in the treatment of impetigo. Adverse reactions are local and include stinging and itching.

ANTIBIOTIC PROPHYLAXIS: THE PREVENTION OF BACTERIAL ENDOCARDITIS

In 1990 the American Heart Association published its current guidelines for antibiotic prophylaxis of the dental patient. Bacteremia is produced by any oral procedure that can cause bleeding and includes most manipulative procedures, periodontal probing, and even wax chewing. If a patient has a damaged or abnormal heart valve he/she is at risk for having bacteria lodge in that area. Therefore, antibiotics are recommended for certain dental procedures.

Dental practitioners should carefully review the literature to determine who should receive antibiotic prophylaxis. They should also have the patient complete a detailed medication/health history and review it with the patient. Remember, medication/health histories may not be complete. Some patients may not know if they have had rheumatic heart disease. Lastly, infective endocarditis may occur even with antibiotic coverage.

Dental Procedures

Many dental procedures can cause bacteremia and they include any dental procedure known to induce gingival or mucosal bleeding, including oral prophylaxis. Endocarditis prophylaxis is not indicated in dental procedures not likely to induce bleeding such as simple adjustments of orthodontic appliances or fillings above the gum line. This list is not all-inclusive and the dental hygienist should continuously review the literature to provide patients with the best possible care. The dental hygienist's clinical judgment will also help to determine whether or not a patient requires prophylaxis.

Medical Conditions

Table 6-8 reviews cardiac situations in which antibiotic prophylaxis is necessary. Cardiac patients at risk for developing bacterial endocarditis include those with prosthetic heart valves, history of bacterial endocarditis, or rheumatic heart disease.

Table 6-8   Endocarditis Prophylaxis Recommendations for Cardiac Patients*

Prophylaxis Recommended
   Prosthetic heart valves
   Previous bacterial endocarditis, even in the absence of heart disease
   History of bacterial endocarditis
   Congenital heart malformations
   Rheumatic heart disease
   Hypertrophic cardiomyopathy
   Mitral valve prolapse with valvular regurgitation

Prophylaxis Not Recommended
   Longer than 6 months after surgical repair of septal defects or patent ductus
     arteriosus
   Previous coronary artery bypass surgery graft
   Mitral valve prolapse without valvular regurgitation
   Heart murmurs
   Rheumatic heart fever without valvular dysfunction
   Cardiac pacemakers and defibrillators

Source: Dajani AS, et al., Prevention of bacterial endocarditis: Recommendations by the American Heart Association. *JAMA* 264:2919–2922, 1990. Copyright 1990, American Medical Association.

Some patients with noncardiac medical problems may also require antibiotic prophylaxis. They include patients taking long-term steroids or any other medication that may immunocompromise the patient. Though there is little evidence for antibiotic prophylaxis in patients with artificial joints, some orthopedic surgeons request it. Table 6-8 reviews situations when antibiotic prophylaxis is not necessary. Again, this list is not all-inclusive and the dental hygienist should continuously review the literature for the most current information.

Antibiotic Regimens

Table 6-9 summarizes the antibiotics of choice for prophylaxis as well as those for patients with penicillin allergies. If there is a question about antibiotic prophylaxis, dental personnel should work closely with the patient's medical doctor to explore all options. One should document in the patient's dental records and send a letter to the patient's physician summarizing the discussions and the final decision. A copy of that letter should be kept in the patient's record. This will help to minimize the suggestion of inappropriate antibiotic use or misuse.

ANTIFUNGAL PHARMACOLOGY

Fungal infections can occur in superficial areas of the body including the oral cavity, mucous membranes, and skin, and can occur systemically. Those of the skin and mucous membranes occur most frequently and systemic infections usually occur in patients who are immunocompromised. This discussion focuses on fungal infections that are treated in the dental office.

Table 6-9   Antibiotic Prophylaxis Dosing Regimens

Drug	Adult Dose	Children's Dose
Amoxicillin	3.0 grams 1 hour before procedure, then 1.5 grams 6 hours after the initial dose	50 mg/kg before the procedure 25 mg/kg after the procedure
If Penicillin Allergic: Erythromycin	Erythromycin stearate* 1 gram 2 hours before the procedure, then 500 mg 6 hours after the initial dose	20 mg/kg before the procedure 10 mg/kg after the procedure
or Clindamycin	300 mg 1 hour before the procedure, then 150 mg 6 hours after the initial dose	10 mg/kg before the procedure 5 mg/kg after the procedure

*Erythromycin ethyl succinate can be used, but there is better bioavailability with erythromycin stearate.

Source: Dajani AS, et. al., Prevention of bacterial endocarditis: Recommendations by the American Heart Association. *JAMA* 264:2919–2922, 1990. Copyright 1990, American Medical Association.

Nystatin

Nystatin (Table 6-10) can be either fungicidal or fungistatic depending on its concentration in contact with fungal cells. Nystatin binds to sterols in the fungal cell membrane and produces a change in cellular permeability, which allows for the loss of potassium and other essential cellular components. Nystatin is not absorbed from intact skin or mucous membranes and it is essentially unabsorbed in the gastrointestinal tract. Adverse reactions are minor and infrequent and include nausea, vomiting, and diarrhea. It is used for the treatment and prevention of oral mucocutaneous infections caused by *Candida albicans* and for the treatment of vaginal yeast infections.

Nystatin Dose Forms. Nystatin is available as a liquid suspension, pastilles, and vaginal tablets; all dose forms can be used to treat oral infections. The suspension contains sugar and the pastilles are licorice flavored and also contain sugar. Patients taking this should be instructed to perform and maintain good oral hygiene. Vaginal tablets can be used to treat oral infections though they do not taste that good. They remain in the oral cavity longer than the suspension and contain no sugar. Nystatin should be taken for a full 2-week course of therapy. Discontinuation prior to this time period may result in another more intense infection.

Clotrimazole

Clotrimazole (Table 6-10) causes leakage of small molecules into fungal cells, which alters cell membrane permeability. The cell membrane loses its function and cellular contents are lost. It is available as an oral lozenge for the treatment of candida. It is also available as a cream or tablet for vaginal infections. It is indicated for the local treatment of oropharyngeal candidiasis.

Patients are instructed to suck on the lozenge, as if they were sucking on a cough drop, which dissolves in about 15–30 minutes. Patients should complete their full course of therapy in order to avoid a relapse. Those patients with xerostomia may have problems dissolving this medication. The most common adverse reactions include abdominal pain, diarrhea, and nausea.

Table 6-10. Antifungal Drugs

Generic Name	Trade Name	Routes of Administration
Nystatin	Mycostatin, Nilstat, others	Aqueous suspension, vaginal tablets, cream, ointment, pastilles
Clotrimazole	Mycelex	Troches, cream, vaginal cream, and tablets
Ketoconazole	Nizoral	Oral tablets
Itraconazole	Sporanox	Oral capsules
Fluconazole	Diflucan	Oral tablets, intravenous

Source: McEvoy GK, ed., Anti-infectives. In *AHFS Drug Information 95*. American Society of Hospital Pharmacists, Bethesda, MD, 1995.

Ketoconazole, Fluconazole, Itraconazole

Ketoconazole, fluconazole, and **itraconazole** (Table 6-10) are azole antifungal drugs that alter cellular membranes and interfere with intracellular synthesis. The azoles inhibit ergosterol synthesis through an interaction with C14 alpha demethylase, which is an enzyme dependent on cytochrome P450 that is necessary for the conversion of lanosterol to ergosterol. The depletion of ergosterol leads to a change in membrane permeability and an inhibition of cell growth and replication. Ketoconazole also inhibits the cytochrome P450 enzymes necessary for the synthesis of adrenal and gonadal steroid hormones. These drugs are used to treat oropharyngeal candidiasis due to *Candida albicans.*

Pharmacokinetic

All three drugs are available as oral dose forms and fluconazole is also available as an intravenous preparation. Ketoconazole absorption is decreased in the presence of food, and food is necessary to increase the absorption of itraconazole. Both ketoconazole and itraconazole are highly protein bound, extensively metabolized by the liver, and excreted almost exclusively in the feces with some urinary excretion. Because so little is excreted in the urine, dose reduction in patients with renal disease is not necessary. However, a dose reduction is recommended in elderly patients and those with liver disease. Ketoconazole and itraconazole are both lipophilic and are well distributed throughout the body.

Fluconazole absorption is not affected by food or gastric acid content. It is hydrophilic and minimally bound to plasma proteins. It has especially high concentrations in cerebrospinal fluid and urine. Approximately 80% of fluconazole is excreted unchanged in the urine with minimal metabolism. The dose of fluconazole should be reduced in patients with renal disease.

Adverse Reactions

These medications are well tolerated and the more common adverse reactions are gastrointestinal and dose related. Gastrointestinal adverse reactions include nausea and vomiting, which are more common with ketoconazole and itraconazole. There have also been reports of abdominal pain and anorexia with ketoconazole. All three azoles can cause asymptomatic elevations in liver enzymes and there have been reports of hepatitis. Ketoconazole can cause adrenal insufficiency, decreased libido, impotence, gynecomastia, and menstrual irregularities, though these are rare. Itraconazole has been reported to cause hypokalemia, hypertension, edema, and impotence. Other adverse reactions include headache, dizziness, drowsiness, photophobia, fever, chills, rash, and insomnia.

Drug Interactions

The drug interactions associated with azoles are either a result of inhibition of absorption or the interference of the cytochrome P450 system. Ketoconazole absorption is decreased in the presence of antacids, H_2-receptor antagonists, and sucralfate. These medications should not be given for at least 2 hours after ketoconazole ingestion. Isoniazid and phenytoin can increase the absorption of ketoconazole and rifampin can increase the concentration of all three azoles. All three azoles can increase the plasma concentrations of cyclosporine, phenytoin, sulfonylureas, and warfarin. Ketoconazole and itraconazole have been reported to cause increases in terfenadine and astemizole levels. There have been several deaths due to cardiac abnormalities associated with the combination of terfenadine and ketoconazole. As a result, the use of either terfenadine or astemizole with ketoconazole and itraconazole is contraindicated. Itraconazole has been reported to increase digoxin levels.

Dental Use

These medications are indicated for the treatment of mucocutaneous and oropharyngeal candidiasis (oral thrush). They are also used to treat many other types of systemic fungal infections. The choice of antifungal drug should be based on practitioner knowledge and experience with the drug, adverse reaction and drug interaction profile, and patient response.

ANTIVIRAL DRUGS

Antiviral drugs used to treat herpes simplex virus are discussed next. Other antiviral drugs are discussed in Chapter 19. Herpes simplex viruses are associated with "cold sores" and patients often ask their dental practitioner for something to treat the "cold sore."

Acyclovir

Acyclovir (Zovirax) is a purine analogue that inhibits DNA (deoxyribonucleic acid) synthesis of the offending virus. It is much less toxic to normal cells because of its preferential ability to be taken up by infected cells.

Pharmacokinetics. Oral absorption is between 15% and 30% and it is not affected by food. It is widely distributed throughout the body and is known to cross the placenta in animals. Drug half-life is prolonged as the patient's creatinine clearance rises. Ten percent of the dose is metabolized in the liver and it is excreted unchanged through the urine.

Spectrum of Activity. Acyclovir is effective against herpes simplex 1 and 2, varicella-zoster (chickenpox, shingles), Epstein-Barr, *Herpesvirus simiae* (B virus), and cytomegalovirus.

Adverse Reactions. Topical administration of acyclovir can produce burning, stinging, or mild pain in about one-third of patients. Itching and skin rashes have also been reported. Adverse reactions associated with the oral dose form include headache, nausea, vomiting, diarrhea, anorexia, and a funny sense of taste has also been reported. Other adverse reactions include acne, accelerated hair loss, arthralgia, fever, menstrual abnormalities, fatigue, insomnia, and irritability. Parenteral administration of acyclovir can cause inflammation and thrombophlebitis at the site of injection. It can also elevate BUN and serum creatinine levels.

Clinical Use. Topical applications of acyclovir are used to treat initial *Herpes genitalis* and limited non-life-threatening initial recurrent mucocutaneous herpes simplex 1 and 2 in immunocompromised patients. Topical treatment has not been proven to be effective in the treatment of recurrent *Herpes genitalis* or *Herpes labialis* in nonimmunocompromised patients.

Oral dose forms are used for prophylaxis and treatment of both initial and recurrent *Herpes genitalis* infections in both immunocompromised and nonimmunocompromised patients. The injectable dose form is used to treat severe initial *Herpes genitalis* in the nonimmunocompromised patient and initial and recurrent mucocutaneous herpes simplex infections in immunocompromised patients.

Summary

There are many different antibiotics available to treat many different infections. Antibiotics can have narrow spectrums and treat only a small number of bacterial infections or they can be broad spectrum and cover large numbers and types of bacteria. Antibiotics are prescribed in a dental office and many dental patients are taking antibiotics for any number of reasons. These drugs can be administered orally, topically, or parenterally. Often, they have adverse reactions that could affect oral hygiene. Many dental patients may require prophylaxis with an antibiotic because of medical health problems or may need antibiotic treatment postdental therapy.

Other patients may be receiving antifungal drugs for a wide variety of illnesses. Some antifungal drugs may be prescribed by a dentist to treat oral thrush. These drugs have different dose forms, which may affect patient compliance. Some antifungal drugs can interact with drugs prescribed by a dentist (e.g., ketoconazole and erythromycin). A sound knowledge of the mechanism of action, spectrum, pharmacokinetics, adverse reactions, drug interactions, and clinical use of antibiotics and antifungal drugs will help to provide the patient with the best possible dental and health care.

Case Study: Kathleen Fitzpatrick

Kathleen Fitzpatrick is 35 years old and has been coming to your practice for many years. She is married, has five children, and works as the secretary at her church. She takes no medication except for occasional cough and cold medicines and acetaminophen or naproxen sodium for aches and pains. Her medication/health history is notable for a history of rheumatic heart disease as a child. Mrs. Fitzpatrick called the office today, as scheduled, for a prescription for her antibiotic because her next dental appointment is in 3 days.

1. Why would Mrs. Fitzpatrick be calling for a prescription for an antibiotic?
2. Under what conditions is antibiotic prophylaxis necessary? Include dental procedures and medical conditions.
3. What antibiotic dose and dosing regimen should be used?
4. What should Mrs. Fitzpatrick be told about the antibiotic?

5. What are the adverse reactions associated with the antibiotic that was chosen? What should Mrs. Fitzpatrick be told about them?
6. What are some reasons that Mrs. Fitzpatrick could be noncompliant with her medication?

Case Study: Hillary Rubenstein

Hillary Rubenstein is an 8-year-old girl who has been coming to your practice since she was three years old. Her mother calls you today because she has noticed that Hillary has "sort of a white milky discharge coming from her mouth." Hillary had a bacterial infection last week and was treated with amoxicillin.

1. What is happening to Hillary?
2. What is the "white milky discharge" and how should it be treated?
3. What are the different dose forms of nystatin and which one would you recommend for Hillary?
4. Is clotrimazole an option for Hillary? Please include mechanism of action, adverse reactions, and dose forms.
5. Compare and contrast ketoconazole, fluconazole, and itraconazole. Can either one of these be given to Hillary? Note that she is taking terfenadine for allergies and nasal congestion.

Review Questions

1. What is the difference between antibacterial and antibiotic?
2. What are the factors that influence antibiotic outcome?
3. What are macrolide antibiotics and what is their role in dentistry?
4. What is clindamycin and what is its role in dentistry?
5. What is the major drug interaction associated with metronidazole? How should patients be counseled about this drug interaction?
6. What are aminoglycoside antibiotics and what are their roles in dentistry?
7. What is the rationale for topical antibiotics in dentistry?
8. What is acyclovir and what is its role in dentistry?

BIBLIOGRAPHY

Bennett JE: Antimicrobial agents. In Goodman Gilman A, Rall TW, Nies A, Taylor P (eds.), *Goodman and Gilman's The Pharmacological Basis of Therapeutics,* 8th ed. Pergamon Press, New York, 1990.

Como JA, Dismukes WE: Oral azole drugs as systemic antifungal therapy. *New Engl J Med* 330:263–272, 1994.

Dajani AS, et al.: Prevention of bacterial endocarditis: Recommendations by the American Heart Association. *JAMA* 264:2919–2922, 1990.

DeSano EA, et al.: Possible interactions of antihistamines and antibiotics with oral contraceptive effectiveness. *Fertil Steril* 37:853, 1982.

Douglas RG, Jr.: Antimicrobial agents. In Goodman Gilman A, Rall TW, Nies A, Taylor P (eds.), *Goodman and Gilman's The Pharmacological Basis of Therapeutics,* 8th ed. Pergamon Press, New York, 1990.

Hussar DA: New therapeutic agents marketed in second half of 1995. *Pharmacy Today* 2:7, 1996.

Mandell GL, Sande MA: Antimicrobial agents, In Goodman Gilman A, Rall TW, Nies A, Taylor P (eds.), *Goodman and Gilman's The Pharmacological Basis of Therapeutics,* 8th ed. Pergamon Press, New York, 1990.

McEvoy GK, ed.: Anti-infectives. In *AHFS Drug Information 95.* American Society of Hospital Pharmacists, Bethesda, MD, 1995.

Orme ML, et al.: Drug interactions with oral contraceptive steroids. *Phamacol Int* 55:33, 1980.

Sande MA, Mandell GL: Antimicrobial agents. In Goodman Gilman A, Rall TW, Nies A, Taylor P (eds.), *Goodman and Gilman's The Pharmacological Basis of Therapeutics,* 8th ed. Pergamon Press, New York, 1990.

CHAPTER 7

Nonnarcotic (Nonopioid) Analgesics

Key Terms

Acetaminophen
Acetylsalicylic Acid
Analgesia
Antiinflammatory

Antipyretic
Nonsteroidal Antiinflammatory Drugs
Pain
Salicylates

LEARNING OBJECTIVES

After completion of this chapter and its learning activities, the student should be able to:

1. Discuss the concept of pain and the different factors that can affect a patient's response to painful stimuli.
2. Describe the salicylates as the prototype of nonopioid analgesics including examples, mechanism of action, pharmacologic effects, pharmacokinetics, and therapeutic effects.
3. Describe the different adverse reactions, drug interactions, and contraindications of salicylates.
4. Describe the dental concerns associated with salicylates.
5. Define nonsteroidal antiinflammatory drugs including examples, mechanism of action, pharmacologic effects, pharmacokinetics, and therapeutic effects.
6. Describe the different adverse reactions, drug interactions, and contraindications of nonsteroidal antiinflammatory drugs.
7. Describe the dental concerns associated with nonsteroidal antiinflammatory drugs.
8. Describe acetaminophen including mechanism of action, pharmacokinetics, pharmacologic effects, and therapeutic effects.
9. Describe the adverse reactions and drug interactions of acetaminophen.
10. Describe, if any, the dental concerns associated with acetaminophen.

INTRODUCTION

Pain is an unpleasant sensory and emotional experience arising from actual or potential tissue damage (International Association for the Study of Pain, 1979; (Merskey, 1964). Pain is what motivates patients to seek help from their physician or dentist; however, fear of a painful procedure may keep them from seeking help.

The reporting of pain is a social transaction between the patient and the health-care provider. The successful assessment and control of pain is, in part, dependent on the development of a positive relationship between the health-care provider, the patient, and the patient's family. The dental hygienist is an important part of this relationship in that he or she already knows the patient. A sound knowledge of the nonnarcotic (nonopioid) pain relievers and their uses will enable the dental hygienist to provide more comprehensive oral health care to the patient. The intent of this chapter is to review nonnarcotic analgesics used in dentistry including mechanisms of action, pharmacology, pharmacokinetics, therapeutic uses, adverse reactions, drug interactions, contraindications, and dental concerns.

PAIN

Pain is a dynamic response to tissue damage or injury. Without treatment, sensory input from the injured tissue to the spinal cord becomes more intense and the pain receptors become more sensitive to the injury. The ultimate goal of the health-care provider is to treat the injured tissue and provide the patient with adequate pain relief.

There are several factors that affect a patient's response to painful stimuli including the patient's perception of and reaction to pain. A patient's perception of pain involves the message that is carried from the injured tissue to the brain. Most people will agree on what will cause pain (Figure 7-1). Patients differ in their reaction

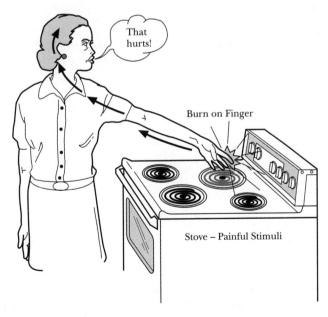

Figure 7-1   *Response to painful stimuli.*

or response to pain. Reaction or response to pain is a psychological component of pain and involves the patient's emotional state at the time of the painful event.

Events that can reduce a patient's pain threshold (greater reaction to pain) include fatigue, emotional instability, anxiety, culture, age, sex, fear, and apprehension. Women, children, and some nationalities tend to have lower pain thresholds. Sleep, sympathy, activity, and analgesics tend to raise the pain threshold (greater tolerance of pain). Analgesic therapy should be based on the individual patient. Some patients may not require analgesics whereas others may require them for the same procedure.

SALICYLATES

The *salicylates,* including **aspirin,** have been used to reduce fever since ancient times. Many salicylates have been synthesized; however, only aspirin is discussed here because it is the most useful salicylate for analgesia and the prototype salicylate. Table 7-1 lists some of the more common oral aspirin preparations and Table 7-2 lists some of the more common oral and topical salicylates other than aspirin.

Chemistry

Aspirin or *acetylsalicylic acid* (ASA) is broken down into acetic acid and salicylic acid. Acetic acid gives broken-down aspirin the smell of vinegar, which lets the patient know that the aspirin is no longer effective and that it may cause gastrointestinal reactions if taken. Salicylic acid is used to remove warts from feet and hands.

Mechanism of Action

The main mechanism of action of aspirin is through its ability to block prostaglandin synthesis in the periphery and in the hypothalamus portion of the brain. Figure 7-2 shows the synthesis of prostaglandins from arachidonic acid and where aspirin exerts its effects. Aspirin irreversibly binds to cyclooxygenase and reduces the patient's perception to pain. Thus, aspirin may be more effective prior to a dental procedure or other painful stimuli. Aspirin is also more effective against throbbing pain (inflammation) rather than stabbing pain (direct effect on nerve ending) because of its ability to block prostaglandin synthesis.

Pharmacokinetics

Aspirin is almost completely and rapidly absorbed from the stomach and small intestine. Buffered aspirin not only protects the patient's stomach but also allows for faster dissolution and absorption. Aspirin can be administered rectally but absorption is erratic. This route should only be used if the oral route is not feasible. Topical application of aspirin to the oral mucosa is not advised because it can cause a severe ulceration of the mucosa.

Aspirin is widely distributed to most body tissues and is poorly bound to plasma proteins. It is hydrolyzed to salicylate in the plasma and on its first pass through the liver and is excreted through the urine.

Table 7-1. Common Oral Aspirin Preparations*

Type of Aspirin	Trade Name	Daily Dose	Comments
Regular	Bayer Empirin St. Joseph	650 mg every 4 hours	Can cause GI irritation and prolong bleeding time
Enteric coated	Ecotrin 325 mg Bufferin 325 mg	650 mg every 4 hours	Less GI irritation Erratic blood levels and absorption May not be good for acute dental pain
Buffered tablets	Bufferin 324 mg Ascriptin 325 mg	650 mg every 4 hours	Contain antacids and cause less GI irritation though they still can prolong bleeding time
Buffered solutions	Alka-Seltzer 324 mg	650 mg every 4 hours	Contains sodium, which is usually contraindicated in patients with high blood pressure
With acetaminophen	Various	250 mg/ASA with 150 mg APAP	Can increase risk of nephrotoxicity
With a sedative diphenhydramine	Excedrin PM	500 mg ASA/38 mg DPH; take 1 or 2 at bedtime	This is okay if anxiety is a major component of pain. The patient is still better off with a separate antianxiety drug
With caffeine	Anacin	400 mg ASA/32.5 mg caffeine; take 1 or 2 every 4 hours	Caffeine potentiates the analgesic effects of aspirin

*Not all-inclusive.

ASA = aspirin, APAP = acetaminophen, DPH = diphenhydramine.

Source: Jacknowitz AI, External analgesic products. In *Handbook of Nonprescription Drugs*, 10th ed. American Pharmaceutical Association, Washington, DC, 1993.

Pharmacologic Effects

Aspirin has a broad range of pharmacologic effects and is very popular and widely used. These therapeutic effects include the following.

Analgesia. Aspirin is used to treat mild to moderate pain such as a headache or toothache. It is not as effective for more intense pain, which is better treated with narcotic or opioid analgesics.

Antipyretic. Aspirin is used to lower body temperature because of its ability to block prostaglandin synthesis in the hypothalamus. It does not lower body temperature if body temperature is normal (98.6°F). It reduces fever by inducing peripheral vasodilation and sweating.

Table 7-2.   Common Oral and Topical Salicylates*

Generic Name	Trade Name	Use
Oral Salicylates		1. All are used to treat mild to
Salsalate	Disalcid	moderate pain
Choline salicylate	Arthrospan	2. They claim to have less GI effects
Magnesium salicylate	Doan's	3. They do not have any effects on
Sodium salicylate	Trilisate	platelets
Diflunisal	Dolobid	4. There is no cross-sensitivity
Topical Salicylates		
Methyl salicylate	Ben Gay	Analgesic cream
Salicylic acid	Compound W	Wart remover
Trolamine	Various	Analgesic cream

*Not all-inclusive.

Source: Jacknowitz AI, External analgesic products. In *Handbook of Nonprescription Drugs,* 10th ed. American Pharmaceutical Association, Washington, DC, 1993.

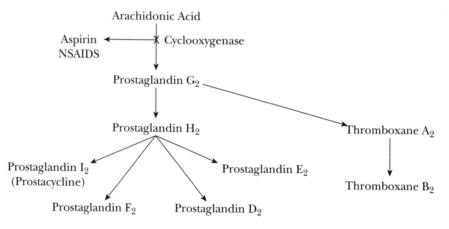

Figure 7-2   *Formation of prostaglandins and thromboxane*

Antiinflammatory Action.   Aspirin's antiinflammatory action is a result of its inhibition of prostaglandin synthesis. It also causes potent vasodilation and increases capillary permeability. Aspirin can decrease the pain, redness, and swelling of inflamed areas such as a toothache or arthritis.

Anticoagulation.   Aspirin administration can prevent blood from clotting by blocking prostaglandin synthesis. Small doses of aspirin are currently used to prevent additional myocardial infarctions or strokes. Aspirin use as an anticoagulant is based on studies in men and its use is currently being studied in women.

Uricosuria. In high doses, aspirin can increase the excretion of uric acid. However, it can antagonize the effects of other drugs (**probenecid** and **colchicine**) used to treat gout.

Therapeutic Effects

Aspirin is used to treat mild to moderate pain and inflammation and is effective against most types of dental-associated pain. It is also used to treat fever and arthritis in adults, and is used to prevent clotting in patients with previous heart attacks or strokes.

Adverse Reactions

The adverse reactions of aspirin may make it an unlikely choice for many patients. Some of the adverse reactions can be minimized but not eliminated.

Gastrointestinal. The most common adverse reactions associated with aspirin use are gastrointestinal (GI) and they include dyspepsia or nausea, vomiting, and increased GI bleeding. GI ulceration and bleeding may be due to a decrease of prostaglandin synthesis in the stomach. Prostaglandins provide protective mechanisms in the stomach.

Bleeding. Aspirin irreversibly binds to platelets and reduces platelet adhesiveness. Bleeding time is prolonged and remains so for about 4–7 days, which is how long it takes for new platelets to form.

Hepatic and Renal Toxicity. Aspirin rarely causes hepatotoxicity and has been reported to cause renal toxicity when taken with **acetaminophen.**

Reye's Syndrome. The use of aspirin has been epidemiologically associated with Reye's syndrome in children and adolescents who took it when they had the chickenpox or influenza. Acetaminophen and nonsteroidal antiinflammatory drugs are now used for fever or pain in children and adolescents.

Hypersensitivity Reaction (Allergy). About 0.2–0.9% of the general population has a true sensitivity to aspirin. This is characterized by bronchospasm, urticaria, edema, and hypotension. Allergic reactions can range from a mild rash to anaphylactic shock. Many patients confuse GI discomfort with allergy, so the dental hygienist should ask patients what happens to them when they take aspirin.

Patients with asthma are more likely to have a hypersensitivity reaction. The aspirin hypersensitivity triad—aspirin hypersensitivity, asthma, and nasal polyps—often occur together. These patients demonstrate cross-sensitivity to other salicylates and nonsteroidal antiinflammatory drugs.

Aspirin Overdose. Toxic blood levels of salicylates are referred to as *salicylism,* which is characterized by tinnitus, headache, nausea, vomiting, dizziness, and dimness of vision. Other symptoms include hyperthermia, electrolyte imbalance, decreases in carbon dioxide (CO_2) levels, hyperventilation, and respiratory and metabolic acidosis. Death can result due to acidosis and electrolyte imbalance. Aspirin overdose is uncommon in adults but occurs more frequently in children. It can be avoided by keeping these products away from children and educating parents about the need for proper storage and handling of aspirin.

Drug Interactions

The drug interactions of aspirin are many and may prohibit some patients from taking it. Some of the more notable interactions are discussed.

Warfarin. **Warfarin** is an oral anticoagulant that is highly plasma protein bound. The concomitant administration of aspirin can displace warfarin from its binding sites and increase its anticoagulant effects. Bleeding and hemorrhage may result.

Probenecid. Aspirin interferes with **probenecid's** uricosuric effects, which may make it ineffective. Aspirin has been reported to precipitate acute gout attacks.

Methotrexate. This drug is used to treat cancers and arthritis. Aspirin can displace **methotrexate** from its binding sites and increase its serum concentration causing toxicity.

Alcohol. Alcohol can cause GI irritation and bleeding and the combination of aspirin and alcohol can result in bleeding and hemorrhage.

Hypoglycemic Medications. Higher doses of aspirin with a sulfonylurea or **insulin** can cause hypoglycemia.

Antihypertensive Effects

Aspirin has been reported to reduce the antihypertensive effects of angiotensin-converting enzyme inhibitors, β blockers, and loop diuretics. This requires continuous dosing of aspirin over several days.

Contraindications

There are several contraindications and precautions to aspirin therapy. Aspirin causes GI irritation and should not be used in patients with ulcers or patients who have problems with alcohol. Aspirin use should also be avoided in patients taking warfarin, probenecid, methotrexate, other nonsteroidal antiinflammatory drugs, or Factor VIII, which is used to treat hemophilia. Aspirin use should also be avoided in patients with the following disorders: hypoprothrombinemia, vitamin K deficiency, glucose-6-phosphate dehydrogenase deficiency, and hemophilia. Aspirin use should be avoided during the last trimester of pregnancy. Aspirin blocks prostaglandin synthesis, which could delay labor, and it could also increase bleeding at the time of delivery.

Dental Concerns

The dental hygienist plays an important role in determining whether or not a patient can take aspirin. A detailed medication/health history will tell if the patient is taking any of the medications discussed in the drug interaction section or has an illness discussed in the contraindications section. The patient should also be questioned about use of aspirin or nonsteroidal antiinflammatory drugs prior to the dental procedure. Prior dosing with aspirin will help to reduce the amount of pain the patient may experience and it may also take longer for the patient's blood to clot. Patients should be instructed to take aspirin with either food or milk or with an antacid, which will help to minimize GI discomfort. They should also call their dentist if pain persists and should not self-medicate without the dentist's advice.

NONSTEROIDAL ANTI-INFLAMMATORY DRUGS

Nonsteroidal antiinflammatory drugs (NSAIDs) are among the fastest-growing class of drugs that are widely used in dentistry. They are similar in mechanism of action, pharmacologic effects, and adverse reactions to aspirin and are used to treat many of the same conditions. Table 7-3 lists the NSAIDs that are available and provides recommended doses for those that are used to treat simple pain.

Mechanism of Action

NSAIDs reversibly bind to the enzyme cyclooxygenase, which results in the breakdown of the formation of prostaglandin precursors and thromboxanes (Figure 7-2, page 109).

Pharmacokinetics

NSAIDs are well absorbed orally and food reduces the rate but not the extent of absorption of NSAIDs. Antacids only reduce the rate of absorption of diflunisal. These drugs are metabolized by the liver and excreted by the kidneys.

Pharmacologic Effects

The analgesic, antipyretic, antiinflammatory effects are the same as aspirin—that is, the inhibition of prostaglandin synthesis. NSAIDs also block prostaglandins in the uterine wall, which make them useful in the treatment of dysmenorrhea (painful menstruation).

Therapeutic Use

NSAIDs are used to treat mild to moderate pain, rheumatoid arthritis, osteoarthritis, acute attacks of gout, dysmenorrhea, and other inflammatory diseases. They are especially useful in the treatment of dental pain.

Table 7-3. Nonsteroidal Antiinflammatory Drugs

Generic Name	Trade Name	Dosage (mg)	Recommended Dose (mg)
Propionic Acids			
Fenoprofen	Nalfon	300–600	200 q4–6h
Flurbiprofen	Ansaid	50–100	—
Ibuprofen	Motrin	200–800	400 q4–6h
Ketoprofen	Orudis, Oruvail	12.5–75	25–50 q6–8h
Naproxen	Naprosyn	250–500	500 stat, 250 q6–8h
Naproxen sodium	Anaprox	275–550	500 stat, 250 q6–8h
Oxaprozin	Daypro	600	—
Acetic Acids			
Diclofenac sodium	Voltaren	50–75	—
Etodolac	Lodine	200–400	200–400 q6–8h
Indomethacin	Indocin	25–50	—
Ketorolac	Toradol		
Oral		10	10 q4–6h
Intramuscular		15–30	—
Nabumetone	Relafin	500–750	—
Sulindac	Clinoril	150–200	—
Tolmetin	Tolectin	200–600	—
Fenamates			
Meclofenamate	Meclomen	50–100	
Mefenamic acid	Ponstel	250	500 stat, 250 q6
Oxicam			
Piroxicam	Feldene	10–20	—

— = not indicated for simple pain.

Sources: McEveoy GK, ed.: Analgesics and antipyretics: General statement. *AHFS Drug Information 94.* American Society of Hospital Pharmacists, Bethesda, MD 1994. Jacknowitz AI, External analgesic products. In *Handbook of Nonprescription Drugs,* 10th ed. American Pharmaceutical Association, Washington, DC, 1993.

Adverse Reactions

Many of the adverse reactions of NSAIDs are similar to those of aspirin. Some of the adverse reactions can be minimized but not eliminated.

Gastrointestinal. GI effects include irritation, pain, and bleeding problems manifested by black, tarry stools, and ulcers. Prostaglandins stimulate the formation of a protective covering in the mucosa of the GI tract and inhibit gastric acid secretion. NSAIDs interfere with those defense mechanisms, resulting in increased acid secretion.

Central Nervous System. Central nervous system (CNS) effects include drowsiness, sedation, dizziness, confusion, headache, mental depression, vertigo, strange dreams, and convulsions.

Blood Clotting. NSAIDs reversibly inhibit platelet aggregation (in contrast to aspirin, which irreversibly inhibits platelet aggregation). Bleeding time is only increased as long as the drug is present in the blood.

Renal. NSAIDs can cause renal failure, cystitis, and an increased incidence of urinary tract infections.

Oral. Oral adverse reactions include ulcerative stomatitis, gingival ulcerations, and dry mouth.

Hypersensitivity Reactions. Hypersensitivity reactions range from mild rashes to anaphylactic reactions similar to aspirin. Other types of hypersensitivity reactions include Stevens-Johnson syndrome, exfoliative dermatitis, and epidermal necrolysis.

Other. Other adverse reactions associated with NSAID use include muscle weakness, tinnitus, hepatitis, hematologic disorders, and blurred vision. NSAIDS can also cause peripheral edema with fluid retention.

DRUG INTERACTIONS

NSAIDs interact with several different medications and conditions.

Lithium. NSAIDs have been reported to increase **lithium** levels, causing toxicity.

Digoxin. NSAIDs increase the effects of **digoxin** which can lead to toxicity.

Methotrexate. As with aspirin, NSAIDs increase the effects of **methotrexate,** which can lead to bone marrow toxicity.

Antihypertensives. NSAIDS can reduce the antihypertensive effects of diuretics, angiotensin-converting enzyme inhibitors, and β blockers, similar to aspirin.

Other Antiinflammatory Drugs. NSAIDs, combined with other antiinflammatory drugs, can increase bleeding and may cause hemorrhage.

Contraindications

NSAIDs should be used with caution in patients with asthma, cardiovascular disease, fluid retention problems, coagulation problems, peptic ulcer disease, and ulcerative colitis if they have to be given at all. Patients at high risk for adverse reactions are those with renal disease, a history of hypersensitivity reactions to aspirin or other NSAIDs, and elderly patients whose liver and kidney functions have declined with age.

Dental Concerns

As with aspirin, the dental hygienist plays an important role in determining whether or not a patient can safely take an NSAID. A detailed medication/health history will determine whether or not a patient is taking a medication or has an illness that is contraindicated or interacts with NSAIDs. Several of the NSAIDs are available without a prescription and it is very important to ask patients about their use of either **ibuprofen, ketoprofen,** or **naproxen sodium.** Many patients forget that these are medications because they can buy them without a prescription. Ask when the patient took her last dose of the NSAID. If it was just prior to the dental procedure, there may be more bleeding because of NSAID ability to prolong bleeding time.

Patients should be instructed to take NSAIDs with a full glass of water and to take them with food to help minimize GI adverse reactions. They should also use caution when driving, operating heavy equipment, or doing anything that requires thought or concentration because of CNS side effects. Patients should always be instructed to call their dentist if the pain has not subsided and should not self-medicate without the advice of the dentist. Patients should avoid the concurrent use of aspirin or other NSAIDs when they are using a particular NSAID.

Over-the-Counter (OTC) NSAIDs

Three OTC NSAIDs are approved for use without a prescription: ibuprofen, naproxen sodium, and ketoprofen. All three are indicated for the treatment of mild to moderate pain—pain associated with colds, flu, muscle aches, headaches, dysmenorrhea, and fever. These drugs are useful in the treatment and management of dental pain.

Ibuprofen. Ibuprofen is the oldest and the most commonly used OTC and prescription NSAID. It is rapidly absorbed orally and food delays its rate but not its extent of absorption. It undergoes hepatic metabolism and is excreted in the kidneys. Ibuprofen has been proven to be effective in the management of dental pain and is usually the drug of choice. Ibuprofen is dosed every 4–6 hours. Adverse reactions include GI upset and some confusion. It is also available in a pediatric dose form in both prescription and OTC strength. Trade names include Motrin IB, Advil, Nuprin, and Children's Motrin.

Naproxen Sodium. Naproxen (Aleve) is similar to ibuprofen but differs in its duration of action and is dosed every 6–8 hours for the prescription product and every 12 hours for the OTC product.

Ketoprofen. Ketoprofen was recently approved for OTC use and the recommended dosing is 12.5 mg tablets; 1–2 tablets every 4–6 hours. It is similar to ibuprofen in terms of mechanism of action, pharmacologic effects, adverse reactions, drug interactions, and contraindications. Trade names include Actron and Orudis KT.

Prescription Strength NSAIDs

Table 7-3, page 112, reviews the different prescription-strength NSAIDS. They are all similar in terms of mechanism of action, pharmacokinetics, pharmacologic effects, adverse reactions, drug interactions, and contraindications. They differ in terms of chemical class and dosing intervals. **Ketorolac** is available as an injectable dose form and is used for short-term management of pain.

ACETAMINOPHEN

Acetaminophen is a nonsalicylate nonnarcotic drug with no antiinflammatory action and is the only member of the *para*-aminophenols used today. **Phenacetin** was the other *para*-aminophenol but was withdrawn from the market because of toxicity. Acetaminophen is extremely popular and one of the most widely used nonnarcotic analgesics when aspirin is contraindicated.

Acetaminophen is available as tablets, capsules, caplets, infant drops, elixirs, suspensions, and suppositories. It is also available in combination with sedatives (**diphenhydramine**), other analgesics, and with **codeine** or **oxycodone.** Trade names include Tylenol, Panadol, and Anacin Free.

Mechanism of Action

Little is known about the mechanism of action of acetaminophen, although its analgesic properties are believed to be in the CNS and not the periphery.

Pharmacokinetics

Acetaminophen is completely and rapidly absorbed following oral ingestion. It is extensively metabolized by the liver by hepatic microsomal enzymes to glucuronide and sulfate conjugates, which are almost entirely excreted by the kidneys within 24 hours. An intermediate metabolite is formed with the ingestion of large doses and is thought to be responsible for the drug's hepatotoxic and nephrotoxic effects.

Pharmacologic Effects

Acetaminophen possesses analgesic and antipyretic effects comparable to aspirin with no clinically significant antiinflammatory effects. Therapeutic doses of acetaminophen have no effects on the respiratory or cardiovascular system and do not interfere with bleeding time (platelet adhesiveness) or cause GI bleeding.

Therapeutic Effects

Acetaminophen is used to treat pain (e.g., headache, dental pain, myalgias, neuralgias, dysmenorrhea) and fever when patients cannot take aspirin. It is used to treat fever in children instead of aspirin because of aspirin's risk of causing Reye's syndrome.

ADVERSE REACTIONS

Acetaminophen, at usual doses, has very few adverse reactions when taken infrequently and for short durations of time. It does not have the GI or bleeding effects associated with aspirin and NSAIDs. Adverse reactions that have clinically significant effects include hepatotoxicity and nephrotoxicity. However, the doses required for these adverse reactions are constant and are usually taken over a long period of time. The usual doses are used in dentistry and the duration is short and should not present a significant problem.

Hepatoxicity

Massive doses (overdose) or usual doses over many days, weeks, or years have been reported to cause liver damage. Massive doses are 10–15 gm and lethal doses are more than 20–25 gm of acetaminophen. The onset of hepatotoxicity occurs within 2–3 days of overdose and is characterized by nausea, vomiting, fever, malaise followed by jaundice, abdominal pain, and signs of liver failure. They include elevated plasma enzyme levels, elevated bilirubin levels, and prolongation of prothrombin time, which can progress to encephalopathy, coma, and death. Patients with liver disease and alcoholics should not receive acetaminophen. Acetaminophen overdose is treated with gastric lavage if ingestion was recent (within 4 hours) followed by the administration of activated charcoal or ipecac, and a full course of sulfhydryl replacement. Sulfhydryl group replacement with the oral administration of **N-acetylcysteine** (Mucomist) can prevent or reduce liver damage if given soon enough after ingestion.

Nephrotoxicity

Nephrotoxicity has been associated with long-term consumption of acetaminophen and includes interstitial nephritis and papillary necrosis. Usually, daily acetaminophen for more than 1 year can place the patient at a very high risk for nephrotoxicity. This risk may be increased even further if the patient is also taking aspirin or an NSAID.

Drug Interactions

Acetaminophen is relatively free of drug interactions at its usual daily dose. Hepatoxicity can be increased by the concurrent administration of barbiturates, **carbamazepine, phenytoin, rifampin,** or any other drug that induces hepatic microsomal enzymes. Alcohol can increase the risk of acetaminophen toxicity.

Contraindications

Acetaminophen should not be used in patients with hepatotoxicity or renal toxicity, nor should it be given to patients with problems with alcohol.

Dental Concerns

The dental hygienist can help patients avoid possible hepatotoxicity and renal toxicity by reviewing with them their instructions for pain management. If the pain is intense or continues longer than 24 hours, patients should be instructed to call the dentist and not self-medicate with additional doses of acetaminophen over a long period of time. The medication/health history will help to determine whether or not the patient has liver, renal, or alcohol problems. Acetaminophen use is contraindicated in these instances.

Summary

Nonnarcotic pain relievers play an important role in helping the patient manage dental pain. Aspirin, NSAIDs, and acetaminophen are effective in treating mild to moderate pain and in lowering fever. Only aspirin and NSAIDs are effective in reducing inflammation. Aspirin and NSAIDs are irritating to the stomach, cause GI bleeding, and prolong bleeding time. Aspirin is contraindicated in children because of the risk of Reye's syndrome and both aspirin and NSAIDs should be avoided in patients with bleeding disorders, ulcers, or problems with alcohol. Some patients can develop aspirin hypersensitivity, characterized by bronchospasm, urticaria, edema, and hypotension. Patients with asthma are more likely to have hypersensitivity reactions to aspirin. Patients who are hypersensitive to aspirin often display this same response to NSAIDs. Acetaminophen is contraindicated in patients with renal, liver, or alcohol problems. Most problems occur with long-term use or large short-term doses of acetaminophen. The doses and durations used in dentistry are usual doses and short in duration and should not present a significant problem.

Case Study: James Smith

James Smith is 45 years old and is new to your practice. This is your first meeting with him and you would like to ask him some questions regarding his medication/health history. During the course of your conversation you learn that he has a history of peptic ulcer disease and is on maintenance therapy for it. His medications include ranitidine 150 mg at bedtime for his ulcer and an occasional acetaminophen for aches and pains. He also likes to have a glass of wine with dinner each night and doesn't mind a few beers when he is watching football. During the course of his examination you and the dentist find two cavities, which are filled that day. Mr. Smith is experiencing some mild pain after the procedure.

1. What is the rationale for using acetaminophen for Mr. Smith?
2. What dose and duration of therapy should be recommended for Mr. Smith?
3. What are the adverse reactions of acetaminophen?

4. Are nephrotoxicity and hepatotoxicity only associated with toxic doses of acetaminophen?
5. How can acetaminophen toxicity be avoided in Mr. Smith?
6. What would increase Mr. Smith's risk of developing nephrotoxicity with acetaminophen?
7. What are the pharmacologic effects of acetaminophen?
8. Compare and contrast acetaminophen to aspirin in terms of pharmacologic and therapeutic effects.
9. Does Mr. Smith have any possible interactions with acetaminophen? If so, what are they and how can they be avoided?
10. What should be said to Mr. Smith during a counseling session on acetaminophen?

Case Study: James Henderson

James Henderson is 52 years old and has a history of high blood pressure. Last year he suffered a heart attack from which he recovered rather well. His medications include enalapril and hydrochlorothiazide for his high blood pressure and one baby aspirin each day for the prevention of future heart attacks. Mr. Henderson is having a crown replaced and would like to know about analgesics after the procedure. He is particularly interested in over-the-counter NSAIDs.

1. What is the role of aspirin in the prevention of heart attacks and stroke?
2. Are there any dental concerns associated with one baby aspirin each day?
3. Can Mr. Henderson take a drug like ibuprofen? Why or why not?
4. Compare and contrast the over-the-counter NSAIDs.
5. When would a prescription NSAID be appropriate?
6. Are there interactions between NSAIDs and antihypertensive drugs?
7. The dentist recommends a short course of over-the-counter ibuprofen. What should Mr. Henderson be told about this drug?

Review Questions

1. What is pain and what is the dental hygienist's role in helping a patient manage pain?
2. What factors help to determine a patient's response to painful stimuli?
3. Explain the mechanism of action of aspirin and NSAIDs.
4. What are the pharmacologic effects of aspirin and NSAIDs?
5. Compare and contrast the therapeutic effects of aspirin and NSAIDs.
6. What are the common adverse reactions of aspirin and NSAIDs?
7. Compare and contrast the different combination products with aspirin.
8. What is the nature and extent of the drug interactions associated with aspirin?

BIBLIOGRAPHY

Butt JH, Barthel JS, Moore RA: Clinical spectrum of the gastrointestinal effects of nonsteroidal anti-inflammatory drugs. *Am J Med* 84(Suppl 2A):5–14, 1988.

Clive DM, Stoff DM: Renal syndromes associated with nonsteroidal anti-inflammatory drugs. *N Engl J Med* 310:563–572, 1984.

Fitch LL, Buchwald H, Matts JP, et al.: Effect of aspirin use on death and recurrent myocardial infarction in current and former cigarette smokers. Program on the Surgical Control of the Hyperlipidemias Group. *Am Heart J* 129:656–662, 1995.

Fleser CR: Newly released therapeutic agents. *Dental Products Report* January: 60–61, 1996.

Flynn BL: Rheumatoid arthritis and osteoarthritis: Current and future therapies. *Am Pharm* NS34:31–42, 1994.

International Association for the Study of Pain: Pain terms: A list of definitions and notes on usage. *Pain* 6:249, 1979.

Jacknowitz AI: External analgesic products. In *Handbook of Nonprescription Drugs,* 10th ed. American Pharmaceutical Association, Washington, DC, 1993.

Lee JB, Katayama S: Inflammation and nonsteroidal antiinflammatory drugs. In Smith CM, Reynard AM (eds.), *Textbook of Pharmacology,* 1st ed. W. B. Saunders, Philadelphia, 1992.

McEvoy GK, ed.: Analgesics and antipyretics: General statement. *AHFS Drug Information 94.* American Society of Hospital Pharmacists, Bethesda, MD, 1994.

Merskey H: An investigation of pain in psychological illness. D.M. thesis, Oxford, England, 1964.

OTC Notes: Ketoprofen. *Am Pharm* NS35:6, 1995.

Perneger TV, Whelton PK, Klag MJ: Risk of kidney failure associated with the use of acetaminophen, aspirin, and nonsteroidal antiinflammatory drugs. *N Engl J Med* 331: 1675–1679, 1994.

Whitcomb DC, Block GD: Association of acetaminophen toxicity with fasting and ethanol use. *JAMA* 272:1845–1850, 1994.

CHAPTER 8

Narcotic (Opioid) Analgesics

Key Terms

Agonist

Agonist-Antagonist

Antagonist

Dynorphins

Endorphins

Enkephalins

kappa

mu

Narcotic

Opioid

sigma

LEARNING OBJECTIVES

After completion of this chapter and its learning activities, the student should be able to:

1. Describe the classification of narcotic analgesics.
2. List the three opioid receptors and their actions.
3. Describe the mechanism of action of opioid analgesics.
4. Describe the pharmacokinetics of opioid analgesics.
5. Describe the pharmacologic effects, therapeutic effects, and dental uses of opioid analgesics.
7. Describe the adverse reactions, drug interactions, contraindications, and dental concerns of opioid analgesics.
8. List specific opioid analgesics including differentiating features.
9. Describe the abuse potential associated with opioid analgesics.
10. Provide a general overview of an opioid addict.

INTRODUCTION

Opioid or narcotic analgesics are used to treat dental pain that does not respond to nonsteroidal antiinflammatory drugs. They differ from nonnarcotic analgesics in that they are more effective against stabbing pain (direct effect on nerve endings) and they relieve most any kind of pain without producing a complete loss of consciousness or loss of any other modality of sensation. The dental hygienist can help the patient by being knowledgeable about the different opioid analgesics, their properties, adverse reactions, drug interactions, and contraindications.

Table 8-1   Classification of Opioid Analgesics and Receptor Activity

Opioid Analgesic	*μ receptor*	*κ receptor*	*σ receptor*
Agonist			
Morphine	Ag	Ag	0
Meperidine	Ag	Ag	0
Hydromorphone	Ag	Ag	0
Hydrocodone	Ag	Ag	0
Oxycodone	Ag	Ag	0
Codeine	Ag	Ag	0
Mixed Agonist/Antagonist			
Buprenorphine	pAg/Ant	?	0
Butorphanol	0	Ag	Ag
Nalbuphine	Ant	Ag	0
Pentazocine	Ant	Ag	0
Antagonist			
Naloxone	Ant	Ant	pAg
Nalorphine	Ant	pAg	Ag

Ag = agonist, pAg = partial agonist, Ant= antagonist, 0 = no effect.

Sources: Smith CM, Opiod analgesics—agonists and antagonists. In Smith CM, Reynard AM (eds.), *Textbook of Pharmacology,* 1st ed. W. B. Saunders Company, Philadelphia, 1992.

HISTORY

Morphine is the major active ingredient of the opium poppy plant and has served as the parent substance for many synthetic compounds. Opioid refers to a morphine-like compound that affects or binds to opiate receptors. The term *narcotic* comes from the Greek word *narcosis,* which means stupor or drugged sleep. The term opiate was used to describe drugs derived from opium and has evolved into the term *opioid,* which refers to synthetic opiate-like drugs.

CLASSIFICATION

Opioid analgesics are classified into three categories based on their interactions with opiate receptors. They include agonists, mixed agonist/antagonists, and antagonists, which can bind to any one of five different opiate receptors. Only three general receptors are discussed: *mu* (μ), *kappa* (κ), and *sigma* (σ). Table 8-1 shows the specific receptor classes pertinent to most of the clinically used opioid analgesics and the effects of certain opioid analgesics.

MECHANISM OF ACTION

The opioids bind to κ, μ, and σ receptors located along the pain-analgesic pathways in the central nervous system (spinal, midbrain, thalamic, and cortical sites of action) and produce altered perceptions and response to pain. The receptors mediate their pharmacologic and adverse reactions to differing degrees based on the stimulating opioid analgesic. Table 8-2 reviews the actions of the κ, μ, and σ receptors. Kappa

Table 8-2   Opioid Receptor Activity

Receptor	Effect
mu (μ)	Respiratory depression, euphoria, analgesia
kappa (κ)	Miosis, sedation, analgesia
sigma (σ)	Dysphoria, hallucinations, anxiety, respiratory and vasomotor stimulation

and mu receptors are responsible for analgesia and sigma receptors are responsible for dysphoria. Opioid analgesics have either agonist, partial agonist, antagonist, or no activity when stimulating these receptors as reviewed in Table 8-1.

The discovery of three naturally occurring groups of neurotransmitters, *endorphins, enkephalins,* and *dynorphins,* has helped to explain the function of opioid receptors. These neurotransmitters have analgesic activity and may help to explain the abuse potential associated with opioid analgesics though their exact function is not known. Continuous physical activity is known to release β endorphins, which can produce a "runner's high."

PHARMACOLOGIC EFFECTS

The primary pharmacologic effects of opioid analgesics are dose related and are discussed next.

Analgesia

The opioid analgesics produce varying degrees of analgesia. Table 8-3 lists the opioid analgesics in order of potency. The analgesic response following administration

Table 8-3   Potency of Selected Opioid Analgesics

Most Potent
   Morphine
   Methadone (Dolophine)
   Meperidine (Demerol)
   Hydromorphone (Dilaudid)

Intermediate
   Oxycodone (Percodan, Percocet, Tylox)
   Nalbuphine (Nubain)
   Pentazocine/naloxone (Talwin-NX)

Least Potent
   Hydrocodone (Vicodin, Lortab, Lorcet)
   Codeine (Tylenol #3)
   Propoxyphene (Darvon, Darvocet)

Source: Rosow CE, The clinical usefulness of agonist-antagonist analgesics in acute pain. *Drug Alcohol Depend* 20:329–337, 1987.

of morphine is characterized by a sense of relief and well-being followed by a decrease in pain perception and reflex response to painful stimuli. Patients may describe the effect as "I have just as much pain, but it doesn't seem to be as bad."

Sedation

Stimulation of κ receptors produces sedation at usual therapeutic doses of opioid analgesics. This may potentiate the analgesic effect and decrease patient anxiety.

Euphoria

Opioid analgesics have the ability to decrease anxiety and induce a feeling of relaxation and tranquility. Some patients may experience euphoria, which is characterized by increased feelings of well-being, energy, and effectiveness. This is due to stimulation of the μ receptor.

Dysphoria

Some patients may experience dysphoria as a result of stimulation of σ receptors, which is characterized by feelings of anxiety or irritability.

Cough Suppression

Opioid analgesics have the ability to decrease or abolish the cough reflex. Cough suppression is mediated by unique opiate receptors that are not stereospecific and include dextromethorphan.

Gastrointestinal (GI) Effects

Opioid analgesics increase smooth muscle tone of the GI tract and decrease propulsive contractions and motility.

Respiration

Opioid analgesics decrease the rate and depth of respiration. All opioid analgesics produce this dose-dependent respiratory depression and it occurs with doses used clinically for analgesia.

PHARMACOKINETICS

The pharmacokinetics of opioid analgesics are similar and are discussed next.

Absorption

Opioid analgesics are well absorbed when administered orally, intramuscularly, subcutaneously, intravenously, nasally, and transdermally. The onset of action is prompt yet peak analgesic response may be delayed for 30–40 minutes. This delay may be partially due to the lipophilicity of the drug and its ability to penetrate the brain. Absorption also occurs from the lungs and from the nasal and oral mucosa. **Butorphanol** is available as a nasal spray and **fentanyl** is available as a transdermal patch and as a lollipop for children.

Distribution

After absorption, opioid analgesics undergo first-pass metabolism in the liver and intestine, which reduces the amount of drug available to produce an analgesic response. The degree of first-pass metabolism differs among patients, so that the dose and frequency of oral preparations should be individualized. The opioids are bound to plasma proteins in varying degrees. They also cross the placenta and are distributed to the fetus.

Metabolism

Opioid analgesics are metabolized in the liver via conjugation with glucuronic acid. The duration of action of opioid analgesics is greater with higher blood levels and pain relief decreases with decreasing blood levels. Maximum pain relief is usually seen within 1 hour followed by a gradual increase in pain over 2–6 hours. Dosing is usually necessary every 4–6 hours. Oral preparations of opioids have similar durations of action.

Excretion

Opioid analgesics are excreted in the kidney via glomerular filtration as the metabolite. Both the metabolite and unchanged drug are excreted in the urine.

ADVERSE REACTIONS

The adverse reactions of opioid analgesics are an extension of their pharmacologic effects. As with their pharmacologic effects, the adverse reactions are proportional to potency.

Respiratory Depression

Morphine and other opioid analgesics reduce the rate and depth of respiration, which is largely due to a decrease in the body's responsiveness to carbon dioxide. This reduced ventilation produces vasodilation, which can increase intracranial pressure. Therefore, these drugs should be avoided in patients with head injuries.

Miosis

Opioids can cause miosis (pupil constriction). This may be advantageous in trying to decide whether or not someone is taking or abusing opioid analgesics.

Nausea and Vomiting

Opioid analgesics stimulate the chemoreceptor trigger zone in the medulla. Repeated dosing will increase morphine or other opioid blood levels, thereby depressing the vomiting center. This adverse reaction is also minimized by having the patient rest and not ambulate.

Constipation

Opioid analgesics decrease propulsive activity in the small and large intestines, which causes constipation. Small, usual doses have this effect and tolerance does not develop with continued use.

Urinary Retention

Opioid analgesics increase the tone of the detrusor muscle, urinary bladder, and vesical sphincter, which can lead to urinary retention. They also stimulate the release of antidiuretic hormone from the pituitary gland, which would also make it difficult for a person to urinate, especially if he has prostatic hypertrophy.

Central Nervous System Effects

Opioid analgesics can produce dysphoria that is characterized by feelings of anxiety, restlessness, and nervousness.

Cardiovascular Effects

In analgesic doses, opioid analgesics have little effect on the cardiovascular system. They may cause orthostatic hypotension and some peripheral vasodilation.

Biliary Tract and Bronchial Constriction

Opioids increase biliary tract tone and pressure and can cause biliary colic. This is of particular concern in patients with gallstones. Opioids can also cause bronchial constriction, which is of importance in patients with asthma.

Histamine Release

Opioids can stimulate the release of histamine, which causes itching and urticaria.

Pregnancy and Nursing

Opioids have not been shown to be teratogenic. They are known to prolong labor and can depress fetal respiration when given near term. Infants born to mothers who are addicted to opioid analgesics have respiratory depression and undergo drug withdrawal. Opioids are present in breast milk but are not a real problem for normal (nonaddicted) infants.

Allergic Reactions

Allergic reactions can and do occur. However, many patients confuse allergic reactions with side effects. It is important for the dental hygienist to determine whether the patient was experiencing nausea and vomiting, which are side effects, or true anaphylactic reactions. The most common types of allergic reactions are skin rashes and urticaria.

DRUG INTERACTIONS

The most common drug interactions with opioid analgesics occur with other medications that produce central nervous system (CNS) effects. Table 8-4 lists some of the more common classes of drugs with CNS effects. If a medication has any type of sedative effect, it will interact with opioid analgesics, which will further increase a person's sedated state and may increase the risk for respiratory depression. Opioid analgesics can also interact with anticholinergic drugs. These drugs are also constipating and the combined effects can be dangerous. Lastly, only **meperidine** can interact with monoamine oxidase inhibitors used to treat depression. This interaction is characterized by CNS excitation, hypertension, and hypotension.

THERAPEUTIC USES

Opioid analgesics are used preoperatively to relieve anxiety, produce analgesia, and reduce the amount of general anesthetic that may be required. They are also used postoperatively to produce analgesia. There are other therapeutic uses of opioids and they are reviewed next.

Use in Dentistry

Their use in dentistry has decreased with the advent of nonsteroidal antiinflammatory drugs (NSAIDs), which can better manage most dental pain. Opioid analgesics are often used in patients who cannot tolerate or have a contraindication to NSAIDs.

Table 8-4   Selected Drugs with Central Nervous System Effects

Drug Class

Alcohol
Anticholinergics
Antidepressants
Antihistamines
Antipsychotics
Antianxiety drugs
Anticonvulsants
General anesthetics
Sedative-hypnotics

Cough Suppressant

Opioid analgesics are used to treat coughs that do not respond to over-the-counter (OTC) preparations. The most common OTC cough suppressant is **dextromethorphan.**

Antidiarrheal Treatment

Opioid analgesics are also effective in treating diarrhea. They are available as prescription and OTC products. Paregoric is a tincture of **opium** containing benzoic acid and is still available over the counter. Other antidiarrheals include **diphenoxylate** with **atropine** (Lomotil) and **loperamide** (Imodium) which is available as an OTC preparation.

DENTAL CONCERNS

The dental hygienist should perform a detailed medication/health history to determine whether or not a patient is allergic to opioid analgesics or may require a dosage reduction. Elderly patients, those with prostatic hypertrophy, and those with liver and kidney disease should have their dosages reduced to minimize or avoid adverse reactions.

These drugs are sedating and the dental hygienist should always remind the patient of this. Patients should be instructed not to drive, operate heavy machinery or equipment, or do anything that requires thought or concentration after taking an opioid analgesic. Patients should also be advised to be careful if they are already taking a CNS depressant drug because this could intensify CNS effects. Patients could become very sedated, agitated, or even psychotic. They should also be advised not to drink alcohol while taking these drugs. The combination of the two could have devastating effects.

Opioid analgesics and anticholinergic drugs could lead to problems with constipation and dry mouth. Patients should be instructed to drink plenty of water and eat fresh fruits and vegetables to help minimize or avoid constipation. This should not be too much of an issue with dental patients because they are only receiving the opioid analgesic for a very short period of time.

The selection of the drug, dose, route, and regimen should be based on the pain being experienced and anticipated. If an opioid analgesic is used, it should be prescribed for no more than 1–2 days. Opioid analgesics should only be given in small amounts, without refills, and only if the patient has had a dental procedure. If the patient's pain persists or intensifies, she should call the dentist and be reevaluated.

SPECIFIC OPIOIDS

The analgesic action of most opioid analgesics is based on their ability to stimulate κ and μ receptors (Table 8-1, page 121). Table 8-5 lists the duration of action, dosing interval, and doses of opioid *agonists,* mixed *agonists/antagonists,* and *antagonists.*

Table 8-5   Selected Opioid Analgesics, Doses, Dosing Interval, and Duration of Action

Generic Name	Trade Name	Dose	Duration of Action (hours)	Dosing Interval (hours)
Morphine		10 mg IM or 60 mg PO	4–5	4–6
Meperidine	Demerol	75–100 mg IM or 50 mg PO	4–5	3–4
Hydromorphone	Dilaudid	1.5 mg IM or 2 mg PO	4–5	4–6
Methadone	Dolophine	10 mg IM or 10-20 mg PO	≥6	4–6
Oxycodone	Percodan (with ASA) Percocet (with APAP) Tylox (with APAP)	5 mg PO	4–5	4–6
Hydrocodone	Vicodin (with APAP) Lortab (with ASA)	5 mg PO	4–5	4–6
Codeine	Tylenol #3 (with APAP) Empirin #3 (with ASA)	30 mg PO	4–5	4–6
Fentanyl	Sublimaze	0.1 mg IM	< 1 hour	NA
Pentazocine	Talwin-NX	50 mg PO	4–6	4–6

NA = dependent on dose form.

Source: McEvoy GK, ed.: Analgesics and antipyretics: General statement. *AHFS Drug Information 94*. American Society of Hospital Pharmacists, Bethesda, MD, 1994.

Opioid Agonists

Morphine. **Morphine** is considered the prototype of opioid agonists and is used to treat or prevent moderate to severe pain. Because it is the prototype, an equivalent strength of each opioid is compared to 10 mg of morphine. Morphine is used intramuscularly to control postoperative pain in hospitalized patients, intravenously to control pain associated with myocardial infarction, and orally for terminally ill patients.

Meperidine. **Meperidine** is one-sixth as potent as morphine and, in sufficient doses, it can produce analgesic activity similar to morphine. It is somewhat shorter acting, less constipating, and without miosis or cough suppression in equianalgesic doses to morphine. It is also available as intramuscular and oral dose forms. Its use is similar to morphine.

Methadone. **Methadone** is a synthetic drug with effects similar to morphine but with a slower onset and longer duration of action. It can be used as an analgesic but is primarily used to gradually withdraw a person from heroin or to maintain opioid dependence.

Hydromorphone. **Hydromorphone** is available orally and intramuscularly. It is more potent than morphine, better absorbed orally, and produces similar adverse reactions. It is highly abusable and its use should be limited and carefully monitored.

Oxycodone. **Oxycodone** is combined with either aspirin or acetaminophen and provides relief from moderate to severe pain. This combination allows for additive analgesic effects with fewer adverse reactions. It is available orally and retains about two-thirds of its analgesic action when given orally.

Codeine. The analgesic effects of **codeine** are similar to morphine. Oral codeine is mostly used, in relatively low doses, for cough suppression or for the relief of mild to moderate pain that does not respond to NSAIDs. It is also used for patients with mild to moderate pain who cannot tolerate NSAIDs. It is often combined with aspirin or acetaminophen, which allows for lower doses and a lower incidence of adverse reactions.

Hydrocodone. **Hydrocodone** is a weak opioid analgesic that produces fewer adverse reactions and has less potential for abuse than morphine. It is also used for cough suppression and for the relief of mild to moderate pain in patients who cannot tolerate NSAIDs or because NSAIDs are ineffective. It is also combined with acetaminophen.

Fentanyl, Sufentanil, and Alfentanil. **Fentanyl, sufentanil, and alfentanil** are short-acting, parenterally administered, potent opioid analgesics that are used perioperatively. They have rapid onset and short duration of action when given parenterally and are shorter acting than morphine or meperidine. Fentanyl is available as a transdermal patch applied to the skin every 3 days to provide pain relief for terminally ill patients. These drugs provide analgesia during and immediately after general anesthesia and are often combined with anesthetics for block or epidural anesthesia, or are combined with neuroleptics to induce or supplement general or regional anesthesia. Postoperative observation is required because of the potential for respiratory depression.

Propoxyphene. **Propoxyphene** has been extensively used as an analgesic for mild to moderate pain and is often combined with acetaminophen or aspirin. It has been claimed that the analgesic efficacy of propoxyphene is more effective than aspirin or acetaminophen. However, there is no general consensus on the validity of this statement. Propoxyphene tends to be overused because of the misconception of a lack of adverse reactions and abuse potential. Its adverse reactions include nausea, vomiting, dizziness, and physical dependence. Its toxic effects are additive or more than other CNS depressants including alcohol. Patients and health professionals should be made aware of this situation. NSAIDs and other drugs make it difficult to justify the use of propoxyphene.

Mixed Opioid Agonists/Antagonists

Mixed opioid agonists/antagonists include opioid analgesics with agonist-antagonist activity and partial agonists. They are used to treat moderate to severe pain and their use in dentistry is unclear.

Pentazocine. **Pentazocine** produces analgesia and drowsiness similar to that produced by morphine, and 30 mg of pentazocine is equivalent to 10 mg of morphine. Pentazocine can produce respiratory depression, some sedation, and patients may experience hallucinations, confusion, or disorientation. Pentazocine can increase blood pressure and heart rate. Chronic administration can lead to tolerance and dependence, which was not thought to be the case when the drug was first introduced. It has become a drug of abuse and is often combined with **pyribenzamine** (antihistamine) or diphenhydramine. This abuse has led to the development of a unique oral preparation, Talwin-NX, which is a combination of pentazocine and **naloxone.** It is unique in that the parenterally administered combination antagonizes the opioid effects of pentazocine. The oral combination product leaves the pentazocine alone to produce analgesic effects and makes it more difficult to abuse.

Nalbuphine and Butorphanol. **Nalbuphine and butorphanol** are effective analgesics with approximately the same potency and duration of action as morphine. Both have proportionately less respiratory depression than morphine. They have agonist activity at κ receptors and antagonist activity at μ receptors. Adverse reactions include sedation, nausea, vomiting, xerostomia, and headache. Their addiction potential is less than other opioid analgesics and butorphanol can produce dysphoria at higher doses. Neither drug is considered a controlled substance.

Buprenorphine. **Buprenorphine** is a partial μ receptor agonist and is unique in that it is long-acting and potent. Peak effects occur in 1 hour and can last for as long as 6 hours. It is effective parenterally and well absorbed after sublingual administration. Physical dependence is low and withdrawal is mild.

Opioid Antagonists

Opioid antagonists are used to counteract the pharmacologic and adverse effects of opioid agonists and mixed opioids.

Naloxone. **Naloxone** is the prototype and works by antagonizing opioid-induced euphoria, analgesia, drowsiness, and respiratory depression. It appears to be less effective against pupillary constriction and smooth muscle contraction. Naloxone is the drug of choice in treating opioid agonist or mixed opioid overdose. It is very short acting and needs to be given repeatedly to manage toxic overdoses. Naloxone should be a part of every emergency kit in a dental office if opioids are used.

Naltrexone. **Naltrexone** is a long-acting oral opioid antagonist that is indicated for maintenance of an opioid-free state in opioid addicts. It should only be administered after the patient has been opioid-free for at least 1 week. It can be dosed daily or even 3 times a week. Patients receiving naltrexone should not receive opioid analgesics.

OPIOID ADDICTION

Chronic administration of opioid analgesics can lead to tolerance, habituation and dependence. Addicts develop tolerance to all side-effects except constipation and miosis. Tolerance can be controlled in terminally ill cancer patients by adjusting the dose of the opioid analgesic. Tolerance is normally not a problem for those who take the opioid analgesic for no more than 1–3 days as is the case with the management of dental pain.

The degree of addiction or dependence is proportional to the analgesic potency of the opioid, which limits the usefulness of such drugs as morphine and meperidine. It is also dependent on the drug's ability to produce euphoria and reduce anxiety. Dependence is also related to the length of administration. Prolonged administration of progressively large amounts of opioids can lead to a withdrawal syndrome following abrupt withdrawal. This is characterized by lacrimation, sweating, rhinorrhea, goose-flesh, vomiting, diarrhea, abdominal cramps, irritability, tachycardia, and chills. Peak severity occurs 36–72 hours after the last dose and gradually wanes over 2–5 weeks. This issue should not be a problem in the short-term management of dental pain.

Dental Concerns

The fear of addiction may prohibit some patients from taking opioid analgesics and adequately managing their pain. The dental hygienist should remind the patient that short-term use should not cause problems with addiction or dependence. The proper use of these medications will provide needed pain management.

The dental hygienist should become suspicious of patients who continuously ask for opioid analgesics. They may not ask outright for the opioid analgesic but in an indirect way. Questions or statements that should send up red flags include:

1. Patient asks for the opioid analgesic by name and says that this is the only drug that will work for him.
2. Patient claims allergies to NSAIDs or lower-potency opioid analgesics.
3. Patient claims that NSAIDs, acetaminophen, or aspirin just don't work for her.
4. Patient calls with a request for an opioid analgesic just as the office is closing or after hours.
5. Patient cancels dental appointment but still requests the opioid analgesic because he will be out of town "on business."
6. Patient often changes dental provider because no one understands his "low pain threshold."
7. Patient claims to experience pain for days after scaling and root planing.

Summary

Opioid analgesics are effective in managing dental pain that is not responsive to NSAIDs or in those patients who cannot tolerate NSAIDs or acetaminophen. Opioid analgesics alter the patient's perception toward painful stimuli. They are also used as cough suppressants and as antidiarrheals. Opioid analgesics exert their pharmacologic effects by binding to any one of three receptors (μ, κ, and σ) located along the pain-analgesic pathways in the CNS. Stimulation results in analgesia, sedation, euphoria, dysphoria, cough suppression, decreased GI motility and propulsive contractions, and decreased respiration. Adverse reactions include sedation, miosis, constipation, nausea and vomiting, urinary retention, and decreased respiration and cardiovascular rates in high doses. These drugs interact with other CNS depressants, nonopioid analgesics that are irritating to the GI tract, and other drugs with anticholinergic activity.

There are many analgesics available and some are beneficial for the management of dental pain. A sound knowledge of opioid analgesics will enable the dental hygienist to effectively work with the dental patient to manage pain and to help her avoid drug interactions and adverse reactions. Unfortunately, there is a segment of the population that abuses opioid analgesics. The dental hygienist can help to reduce abuse in his practice by carefully screening patients with detailed medication/health histories and by paying attention to red flags sent up by substance abusers.

Case Study: Sam Smith

Sam Smith is a 25-year-old who is new to your practice. He presents today with vague complaints of pain that he associates with a cleaning that he had last week from another dental practice. You attempt to complete a medication/health history and learn that he has had problems with chronic pain since a work-related injury about 3 years ago. He takes no medications and tells you that NSAIDs do not "touch his pain." He also tells you that acetaminophen with codeine is not very effective. He would like for you to review what was done to him at his other visit and hopefully have the dentist prescribe some Vicodin for the pain.

1. What are the concerns associated with this patient? What should be done?
2. What are some other red flags associated with opioid addiction?
3. Is any one opioid more addicting than the other? If so, upon what is this fact based?
4. Is there a need for concern with opioid addiction for patients taking these drugs to treat or manage dental pain? Why or why not?
5. What is hydrocodone and how effective is it in treating or managing dental pain?
6. What should be recommend for this patient?

Case Study: Paula Barnes

Paula Barnes is a 32-year-old woman with a history of poor teeth despite the use of fluoride toothpaste, brushing, and flossing. Her medication/health history reveals a healthy woman whose only medications include oral contraceptives and occasional over-the-counter analgesics and cough and cold products. She is in your office today for a root cannel and new crown. Ms. Barnes experienced a lot of pain with her last root cannel and crown. Ibuprofen did not help with the pain and she required something stronger. The dentist decides to give Ms. Barnes a prescription for hydrocodone with acetaminophen (Vicodin).

1. What is hydrocodone and how effective is it in treating or managing dental pain?
2. Compare and contrast hydrocodone with ibuprofen.
3. What are the adverse reactions associated with hydrocodone?
4. Are there any drug interactions that Ms. Barnes should be aware of?
5. What are the dental concerns associated with hydrocodone?
6. What should Ms. Barnes be told about this medication?

Review Questions

1. What are the different opioid receptors and what happens to them when they are stimulated by opioid analgesics?
2. What are the different classifications of opioid analgesics and what do they mean?
3. What are the pharmacologic effects of opioid analgesics?
4. What are the adverse reactions of opioid analgesics?
5. Describe the therapeutic uses of opioid analgesics.
6. How do opioid analgesics differ from each other?
7. What is the rationale for using propoxyphene and what is its degree of clinical effectiveness?
8. Why is pentazocine combined with naloxone?
9. When would opioid use be contraindicated or used with caution? What would you tell the patient?
10. What should a patient be told about the concerns associated with opioid analgesics?

BIBLIOGRAPHY

Hoffert MJ: The neurophysiology of pain. *Neurol Clin* 7:183–203, 1989.
Jaffe JH, Martin WR: Opioid analgesics and antagonists. In Goodman Gilman A, Rall TW, Nies AS, Taylor P (eds.), *Goodman and Gilman's The Pharmacological Basis of Therapeutics,* 8th ed. Pergamon Press, New York, 1990.

Martin WR: Clinical evidence for different narcotic receptors and relevance for the clinician. *Ann Emerg Med* 15:1026–1029, 1986.

Rosow CE: The clinical usefulness of agonist-antagonist analgesics in acute pain. *Drug Alcohol Depend* 20:329–337, 1987.

Smith CM: Opioid analgesics—agonists and antagonists. In Smith CM and Reynard AM (eds.), *Textbook of Pharmacology,* 1st ed. W. B. Saunders Company, Philadelphia, 1992.

CHAPTER 9

Sedative-Hypnotic Medications

Key Terms

Anxiety
Barbiturates
Benzodiazepines
Buspirone

Chloral Hydrate
Insomnia
Nonbarbiturate/nonbenzodiazepine
Zolpidem

LEARNING OBJECTIVES

After completion of this chapter and its learning activities, the student should be able to:

1. Describe the antianxiety drugs as a group.
2. Describe the impact that dental treatment has on anxiety and insomnia.
3. Discuss the benzodiazepines as sedative-hypnotics, including mechanism of action, pharmacokinetics, clinical use, adverse reactions, dependence, contraindications, potential for abuse, and dental concerns.
4. Describe the barbiturates as sedative-hypnotics, including mechanism of action, pharmacokinetics, clinical use, adverse reactions, dependence, contraindications, potential for abuse, and dental concerns.
5. Discuss the nonbarbiturate sedative-hypnotics, along with their sedative effects, adverse reactions, clinical use, and potential for abuse.
6. Discuss the nonbenzodiazepine-nonbarbiturate antianxiety agent, including mechanism of action, clinical use, adverse reactions, and potential for abuse.
7. Discuss the drug interactions that can occur with all classes of sedative-hypnotic drugs.
8. Effectively counsel the patient about the adverse reactions associated with sedative-hypnotic drugs and any drug interactions that can occur.
9. Discuss both the pharmacologic and nonpharmacologic treatments of insomnia.

INTRODUCTION

Anxiety and insomnia are common problems that affect a significant percentage of the population, and a great number of dental patients will be receiving medications to treat these disorders. Some patients who experience anxiety or insomnia in anticipation of a dental office visit may be successfully treated with medication just prior to or the night before their appointment. Both the dental hygienist and the dentist recognize the fact that a calm patient is much easier to treat. Most patients can be calmed by the reassurance of an understanding dental hygienist, although some patients may require medication.

There are several different classes of medication to treat anxiety and insomnia and dental hygienists should familiarize themselves with one or two medications and know them well. The intent of this chapter is to review medications used to treat anxiety and insomnia, including mechanism of action, pharmacokinetics, clinical use, adverse reactions, drug interactions, and advice for the patient.

ANXIETY DISORDER

Anxiety has been defined as an unpleasant emotional state characterized by apprehension and nervousness. Everyone experiences a certain degree of anxiety when faced with a stressful situation and most adapt to that situation. However, other people experience irrational, excessive, unremitting, or unwarranted fears. Anxiety can be a symptom of a physical illness, the result of a psychosocial, dental, or medical stressor, or a psychiatric illness.

Most patients can adapt to the stress associated with dentistry and do not require medication or only require psychosedation. There is a group of patients that will require medication prior to a dental appointment. The dental hygienist plays an important role in determining the level of patient anxiety by observing and questioning the patient and then determining if he requires medication.

Pharmacotherapy

There are several different agents available to treat anxiety and they are referred to as either sedative-hypnotics or antianxiety drugs. They differ in terms of duration of action, adverse reaction profile, and potential for abuse and suicide. The dose required to alleviate a patient's symptoms will depend on the patient and her level of anxiety and the procedure to be performed.

BENZODIAZEPINES

The *benzodiazepines* were first discovered in the 1930s but were not marketed until the 1960s. More than 30 benzodiazepines are available worldwide and eight are indicated for the treatment of anxiety in the United States. Table 9-1 reviews those medications.

Mechanism of Action

Benzodiazepines are thought to work by binding to benzodiazepine receptors in the central nervous system (CNS) and potentiating the activity of γ-aminobutyric acid

Table 9-1 Benzodiazepines Used to Treat Anxiety

Generic Name	Trade Name	Onset of Action (minutes)	Dose Range
Long Acting			
Chlordiazepoxide	Librium	15–45	15–100 mg/day
Clorazepate	Tranxene	15–45	15–60 mg/day
Diazepam	Valium	15–45	4–40 mg/day
Prazepam	Centrax	15–45	60–160 mg/day
Intermediate Acting			
Lorazepam	Ativan	30–55	2–6 mg/day
Alprazolam	Xanax	30–45	0.75–4 mg/day
Oxazepam	Serax	45–90	30–120 mg/day
Halazepam	Paxipam	15–45	20–60 mg/day
Short Acting			
Midazolam	Versed	15	0.07–0.08 mg/kg of body weight for preoperative sedation
Triazolam	Halcion	2–30	0.125–0.5 mg/day

Sources: Ashton H, Guidelines for the rational use of benzodiazepines: When and what to use. *Drugs* 48:25–40, 1994; Dommisse CS, Hayes PE, Current concepts in clinical therapeutics; Anxiety disorders, part 2. *Clin Pharm* 6:196–215, 1987; Smith CM, Antianxiety drugs. In Smith CM, Reynard AM (eds.), *Textbook of Pharmacology,* 1st ed. W. B. Saunders Company, Philadelphia, 1992.

(GABA). GABA is the major inhibitory neurotransmitter in the CNS. The benzodiazepine-GABA receptor interaction allows chloride to flow freely into the cells. This results in a more negatively charged cell membrane, which attenuates subsequent depolarizing excitatory neurotransmitters.

Pharmacokinetics

The benzodiazepines are well absorbed from the oral route and are available as tablets and capsules. The intramuscular (IM) route is unpredictable, slow, and erratic. The intravenous (IV) route produces a rapid, predictable response. Once a benzodiazepine is absorbed, the rate at which it crosses to the CNS is dependent on lipid solubility, protein binding, and the degree of ionization. Most benzodiazepines are highly protein bound, lipid soluble, and present in the unionized form. As a result, they readily cross the blood-brain barrier.

Benzodiazepines undergo two primary metabolic pathways: oxidation and glucuronide conjugation. Conjugation is a very simple process that is affected very little by liver disease or advanced age. Oxidation is the rate-limiting step in the metabolism of benzodiazepines and can be impaired by liver disease or advancing age. The metabolites of some of the benzodiazepines are active. The metabolites are renally excreted with half-lives that range from 2 to 200 hours. The biologic half-lives do not correlate with duration of action.

Adverse Reactions

Despite what one may have learned from the lay press, the benzodiazepines, when used appropriately, have a wide margin of safety. The most common adverse reactions result from CNS depression and include drowsiness, sedation, blurred vision, ataxia (unsteady gait), and psychomotor impairment. Disorientation, confusion, aggressive behavior, and excitement can occur, especially in elderly patients. Cardiovascular and respiratory depression are minimal though respiratory depression can occur in a person with compromised pulmonary function.

The amnestic properties of benzodiazepines have been well documented (Scharf et al., 1984; Roehrs et al., 1983; Mac et al., 1985). Lorazepam appears to produce a more profound amnesia (up to 4 hours after a single 2-mg oral dose) than other benzodiazepines (Scharf et al., 1983). The memory loss is limited to events occurring after drug administration (anterograde amnesia) and most likely results from impaired consolidation processes that store information (Roth et al., 1980). The amnesia may actually be a therapeutic advantage especially if the patient is scheduled for a long and unpleasant dental procedure.

There have been reports of benzodiazepines producing xerostomia, swollen tongue, increased salivation, and a metallic or bitter taste. Other adverse reactions include diplopia, nystagmus, and malfunctioning in the gastrointestinal (GI) and genitourinary (GU) tracts.

The parenteral dose form of diazepam can produce phlebitis especially when given in the dorsum of the hand rather than the antecubital space. The phlebitis is actually due to propylene glycol, which is used to solubilize the **diazepam.** This does not happen as frequently with **midazolam** which may be attributed to the fact that midazolam is water soluble.

Cardiovascular and respiratory adverse reactions are more common with rapid administration of parenteral benzodiazepines. Emergency equipment should be on hand if these agents are used for conscious sedation in the office.

There is an increased risk for congenital malformations to infants whose mothers are taking benzodiazepines when they are pregnant. The benzodiazepines are categorized as Food and Drug Administration (FDA) pregnancy category D except for **triazolam** and **temazepam,** which are category X. A woman of childbearing age should always be asked if she may be pregnant in order to avoid complications due to the use of these medications.

Though the benzodiazepines are considered to be safe medications, some patients can overdose on them. Should this occur there are several steps to follow. Supportive measures should be initiated immediately. Emesis may be induced if ingestion has been recent and one can administer either activated charcoal or a saline cathartic. Always monitor the patient's respiration and pulse. A new medication, **flumazenil,** is now available for benzodiazepine overdose. Flumazenil is a benzodiazepine antagonist that reverses the CNS depression associated with benzodiazepines. Adverse reactions include pain at the site of injection, agitation, and anxiety.

Dependence

There has been much concern about the abuse potential of benzodiazepines. Physiologic addiction usually occurs after an extended period of large doses. It has also been reported that some patients may experience withdrawal symptoms after taking therapeutic doses for as little as 4–6 weeks (Fontaine et al., 1984). Symptoms include anxiety, insomnia, malaise, anorexia, diaphoresis, strange smells, metallic taste, and in more severe cases, tremor, orthostasis, nausea, vomiting, seizures, and psychosis. However, the abuse and addiction potential of benzodiazepines is less than barbiturate and nonbarbiturate sedative hypnotics.

Whether benzodiazepines lose their anxiolytic effects over time is unclear. Tolerance has been clearly demonstrated to the sedative, muscle relaxant, and anticonvulsant properties of benzodiazepines.

Drug Interactions

Benzodiazepines interact with other CNS medications such as barbiturates, antipsychotics, antidepressants, opioid analgesics, and alcohol. Patients taking a benzodiazepine with any one of these types of medication can experience increased CNS depressant effects. Medications such as **cimetidine, disulfiram, isoniazid,** and **omeprazole** have been reported to inhibit the metabolism of such benzodiazepines as **diazepam** and **chlordiazepoxide.** Benzodiazepines may reduce the effectiveness of **levodopa** and may increase the effects of **digoxin, phenytoin,** and **probenecid.**

Clinical Use

Benzodiazepines are used to treat situational anxiety (dental appointment), generalized anxiety disorders, panic attacks, and insomnia.

Dental Concerns

If a benzodiazepine is prescribed, the patient should be counseled about the additive CNS depressant effects with alcohol, opioid analgesics, and other CNS depressant medications. The dose of a benzodiazepine should be lowered in elderly patients, patients with liver disease, and patients with renal failure. Benzodiazepines are lipid soluble and can accumulate in the adipose tissue of elderly patients which can lead to CNS changes because the medication is erratically released into the body. All patients should be counseled about the sedative and amnestic qualities of the medication. They should be instructed not to operate heavy machinery or equipment and they should avoid any activity that requires thought or concentration. Lastly, patients should have someone drive them to and from their appointment if a benzodiazepine is prescribed.

BARBITURATES

Barbiturates were originally used to treat situational anxiety and insomnia and are reviewed in Table 9-2. The barbiturates have a long history and are effective sedative-hypnotics. However, they cause significant motor and intellectual impairment, interact with many drugs, have a high fatality rate with overdose, and have a high addiction potential. Their use as antianxiety agents has been supplanted by the benzodiazepines which have been found to be superior in clinical studies (Goldberg, 1984).

Table 9-2   Barbiturates Used to Treat Anxiety

Generic Name	Brand Name	Onset of Action (minutes)	Duration of Action (hours)
Amobarbital	Amytal	40–60	6–8
Butibarbital	Butisol	40–60	6–8
Pentobarbital	Nembutal	30	3–4
Secobarbital	Seconal	30	3–4

McEvoy GK, ed., Barbiturates: General statement. *AHFS Drug Information 94.* American Society of Hospital Pharmacists, Bethesda, MD, 1994.

Mechanism of Action

Barbiturates are thought to produce their effect by interacting with GABA receptors, thereby prolonging the opening of the chloride channel. They may also act on chloride channels without affecting GABA at higher doses.

Pharmacokinetics

The barbiturates are well absorbed orally, intravenously, and rectally. The short- and intermediate-acting barbiturates are completely and rapidly metabolized by the liver. The long-acting barbiturates are excreted renally. Caution should be used with these medications in a person with renal or liver disease. The dose should also be lowered in an elderly patient.

Adverse Reactions

The adverse reactions of barbiturates range from mild sedation to complete CNS depression or mental stimulation in elderly patients. Their potential lethality is well documented in that they are commonly used in successful suicides (Gary and Tresnewsky, 1983). Barbiturates are absolutely contraindicated in patients with intermittent porphyria or with a family history of porphyria.

Dependence

Chronic use of barbiturates can lead to physical and psychological dependence. Tolerance develops to the therapeutic dose but not to the lethal dose.

Drug Interactions

As with the benzodiazepines, the use of barbiturates with alcohol, other CNS depressant medications, and opioid analgesics produce enhanced or additive CNS depressant effects. Barbiturates can reduce the efficacy of β blockers, birth control pills, estrogens, phenytoin, **doxycycline,** and tricyclic antidepressants. Disulfiram, monoamine oxidase inhibitors, and **propoxyphene** all increase the effects of barbiturates.

Clinical Use

The barbiturates are classified as ultra-short-acting, short-acting, intermediate-acting, and long-acting and differ in their onset and duration of action. The ultra-short-acting barbiturates are used for anesthesia and the long-acting barbiturates are used to treat seizure disorders. The short-acting and intermediate-acting agents are used to treat anxiety disorders and insomnia.

Dental Concerns

The dental concerns of the barbiturates are similar to those of the benzodiazepines. Patients should be counseled in the same manner as if they were taking a benzodiazepine. This information is reviewed in the discussion about benzodiazepines.

NONBARBITURATE/NONBENZODIAZEPINE SEDATIVE HYPNOTICS

Chloral hydrate is an inexpensive therapeutic option for the treatment of dental anxiety and insomnia. It has an onset of 20–30 minutes with a duration of action of approximately 4 hours. In the usual therapeutic doses, chloral hydrate does not produce pronounced respiratory and cardiovascular depression. However, this condition may be observed in patients with renal or liver disease. The major adverse reaction associated with chloral hydrate is gastric irritation, which can be minimized by taking it with food or milk. The disagreeable odor and taste of the liquid preparation can be masked by mixing it with a flavored syrup, juice, or punch. Chloral hydrate is used in young children and the child's dose is 50 mg/kg of body weight up to a maximum of 1 gm.

Meprobamate was developed in order to reduce the tolerance and addiction problems that were occurring with the barbiturates. It was promoted as being different from the barbiturates, it produced anxiety relief, and it was less dangerous. However, it was just as addicting and dangerous as the barbiturates. Meprobamate is being reviewed in this chapter for the sake of completeness.

CNS depression, cardiovascular collapse, respiratory depression, and death can result from an acute overdose of meprobamate. Chronic use can lead to CNS tolerance, physical dependence, and abuse. The use of this medication with other CNS depressant drugs can lead to additive depressant effects.

Buspirone

Buspirone relieves the symptoms of anxiety without producing significant sedation, drowsiness, or amnesia. CNS depression is not observed even at doses higher than those necessary to treat anxiety.

Buspirone's mechanism of action is unknown but may be related to its ability to bind to serotonin and dopamine receptors. It has no additive CNS depressant effects and does not interact with alcohol or other CNS depressant medications. However, it takes about 2–4 weeks for buspirone to be effective which would not make it very practical for the person experiencing situational anxiety (dental).

INSOMNIA

Approximately 95% of the U.S. population has problems falling or staying asleep at one time or another. About 20–40% of adults experience *insomnia* each year and only 5–15% seek professional help. Insomnia can be caused by a medical illness, psychiatric disorders, alcohol or substance abuse, or psychosocial stressors (Gillin, 1992).

Insomnia is defined as insufficient or nonrestorative sleep and is further defined as transient it if lasts no longer than a few nights, short-term if it lasts less than 3 weeks, and chronic if it persists for longer than 3 weeks. Table 9-3 reviews the physiology of sleep, which can be altered by medication. Most adults require 8 hours of sleep; children and adolescents generally require more. Insomnia can disrupt daytime functioning and adversely affect a sense of well-being and quality of life. Chronic fatigue and drowsiness associated with insomnia can impair cognitive abilities and may play a role in many traffic and industrial accidents (Rakel, 1993).

Pharmacotherapy

The medications used to treat insomnia are similar to those used to treat anxiety disorders. In some instances, the medications are the same but the dose is different, and in other instances the medications are different but from the same class of drugs. Classes of medications used to treat insomnia include the benzodiazepines, barbiturates, and the nonbarbiturate sedative-hypnotics; they are reviewed in Table 9-4.

Benzodiazepines

Benzodiazepines are widely used because of their efficacy, wide margin of safety, low abuse potential, and low number of drug interactions. Short-acting benzodiazepines are ideal for people who have trouble falling asleep and they also cause less daytime sedation, fatigue, and psychomotor impairment than long-acting agents. Long-acting

Table 9-3 Physiology of Sleep

Sleep Stage	Description
Non-REM Sleep	
Stage 1	Transition between wakefulness and sleep
Stage 2	Light sleep
Stages 3 and 4	Deep, restful, restorative sleep (slow-wave or delta sleep)
REM Sleep	Characterized by rapid eye movement
	Patient dreams during this time period
	Increase in blood pressure, heart rate, respiratory rate, and oxygen consumption

Rall, TW, Hypnotics and sedatives: Ethanol. In Goodman Gilman A, Rall TW, Nies AS, Taylor P (eds.), *Goodman and Gilman's The Pharmacological Basis of Therapeutics,* 8th ed. Pergamon Press, New York, 1990.

Table 9-4   Medications Used to Treat Insomnia

Generic Name	Trade Name	Dose (mg/day) at bedtime
Benzodiazepines		
Long Acting		
Flurazepam	Dalmane	15–30
Quazepam	Doral	7.5–15
Intermediate Acting		
Estazolam	ProSom	1–2
Temazepam	Restoril	15–30
Short Acting		
Triazolam	Halcion	0.125–0.25
Barbiturates		
Amobarbital	Amytal	65–200
Pentobarbital	Nembutal	100–200
Secobarbital	Seconal	100–200
Others		
Choral hydrate	Noctec	500–100, 15–30 minutes before bedtime
Zolpidem	Ambian	10

Sources: Anon, Zolpidem for insomnia. *Med Let Drugs Ther* 35:35–36, 1993; Ashton H, Guidelines for the rational use of benzodiazepines: When and what to use. *Drugs* 48:25–40, 1994; Gillin JC, Relief from situational insomnia: Pharmacologic and other options. *Postgraduate Med* 92:157–170, 1992; McEvoy GK, ed., Barbiturates: General statement. *AHFS Drug Information 94*. American Society of Hospital Pharmacists, Bethesda, MD, 1994; Smith CM, Antianxiety drugs. In Smith CM, Reynard AM (eds.), *Textbook of Pharmacology*, 1st ed. W. B. Saunders Company, Philadelphia, 1992.

benzodiazepines are good for people who have problems staying asleep or who awaken in the early morning. Patients can experience daytime sedation, fatigue, and psychomotor impairment while taking these medications. Rebound insomnia has been noted after discontinuation of benzodiazepine therapy (Lader, 1992).

Barbiturates

Barbiturates suppress non-REM stages 3 and 4 and REM sleep. REM rebound, increased dreaming, insomnia, and nightmares can occur upon discontinuation of therapy. These medications can also cause daytime sedation, fatigue, and psychomotor impairment.

Chloral Hydrate

Chloral hydrate is thought to cause less paradoxical excitement than the barbiturates but it does cause GI irritation. Tolerance and physical and psychological dependence have been associated with chloral hydrate use. It is inexpensive and is often used in elderly patients.

Zolpidem

Zolpidem is a nonbenzodiazepine sedative-hypnotic that decreases sleep latency and the number of nocturnal awakenings, and increases sleep duration. Zolpidem appears to have a minimal effect on sleep stages and there is limited evidence of rebound insomnia after the discontinuation of the drug. Adverse reactions include dizziness and diarrhea. It is also associated with memory problems and patients should not perform any activities that require thought or concentration after taking this medication. They should also avoid alcohol or any other CNS depressant medication because of the potential for increased CNS depressant effects.

Nonpharmacological Therapy

Insomnia can also be treated with improved sleep hygiene. Different means of improving sleep hygiene include:

- Exercise moderately early in the evening
- Establish a regular sleep time and wake-up time regardless of the day of the week or holidays
- Avoid daytime napping
- Use the bedroom for sleep and sexual activity
- Use earplugs to reduce noise
- Use dark window treatments to block out sunlight
- Take a warm bath
- Listen to relaxing music
- Avoid cigarette smoking and reduce alcohol and caffeine consumption at least 6 hours before bedtime
- Avoid heavy meals just before bedtime

Patients with insomnia should practice these suggestions whether or not they are taking medication to treat their insomnia.

Summary

Anxiety disorders and insomnia are among the more common illnesses seen in clinical practice and the dental hygienist will treat patients receiving medication for anxiety or insomnia. Symptoms may be precipitated by a known event, such as a visit to a health professional's office, or unknown causes. Dental patients may require a sedative-hypnotic medication prior to their dental appointment in order to help minimize the symptoms of stress. Treat the patient so that the office visit is as stress-free as possible.

There are many medications available to treat anxiety or insomnia. The benzodiazepines appear to be well suited for stress associated with a dental appointment. Benzodiazepines range from very short acting to long acting, have a low potential for abuse, and have a good adverse reaction profile. Chloral hydrate is a short-acting non-barbiturate sedative-hypnotic that is good for the elderly and young children. The older nonbarbiturate sedative-hypnotics and the barbiturates are not used as much today. These medications have a high potential for abuse and can lead to successful suicide. The benzodiazepines are much safer to use. Buspirone is not indicated for short-term use associated with dental stress. This medication requires 2–4 weeks before the patient experiences a decrease in anxiety. Medications that are sedating can interact with the opioid analgesics and cause an increase in sedation and drowsiness. The dental hygienist should be aware of this and counsel the patient appropriately.

Case Study: Mario DePasquale

Mario DePasquale is 72 years old and has been coming to this practice for close to 20 years. He has a remarkable health history. His only medications include one baby aspirin each day, chloral hydrate for his insomnia, and an occasional acetaminophen for aches and pains. Mr. DePasquale has had problems sleeping since his wife passed away 6 months ago. He comes in today for his regular oral examination and cleaning.

1. What is chloral hydrate and what is its role in the treatment of insomnia?
2. Is chloral hydrate effective in treating anxiety or insomnia associated with dental therapy?
3. Would Mr. DePasquale's age and health status determine what dose of chloral hydrate he is given?
4. Compare chloral hydrate to zolpidem.
5. What are the dental concerns associated with chloral hydrate?
6. What should Mr. DePasquale be told about the dental concerns if a sedating drug is prescribed?

Case Study: Leslie Fitzsimmons

Leslie Fitzsimmons is 33 years old and has been coming to your practice for several years. She has always been somewhat anxious and her dental appointments seem to intensify her level of anxiety. Her medications include the occasional use of lorazepam when her anxiety "gets the best of her." She does not like taking benzodiazepines because they make her tired and she cannot drive. She comes in today and tells you that her doctor placed her on buspirone for her anxiety.

1. What is buspirone?
2. How does buspirone differ from benzodiazepines?
3. Is buspirone appropriate for the treatment of dental anxiety?
4. What are the adverse reactions associated with buspirone?
5. Would there be a problem if the dentist had to prescribe or use a sedating medication on Ms. Fitzsimmons while she was taking buspirone?

Review Questions

1. What is the physiology of sleep?
2. Are barbiturates appropriate for the treatment of insomnia? Why or why not?
3. Should barbiturates be given to a person with a history of suicide? Why or why not?
4. Which benzodiazepines are more appropriate for insomnia? Discuss your response in terms of having problems falling asleep and problems staying asleep.
5. Compare and contrast the benzodiazepines and barbiturates as sedative-hypnotics.
6. What is the role of meprobamate in the treatment of anxiety?
7. What are some of the drug interactions associated with benzodiazepines and barbiturates? What would you tell the patient about these interactions?

BIBLIOGRAPHY

Anon: Zolpidem for insomnia. *Med Let Drugs Ther* 35:35–36, 1993.

Ashton H: Guidelines for the rational use of benzodiazepines: When and what to use. *Drugs* 48:25–40, 1994.

Dommisse CS, Hayes PE: Current concepts in clinical therapeutics: Anxiety disorders, part 2. *Clin Pharm* 6:196–215, 1987.

Fontaine R, Chouinard G, Annable L: Rebound anxiety in anxious patients after abrupt withdrawal of benzodiazepine treatment. *Am J Psychiatry* 141:848–852, 1984.

Gary NE, Tresnewsky O: Clinical aspects of drug intoxication: Barbiturates and a potpourri of other sedatives, hypnotics, and tranquilizers. *Heart Lung* 12:122–127, 1983.

Gillin JC: Relief from situational insomnia: Pharmacologic and other options. *Postgraduate Med* 92:157–170, 1992.

Goa KL, Ward A. Buspirone. *Drugs* 32:114–129, 1986.

Goldberg HL: Benzodiazepines and nonbenzodiazepine anxiolytics. *Psychopathology* 17(Suppl): 45, 1984.

Lader M. Rebound insomnia and newer hypnotics. *Psychopharmacology* 108:248-255, 1992.

Mac DS, Kumar R, Goodwin DW: Anterograde amnesia with oral lorazepam. *J Clin Psychiatry* 46:137–138, 1985.

McEvoy GK, ed.: Analgesics and antipyretics: General statement. *AHFS Drug Information 94.* American Society of Hospital Pharmacists, Bethesda, MD, 1994.

McEvoy GK, ed.: Barbiturates: General statement. *AHFS Drug Information 94.* American Society of Hospital Pharmacists, Bethesda, MD,1994.

Rakel RE. Insomnia: Concerns of the family physician. *J Fam Pract* 36:551–558, 1993.

Rall TW: Hypnotics and sedatives: Ethanol. In Goodman Gilman A, Rall TW, Nies AS, Taylor P (eds.), *Goodman and Gilman's The Pharmacological Basis of Therapeutics,* 8th ed. Pergamon Press, New York, 1990.

Roehrs T, Zorick FJ, Sicklesteel JM, et al.: Effects of hypnotics on memory. *J Clin Psychopharmacol* 3:310–313, 1983.

Roth T, Hartse KM, Saab PG, et al.: The effects of flurazepam, lorazepam, and triazolam on sleep and memory. *Psychopharmacology* 70:231–237, 1980.

Scharf MB, Khosla N, Lysaght R, et al.: Anterograde amnesia with oral lorazepam. *J Clin Psychiatry* 44:362–364, 1983.

Scharf MB, Khosla N, Brocker N, et al.: Differential amnestic properties of short- and long-acting benzodiazepines. *J Clin Psychiatry* 45:51–53, 1984.

Shader RI, Greenblat DJ: Use of benzodiazepines in anxiety disorders. *New Engl J Med* 328:1398–1405, 1993.

Smith CM: Antianxiety drugs. In Smith CM, Reynard AM (eds.), *Textbook of Pharmacology*, 1st ed, W. B. Saunders Company, Philadelphia, 1992.

CHAPTER 10

Fluorides

Key Terms

Dental Caries
Dentrifice
Fluoridation
Fluorides

Fluorosis
Gels
Solutions

LEARNING OBJECTIVES

After completion of this chapter and its learning activities, the student should be able to:

1. Describe the relationship between fluoride and dental caries.
2. List the different sources of fluoride.
3. Describe the mechanism of action, pharmacokinetics, toxicity, and dental concerns of fluoride.
4. Describe the relationship between water fluoridation and dental caries.
5. List the professionally applied systemic fluoride preparations.
6. List the professionally applied topical fluorides including solutions and gels.
7. List some of the patient/home-applied fluoride products.
8. Describe the relationship between fluorides in dentifrices and dental caries.

INTRODUCTION

Fluorides are used both systemically and topically to help prevent *dental caries*. Their effectiveness has been long recognized and accepted by the dental profession.

Fluoride therapy begins at home. This therapy includes fluoridated water, oral home-care products, and/or systemic fluoride, which is a combination of low-concentration and high-frequency use of fluoride. Through patient education, effective oral hygiene techniques, and the use of fluoride, the dental hygienist can help the patient prevent or minimize dental caries.

The intent of this chapter is to review the mechanism of action, pharmacokinetics, toxicity, and dental concerns of fluoride. It also reviews those products that have received the American Dental Association (ADA) Seal of Acceptance. This approval is based on the safety and efficacy of the fluoride product in preventing dental caries.

SOURCES OF FLUORIDE

Fluoride (F) is found in most foods and water supplies and is the thirteenth most common element found in the earth's crust. Water levels of fluoride are dependent on the climate, which also regulates the amount ingested. The optimum fluoride level in moderate climates is 1 part per million (ppm) F, 1.2 ppm F in cold climates, and 0.6–0.8 ppm F in warm climates. Tea leaves, processed fish products with bones, and seafood are also rich in fluoride.

Fluoride is also found in green, leafy vegetables and fruit and its concentration is dependent on soil, watering conditions, and the fluoride content of the water that was used in preparing them. These foods are not a major source of fluoride but they do contribute to the total daily intake.

MECHANISM OF ACTION

Though the exact mechanism of action of fluoride is unknown, there are several different mechanisms of action that may be responsible for its anticariogenic effects. Systemic application of fluoride is known to exert its action upon hydroxyapatite crystals of enamel, which results in an improved crystalline structure and a decrease in the solubility of enamel in acid. Topical application promotes remineralization or hardening of the enamel surface of the teeth. Also, topical fluoride is taken up by dental plaque and inhibits vital microbial enzymes, thus altering the usual pattern of growth and acid production that leads to tooth decay. Topical fluoride is bactericidal and the correct application of fluoride-containing pastes has been shown to reduce *Streptococcus mutans,* which is responsible for dental caries.

PHARMACOKINETICS

As with any drug, fluoride must be absorbed and distributed before it can exert its pharmacologic effect. This section discusses the absorption, distribution, and excretion of fluoride.

Absorption

Ingested fluoride is absorbed from the gastrointestinal (GI) tract by simple diffusion, with more being absorbed in the upper small intestine. More than 80% of fluoride is absorbed within 90 minutes after oral administration. Absorption into the body is also dependent on the amount, type, and solubility of fluoride in the drinking water. In areas where there is less than 0.1 ppm fluoride in the drinking water, only 1 mg is absorbed. In areas where the concentration of fluoride is between 0.8 to 1.2 ppm, approximately 2.5 mg are absorbed. There is also a wide variation in the amount of fluoride absorbed between persons in any given community.

Distribution

Fluoride is absorbed into the circulating blood and body tissues and is distributed to bones and teeth. The amount of fluoride distributed to bones and teeth is dependent on the patient's age and prior ingestion of fluoride. More fluoride will deposit in growing bones and mineralizing teeth of children than in mature adults.

Excretion

Fluoride is excreted from the body by the kidneys, feces, and sweat, with the kidneys being the major route.

TOXICITY

As with any drug, fluoride has the ability to produce both therapeutic and toxic effects. Toxicity is related to the dose or concentration of the drug and produces a harmful response or death. Fluoride toxicity can be due to a large, single dose or long-term ingestion.

Acute Toxicity

Acute toxicity is due to the ingestion of a lethal dose of fluoride and the patient can die if not treated immediately. The lethal dose of fluoride is estimated to range between 50 and 225 mg/kg of body weight and the toxic dose has been reported to be as low as 4 mg/kg of body weight (Christensen, 1973). Signs of acute toxicity include nausea, salivation, abdominal pain, vomiting, and diarrhea. Other symptoms include muscle hyperirritability or convulsions, sweating, thirst, followed by cardio-vascular collapse, coma, and death. If acute toxicity is suspected, the patient must receive emergency care immediately. Death can occur within 1–4 hours after inges-tion of large toxic doses of fluoride. One should have the patient drink milk, which acts as a demulcent, and then perform gastric lavage repeatedly with a 0.15% calci-um chloride solution.

Chronic Toxicity

Chronic toxicity is the result of long-term exposure to fluoride preparations. A flu-oride ion concentration of more than 2 ppm in the drinking water can lead to *fluo-rosis* or mottled enamel during the time of crown formation of the permanent teeth. It is characterized by white opaque lines, brown discoloration of the tooth surface, or enamel hypoplasia as the water concentration of fluoride increases.

Mild fluorosis has been noted in children drinking water with 1 ppm fluoride and it has been estimated that at levels of 4–6 ppm fluoride in drinking water, 100% of children will develop mottled enamel (Haynes, 1990). Thus, it is important to deter-mine the usual daily ingestion of fluoride by the patient if a dental practitioner is thinking about prescribing fluoride.

DENTAL CONCERNS

The dental hygienist should review with patients the importance of home and office fluoride treatments. He should also question patients as to whether or not their water supply is fluoridated. This is of great importance and will help to determine if a systemic or topical fluoride preparation should be prescribed. If a fluoride preparation is prescribed, the dental hygienist should always ask patients if there has been any change in their drinking water supply. For example, some patients may move or public drinking water may become fluoridated. This will help to avoid fluoride toxicity.

Once a preparation is prescribed, the dental hygienist should review with the patient how to use the product. This will help to minimize both acute and chronic toxicity. Acute toxicity can be avoided by explaining to parents that fluoride is a drug and that it should be kept away from children. The oral preparations smell good, look like candy, and are well accepted by the pediatric population. Young children should be taught that this is medicine and can only be taken under the supervision of a parent or guardian.

The dental hygienist should review with the patient how to use dentrifices (toothpaste). Parents should be instructed to place a very small amount (size of a pea) on the child's toothbrush. Acute toxicity could occur if the child ingested a full tube of toothpaste or fluoride gel or a systemic preparation. Always instruct patients to have themselves or their children receive immediate medical attention if toxicity is suspected.

FLUORIDE PREPARATIONS

The addition of fluoride, at a concentration of 1 ppm, to community drinking water has helped to decrease the rate of dental caries. This addition is an economically feasible, reliable, and effective means of ensuring that patients from at least birth through 13 years of age will be exposed to the proper dietary level of fluoride. Lifelong exposure to water *fluoridation* reduces the number of dental caries in permanent teeth, which increases with age.

Though approximately 50% of the people in the United States drink fluoridated water, there still remains a segment of the population that does not. These people will benefit from the prescription and nonprescription fluoride preparations that are available. The next section reviews prescription systemic fluoride supplements, professionally applied topical fluoride supplements, and self-applied fluoride supplements.

Prescription Systemic Fluoride Supplements

Supplemental systemic or oral preparations should be considered for those people living in areas with less than 1 ppm of fluoride in the drinking water. Table 10-1 reviews the daily fluoride supplementation based on water fluoridation levels and the child's age. Supplemental fluoride preparations show a beneficial reduction in tooth decay (50–75%) when begun early. Only a trace amount of fluoride is found in breast milk, and infants who are solely breast-fed, or whose formulas are not prepared with fluoridated water, should probably receive supplementation based on the recommendations in Table 10-1.

Systemic or oral fluoride supplements are available as tablets, liquid drops, or in vitamin supplements (Table 10-2). The choice of preparations is based on the child's

Table 10-1   Recommended Daily Fluoride Supplementation Based on Water Fluoridation Levels and the Child's Age

| Child's Age | *Fluoride Ion Concentration of Drinking Water* | | |
	< 0.3 ppm	*0.3-0.6 ppm*	*> 0.6 ppm*
Newborn–6 months	0	0	0
6 months–3 years	0.25	0 (Drinks water)	0 (Drinks water)
3–6 years	0.5	0.25	0 (Drinks water)
6–16 years	1	0.5	0 (Drinks water)

Adapted from the American Academy of Pediatrics Committee on Nutrition, Fluoride supplementation for children: Interim policy recommendations. *Pediatrics* 95:777, 1995. Reproduced by permission.

Table 10-2   Selected Oral, Systemic Fluoride Preparations

Trade Name	*Dose Form*
Fluoritab	Liquid
	Tablets
Flura-Drops	Liquid
Flura-Loz	Lozenge
Flura-Tablets	Tablet
Luride Drops	Liquid
Luride Lozi-Tab	Tablets
Pediaflor	Liquid
Phos-Flur	Liquid

age and ability to chew and swallow an oral preparation. Fluoride supplements show best results when given just before bedtime after brushing and flossing. The patient should first swish liquid preparations and then swallow them. Tablets should be chewed and swallowed. The patient should not rinse after swallowing an oral preparation.

Professionally Applied Topical Fluoride Preparations

The fluoride compounds available for professional office use include neutral 2% sodium fluoride (NaF), 8% stannous fluoride (SnF_2), and 1.23% acidulated phosphate-fluoride (APF). Table 10-3 lists some of the different products available for use.

In areas that do not have the benefit of fluoridated water, the topical application of fluoride on erupted crowns can reduce dental decay. Even in those areas with fluoridated water, some adults may benefit from the scheduled topical application of fluoride to erupted crowns. Included are those with rampant tooth decay, xerostomia, orthodontic appliances, overdentures, and exposed root surfaces.

Neutral 2% Sodium Fluoride. Sodium fluoride *solutions* are relatively stable, have an agreeable taste, are nonirritating to soft tissue, and do not discolor the teeth or re-

Table 10-3 Selected, Professionally Applied Topical Acidulated Fluoride Preparations

Trade Name	Dose Form
Fluorident	Solution
Flura-Gel	Gel
Fluor-O-Kote	Gel
Karidium Phosphate Fluoride	Gel, solution
Luride Phosphate	Gel, solution

storative materials. Their disadvantage is that they must be used at 1-week intervals for 4 weeks. Sodium fluoride solutions are applied after an initial prophylaxis of the crowns. The teeth are isolated and air-dried and fluoride is applied for 3 minutes. The complete series is carried out at ages 3, 7, 11, and 13.

8% Stannous Fluoride. The aqueous solution of 8% stannous fluoride is not stable and must be made up immediately before application. The 8% solution has a disagreeable taste, is astringent, causes gingival blanching, and causes discoloration of the teeth. This discoloration is due to the tin and not the fluoride.

1.23% Acidulated Phosphate Fluoride (APF). APF solutions and *gels* are commonly preferred because of patient acceptability and greater uptake of the fluoride by the surface enamel of the tooth. They are not irritating to soft tissue, do not discolor teeth or restorative material, and are slightly astringent. They are stored in plastic containers because they become more acidic when stored in glass. The application procedure involves prophylaxis, isolation, and drying of teeth, and then application of the solution or gel for 4 minutes. The single application is repeated at either 6- or 12-month intervals. The choice of solution or gel is up to the individual practitioner and gels appear to be more popular at this time.

Prophylactic Pastes

Fluorides are also applied topically in fluoride-containing prophylactic pastes used by the dental hygienist or dentist during the routine cleaning of a patient's teeth. Fluoride-containing prophylactic paste should not be used in place of topical fluoride gels or solutions. Oral cleaning is usually followed by the application of topical fluoride gels or solutions to replace mineralized fluoride-containing enamel lost due to the abrasiveness of the cleaning agent.

SELF-APPLIED FLUORIDE PREPARATIONS

Self-applied fluoride preparations include dentifrices, rinses, and gels. Table 10-4 reviews several of those products approved by the ADA's Council on Dental Therapeutics.

Table 10-4   Selected Home Fluoride Preparations

Fluoride Preparations	Trade Name
Dentrifices	Aim
	Aqua-Fresh and Aqua-Fresh Tartar Control
	Colgate with MFP, Colgate Gel with MFP, and both with Tartar Control
	Crest, Crest Gel Formula and Crest Tartar Control
	Macleans Fluoride Toothpaste
Nonprescription Mouth Rinses	Act
	Fluorigard
	Reach Fluoride
	Listermint with Fluoride
Prescription Mouth Rinses	Fluorinse
	Phos-Flur
	Previ-dent
Gels	Activus
	Control
	Flo-Gel
	Gel-Kam
	Stan-Gard
	Stop

Source: Flynn AA, Oral health products. In *Handbook of Nonprescription Drugs,* 10th ed. American Pharmaceutical Association, Washington, DC, 1993.

Dentrifices

Only those *dentrifices* with the ADA's Council on Dental Therapeutics seal of acceptance have demonstrated clinically significant anticaries effects. This seal is displayed on the outside of the dentrifice package to make the consumer aware that the anticaries claim is valid. Several examples include Aim, Aqua-Fresh, Colgate with MFP Fluoride, Colgate Gel with MFP, Macleans Fluoride Toothpaste, Crest Toothpaste, and Gel Formula Crest.

Sodium monofluorophosphate (MFP) 0.4% is the most common fluoride compound and has been associated with caries reduction when compared to nonfluoride dentrifices. The other fluoride compound is NaF 0.22%. Studies have demonstrated that sodium fluoride dentrifices have a clinically significant anticaries effect when compared to sodium monofluorophosphate–containing dentrifices (Gerdin, 1972; Koch et al., 1982).

A home oral-care program is a must for all people whether or not they live in fluoridated water areas. A single, thin strip on the head of the toothbrush provides the adult patient with 1 mg of fluoride, which has been proven to reduce dental caries when used at least once a day. Young children should be supervised to carefully monitor the amount of dentrifice used. A mild mottling of tooth enamel may occur because of the chronic toxicity if the child swallows the toothpaste at each brushing over a long period of time.

Mouth Rinses

The most commonly used mouth rinses contain sodium fluoride in concentrations of either 0.05% over-the-counter products for daily use or 0.2% prescription products for weekly use and are of benefit for individuals who live in fluoridated as well as nonfluoridated communities. Those products approved by the ADA include ACT, Fluorigard, and Listermint with Fluoride, and they contain anywhere from 100 to 250 ppm of fluoride. Studies have shown a 16–49% reduction in dental caries when a 0.05% sodium fluoride preparation was used once a day, especially when used in children living in an area with nonfluoridated water supplies (Rugg-Gunn et al.,1973; Driscoll et al., 1982). Patient instructions for these mouth rinses should read as follows: After brushing, a 10-ml (2 teaspoonful) dose should be swished around and between teeth for 1 minute, then spit out. *Do not swallow.* Use once or twice daily (Listermint with Fluoride) and do not eat or drink for 30 minutes afterward. One should use caution with young children because they tend to swallow a significant amount of mouth rinse. Children older than 6 years of age should only use these rinses under direct adult supervision and they should not be used in children under 6 years of age.

Several fluoride mouth rinses are available by prescription only and contain concentrations of 1,000 ppm of fluoride. These mouth rinses are used daily or biweekly and are as effective as once or twice daily over-the-counter rinses.

Gels

Several fluoride gels are available for home use and contain either 0.5% acidulated phosphate-fluoride or 1.19% sodium fluoride. The Food and Drug Administration has recently approved the use of 0.4% stannous fluoride gel for over-the-counter use because it delivers the same amount of fluoride that is present in most fluoride dentifrices. Fluoride gels are available as both prescription and nonprescription preparations and are indicated in patients with xerostomia, radiation therapy, overdentures, rampant or recurrent tooth decay, exposed root surfaces, or orthodontic appliances. They should not be used in children under 6 years of age.

Summary

Fluoride supplementation is known to play an important role in preventing dental caries. Maximum anticaries effectiveness is carried out through frequent exposure of the teeth to low levels of fluoride both systemically and topically. Most Americans live in areas that have well-fluoridated water supplies and usually do not need systemic fluoride supplementation. Others require either systemic or topical applications based on the patient's age, caries history, caries susceptibility, and fluoride history.

The primary place for frequent exposure is the home and the dental hygienist plays an important role in helping the patient achieve the right balance of fluoride supplementation. A sound knowledge of the mechanism of action, pharmacokinetics, and toxicity of fluoride allows the dental hygienist to choose the appropriate home or professionally applied preparation.

There are many different products available that claim to reduce the incidence of dental caries. Only products that have received the ADA's Seal of Acceptance have been officially reviewed and evaluated as safe and effective in reducing dental caries. The dental hygienist should periodically check for the most current list of products accepted by the ADA in order to provide the patient with optimal oral health care.

Case Study: Destiny Savoy

Destiny Savoy is 2 years old and is new to your practice. This is her first visit to the dentist's office and she is very curious about you and the dentist. Through the medication/health history you learn that she and her mother were living in an area in which the water supply was fluoridated and Destiny drank plenty of water. They have recently moved to the country and rely on well water that is not fluoridated. Destiny does not take any medications except for a daily multivitamin that is not supplemented with fluoride. Her teeth appear to be in good condition and she has all but her last set of molars. Destiny informs you that she brushes her teeth every day.

1. What are your concerns regarding the new living arrangements?
2. Would Destiny benefit from a fluoride supplement? Which would you pick and why?
3. What are the acute and chronic toxicities associated with fluoride supplements? Review your concerns with Miss Savoy's mother.
4. What are your concerns regarding Destiny's eagerness for brushing her teeth every time that she has eaten? Counsel Destiny and her mother on the proper use of dentrifice in young children.
5. Should Destiny's mother receive fluoride supplements since she is drinking from the same water supply?
6. What would you choose and why?

Case Study: Sandra Smith

Sandra Smith is a 47-year-old woman who has been receiving successful cancer chemotherapy for close to 1 year. Her major complaint is the constant xerostomia that she experiences after each chemotherapy. She has tried many products, drinks plenty of water, and keeps tart, sugarless candy around. Mrs. Smith is also concerned that she may increase her risk for caries since her mouth is so dry. She is at the office today for a scheduled oral examination and would like to know what she can do about her dry mouth.

1. What can be done to reduce Mrs. Smith's chances of developing caries?
2. Compare and contrast the different fluoride gels.
3. Would Mrs. Smith be a candidate for home, self-applied fluoride treatments?
4. Compare and contrast the home, self-applied fluoride gels.
5. Would a fluoride mouth rinse be useful for Mrs Smith. Why or why not?

Review Questions

1. What is the relationship between fluoride and dental caries?
2. What are the different sources of fluoride and how are they related to daily intake?
3. What is the rationale for adding fluoride to community water supplies?
4. What is the mechanism of action of fluoride related to the prevention and control of dental caries?
5. Describe the pharmacokinetics of fluoride.
6. What is the active ingredient of dentrifices and which ones are approved by the ADA?

BIBLIOGRAPHY

American Academy of Pediatrics Committee on Nutrition: Fluoride supplementation for children: Interim policy recommendations. *Pediatrics* 95:777, 1995.

Brown WE, Konig KG (eds.): Cariostatic mechanisms of fluorides. *Caries Res* 11 (Suppl. 1), 1977.

Christensen HE (ed.): *The Toxic Substances List,* 1973 edition. U.S. Department of Health, Education, and Welfare, Rockville, MD.

Driscoll WS, Swango PH, Horowitz AM, Kingman A: *J Amer Dent Assoc* 105:1010, 1982.

Flynn AA: Oral health products. In *Handbook of Nonprescription Drugs,* 10th ed. American Pharmaceutical Association, Washington, D.C., 1993.

Gerdin PO: Studies in dentrifices on dental caries. *Swedish Dent J* 65:521, 1972.

Haynes RC Jr: Agents affecting calcification. In: Goodman Gilman A, Rall TW, Nies AS, Taylor P (eds.), *Goodman and Gilman's The Pharmacological Basis of Therapeutics,* 8th ed. Pergamon Press, New York, 1990.

Koch G, Peterson LG, Kling L: Effect of 250 and 1,000 ppm fluoride dentrifices on caries: A three-year clinical study. *Swedish Dent J* 6:233, 1982.

Picozzi A, Smudski J (eds.): *Pharmacology of Fluoride.* Symposium of the Pharmacology, Therapeutics, and Toxicology Group, International Association for Dental Research, Atlanta, GA, March 21, 1974.

Ripa LW (ed.): *A Guide to the Use of Fluorides for the Prevention of Dental Caries,* 2nd ed. American Dental Association, Chicago, 1986.

Rugg-Gunn AJ, Holloway PJ, Davies TGH: Caries prevention by daily fluoride mouth rinsing: Report of a three year clinical trial. *Br Dent J* 135:353, 1973.

Wei WH, Kanellis MJ: Fluoride retention after sodium fluoride mouth rinsing by preschool children. *J Amer Dent Assoc* 106:626, 1983.

Yamamoto J, Fannon ME, McKenzie M: Dental hygiene care: Caries, prevention, and control. In Darby ML, Walsh MM (eds.), *Dental Hygiene Theory and Practice,* 1st ed. W.B. Saunders Company, Philadelphia, 1995.

CHAPTER 11

Vitamins and Minerals

Key Terms

Beriberi
Fat Soluble
Pellagra
Pernicious Anemia
Recommended Dietary Allowances

Rickets
Scurvy
Vitamins
Water Soluble

LEARNING OBJECTIVES

After completion of this chapter and its learning activities, the student should be able to:

1. Review the requirements of recommended dietary allowances.
2. Describe the two classes of vitamins.
3. List the sources and recommended dietary allowances of both water-soluble and fat-soluble vitamins.
4. Describe the clinical use, deficiencies, toxicities, and dental considerations of water-soluble and fat-soluble vitamins. Also include the function of vitamin A.
5. List the sources and recommended dietary allowances of iron, zinc, and calcium.
6. Describe the clinical use, deficiencies, toxicities, and dental considerations of iron, zinc, and calcium.
7. List drugs that can cause vitamin deficiencies.
8. List selected drug-induced vitamin deficiencies.

INTRODUCTION

Vitamins are organic compounds that are necessary for the maintenance of normal metabolic functions but are not synthesized by the body. Thus, vitamins are supplied from exogenous sources. They are used to treat vitamin deficiencies and may be used to treat health problems not related to deficiencies. Many vitamin deficiencies have oral manifestations and the dental hygienist plays an important role in recognizing those signs and symptoms and ensuring that the patient receives proper treatment.

The intent of this chapter is to briefly review the sources, recommended dietary allowances, function, deficiencies, and dental concerns of fat-soluble vitamins, water-soluble vitamins, and selected minerals. This chapter also reviews vitamin deficiencies that are drug induced.

RECOMMENDED DIETARY ALLOWANCE

Humans have specific vitamin requirements that are influenced by age, sex, physical health, types of activities, dietary habits, pregnancy, and lactation. This is made evident by the wide range in present-day requirements. The *recommended dietary allowances* (RDAs) (Table 11-1) were developed to provide the vast majority of the population with the amounts required to meet certain criteria.

Healthy adults with well-balanced diets will usually get the necessary amount of vitamins necessary to maintain basic body requirements through food intake. Vitamin supplementation may be necessary for those with improperly balanced diets (fad dieters, teenagers, elderly, toddlers), those living in poverty, or those with decreased food consumption (alcohol-troubled persons, elderly, teenagers, toddlers, dieters). They may also be necessary for people with chronic diseases, malabsorption problems, or those taking medications that inhibit vitamin absorption. The RDAs are used to plan and obtain nutritionally adequate diets and food supplies for individuals or institutions (schools, hospitals, nursing homes).

CLASSIFICATION OF VITAMINS

Vitamins can be classified as *fat-soluble* or *water-soluble* vitamins. Fat-soluble vitamins are absorbed in the gastrointestinal tract (GI) and are distributed to the fat and liver where they are stored. Fat- soluble vitamins are excreted by biliary excretion. Extended administration of high doses of fat-soluble vitamins can lead to toxicity. On the other hand it may take a long time before signs of deficiency are noted because they are well-stored in the body. Water-soluble vitamins are well absorbed from the GI tract and are well distributed throughout the body. They are not readily stored in the body and are readily excreted through the kidneys. Lack of storage and rapid excretion make them less susceptible to toxicty, and signs of deficiency are seen almost immediately.

FAT-SOLUBLE VITAMINS

The fat-soluble vitamins include vitamins A, D, K, and E and they will be reviewed next.

Vitamin A (Retinoids and Carotenoids)

Vitamin A plays an important role in maintaining the integrity of epithelial cells, the formation of tooth enamel, and the function of the retina. The term *vitamin A* represents retinol (vitamin A_1), 3-dehydroretionol (vitamin A_2), retinoic acid, and β carotene.

Table 11-1   Recommended Dietary Allowances

	Fat-Soluble Vitamins			Water-Soluble Vitamins							Minerals			
	A	D	E	K	C	B_1	B_2	Niacin	B_6	Folate	B_{12}	Calcium	Iron	Zinc
	$(\mu g\,RE)^*$	$(\mu g)^{**}$	$(mg\,\alpha\text{-}TE)^\dagger$	(μg)	(mg)	(mg)	(mg)	$(mg\,NE)^\ddagger$	(mg)	(μg)	(μg)	(mg)	(mg)	(mg)
Infants (Age)														
Newborn to 5 months	375	7.5	3	5	30	0.3	0.4	5	0.3	25	0.3	400	6	5
5 months to 1 year	375	10	4	10	35	0.4	0.5	6	0.6	35	0.5	600	10	5
Children (Age)														
1–3 years	400	10	6	15	40	0.7	0.8	9	1.0	50	0.7	800	10	10
4–6 years	500	10	7	20	45	0.9	1.1	12	1.1	75	1.0	800	10	10
7–10 years	700	10	7	30	45	1.0	1.2	13	1.4	100	1.4	800	10	10
Males (Age)														
11–14 years	1000	10	10	45	50	1.3	1.5	17	1.7	150	2.0	1200	12	15
15–18 years	1000	10	10	65	60	1.5	1.8	20	2.0	200	2.0	1200	12	15
19–24 years	1000	10	10	70	60	1.5	1.7	19	2.0	200	2.0	1200	10	15
29–50 years	1000	5	10	80	60	1.5	1.7	19	2.0	200	2.0	800	10	15
> 50 years	1000	5	10	80	60	1.2	1.4	15	2.0	200	2.0	800	10	15
Females (Age)														
11–14 years	800	10	8	45	50	1.1	1.3	15	1.4	150	2.0	1200	15	12
15–18 years	800	10	8	55	60	1.1	1.3	15	1.5	180	2.0	1200	15	12
19–24 years	800	10	8	60	60	1.1	1.3	15	1.6	180	2.0	1200	15	12
29–50 years	800	5	8	65	60	1.1	1.3	15	1.6	180	2.0	800	10	12
> 50 years	800	5	8	65	60	1.0	1.2	13	1.6	180	2.0	800	10	12
Pregnancy	800	10	10	65	70	1.5	1.6	17	2.2	400	2.2	1200	30	15
Lactation														
Birth–6 months	65	10	10	65	95	1.6	1.8	20	2.1	280	2.6	1200	15	19
6 months–1 year	62	10	10	65	90	1.6	1.7	20	2.1	260	2.6	1200	15	16

Adaptation of RDA's foldout table from *Recommened Dietary Allowances,* 10th ed. National Academy of Sciences, National Academy Press, Washington, DC, 1989. Reprinted with permission.

*RE = retinol equivalents, 1 retinol equivalent = μg retinol or 6 μg β-carotene

**as cholecalciferol, 10 μg cholecalciferol = 400 IU vitamin D

†α-locopherol equivalents, 1 mg d-α tocopherol = 1α-TE

‡Niacin equivalent, 1 NE = 1 mg or niacin or 60 mg of dietary tryptophan

Sources. Vitamin A_1 occurs naturally in saltwater fish and animal tissue and vitamin A_2 is found in freshwater fish. Liver, milk, and some cheeses contain preformed vitamin A and some margerines are fortified with vitamin A. β carotene provides individuals with the greatest source of vitamin A. It is found in pigmented fruits such as apricots, peaches, watermelons, and tomatoes and in vegetables such as carrots, pumpkins, broccoli, spinach, and sweet potatoes.

Function. Vitamin A plays a key role in maintaining normal vision, the integrity of epithelial cells of the mucous membranes of the eye, and the mucosa of the respiratory, gastrointestinal (GI), and genitourinary (GU) tracts. Vitamin A is also important for bone and teeth foramtion.

Deficieny. Vitamin A deficiency can be caused by low intake or fat malabsorption due to cystic fibrosis, cholestasis, pancreatic insufficiency, chronic diarrhea, or severe disease. However, it may be a year or more before signs of deficiency are noted because of the ability of the human liver to store sufficient quantities of vitamin A. Signs and symptoms of vitamin A deficiency include night blindness (impaired vision in dim light), corneal and mucosal keratinization. Corneal keratinization can lead to xerophthalmia, which is an abnormal dryness and thickening of the conjunctiva and cornea. Kerotomalacia can also occur and it is characterized by irritation and inflammation on the cornea. Keratinization can also occur in gingival tissue and mucosa. Vitamin A deficiency can lead to a loss of taste and smell. Vitamin A deficiency during pregnancy and infancy can result in enamel hypoplasia and caries in primary teeth.

Toxicity. Vitamin A toxicity results in a toxic syndrome characterized by irritability, loss of appetite, headache, sloughing of the skin, fatigue, myalgia, gingivitis, fissures of the oral mucosa, increased intracraneal pressure, and neurologic symptoms. This condition is called hypervitaminosis A.

Vitamin D (Calciferol)

Vitamin D is formed from the irradiation of certain sterols and plays an important role in the regulation of calcium and phosphate metabolism. It increases the intestinal absorption of calcium and, in high doses, mobilizes calcium and phosphate from old bones to the formation of new bones.

Source. The two major vitamin D compounds are vitamin D_2 and vitamin D_3 (cholecalciferol). Vitamin D_3 is produced by sunlight exposure of mammal skin on its precursor 7-dehydrocholesterol, which is then converted to previtamin D_3 in the skin. Vitamin D_2 is produced by commercial irradiation and is added to vitamin supplements.

Clinical Use. Vitamin D is essential for the normal development of bones and teeth. It is also used to treat chronic hypocalcemia, hypophosphatemia, osteodystrophy, and osteomalacia.

Deficiency. Vitamin D deficiency in children results in a syndrome called *rickets,* which is a result of inadequate absorption of calcium and phosphate with decreased calcium in plasma. It is characterized by bones that are unusually soft, easily bent, compressed, or fractured, resulting in gross abnormalities in the formation of the skeleton. In adults, vitamin D deficiency produces osteomalacia, which is characterized by deformities of weight-bearing bones. It occurs most often during times of increased calcium needs, malabsorption syndromes, in low-fat dieters, strict vegetarians, and those taking anticonvulsants or sedative-hypnotics.

Toxicity. Chronic administration of excessive doses of vitamin D can result in a toxic condition known as hypervitaminosis D. It is characterized by weakness, fatigue, GI disturbances, headache, and impaired renal, cardiovascular, and respiratory function.

Vitamin E (Tocopherols)

Vitamin E is an antioxidant and is known chemically as tocopherol. It prevents the formation of toxic oxidation materials and the oxidation of essential cellular constituents. Its exact metabolic function as a vitamin is not known though it increases the absorption and use of vitamin A.

Source. Vitamin E is found in such vegetable oils as corn, cottonseed, and soybean. It is also found in fresh greens and other vegetables.

Clinical Use. Vitamin E has been recommended for and is used to treat or prevent a wide variety of human diseases. It is thought to help prevent cancer and has been used to treat Parkinson's disease, β thalassemia, and sickle-cell anemia. It has been used as an antioxidant in premature infants exposed to high concentrations of oxygen to reduce the severity of retinopathy and bronchopulmonary dysplasia.

Deficiency. Vitamin E deficiency can occur in humans with malabsorption syndromes and premature infants are at risk of vitamin E deficiency because of low placental transfer, low body fat, poor fat absorption, and rapid growth.

Toxicity. Vitamin E has no significant toxic effects though nausea, diarrhea, fatigue, weakness, and rash have occurred.

Vitamin K (Phylloquinone or Phytonadione)

Vitamin K is essential for the normal biosynthesis of prothrombin and of blood-clotting factors VII, IX, and X. It is synthesized by intestinal bacteria.

Source. Green leafy vegetables such as spinach, cabbage, and alfalfa are good sources of vitamin K. Other sources include egg yolk, soybean oil, and liver.

Clinical Use. Vitamin K injections are given to newborns whose intestinal organisms have not yet been established to produce vitamin K. Vitamin K_1 is also used to treat excessive hypoprothrombinemia due to warfarin toxicity.

Deficiency. Vitamin K deficiency can cause severe bleeding. Even the smallest trauma can cause hemorrhaging. The most common sites of hemorrhage include wounds, skin, mucous membranes in the intestinal tract, and serosal surfaces. Vitamin K deficiency is usually due to malabsorption syndromes, inadequate intake, or decreased normal bacterial flora due to prolonged antibiotic use.

Toxicity. The naturally occurring vitamins K_1 and K_2 are essentially nontoxic. Vitamin K_3, which is synthetic, can cause hemolytic anemia in newborns and hemolysis in persons with glucose-6-phosphate dehydrogenase when given in large doses.

Dental Concerns

The dental hygienist can help to evaluate patients for vitamin deficiencies. Fat-soluble vitamin deficiencies, except for vitamin E, have oral manifestations. Delayed tooth development may be a result of a vitamin deficiency. The dental hygienist should ask patients about their dietary intake or any health problems. Patients should be referred to their health-care provider for appropriate therapy.

WATER-SOLUBLE VITAMINS

The water-soluble vitamins include vitamin C and the B-complex vitamins.

Vitamin C (Ascorbic Acid)

Vitamin C is thought to play a major role in oxidation-reduction reactions and is essential for the normal synthesis and maintenance of collagen, which is necessary for wound healing.

Source. Vitamin C is found in citrus fruits, green peppers, tomatoes, strawberries, broccoli, raw cabbage, potatoes, and papaya. Many other foods are fortified with vitamin C. However, as much as 59% of vitamin C content in foods can be destroyed during cooking.

Clinical Uses. Vitamin C has no significant pharmacologic actions though it has been used to prevent and treat the common cold. It has also been used to manage some types of cancer but well-controlled clinical trials are needed to truly determine its use in treating both conditions.

Deficiency. Signs and symptoms of vitamin C deficiency *(scurvy)* include gingival swelling, capillary fragility and bleeding, resorption of dentin, decrease in odontoblastic activity, degeneration of alveolar bone, and loss of teeth. Other signs of vitamin C deficiency include poor wound healing, lack of collagen, and an inadequate response to infections. It is usually a result of a lack of fresh fruits and vegetables and tends to occur more frequently in the winter months when these foods are not as available.

Toxicity. Megadoses (greater than 1 gm/day) of vitamin C can precipitate oxalate stones in the urinary tract. Megadoses can also destroy vitamin B_{12}, reduce copper absorption, and increase plasma cholesterol.

Vitamin B_1 (Thiamine)

Thiamine acts as a coenzyme in carbohydrate metabolism and is converted in the liver to its active coenzyme form, thiamine pyrophosphate (TPP).

Source. Thiamine is found in pork, whole-grain and enriched breads, cereals and pastas, peas, dried brewer's yeast, wheat germs, and other legumes.

Clinical Use. Thiamine is used to treat beriberi, Wernicke's encephalopathy, and peripheral neuropathies.

Deficiency. Thiamine deficiency is characterized by neurological and circulatory disorders and is called *beriberi*. Neurological symptoms include peripheral neuritis, muscle weakness, and limb paralysis. Circulatory symptoms include heart enlargement, edema, and tachycardia. GI effects include loss of appetite, intestinal atony, and constipation. Possible oral symptoms include burning tongue, loss of taste, and hyperesthesia of the oral mucosa. Thiamine deficiency tends to occur most often in persons with alcoholism in the United States.

Toxicity. Thiamine has no significant toxic effects.

Vitamin B$_2$ (Riboflavin)

Riboflavin acts as an essential part of the coenzymes flavin mononucleotide and flavin adenine dinucleotide, which are involved in many oxidation-reduction reactions.

Source. Riboflavin is found in dairy products and meat and is heat stable. It is also found in many plants and animals.

Clinical Use. Riboflavin is used in combination with other B vitamins to treat vitamin B deficiency. Those with vitamin B deficiencies include alcoholics, economically deprived persons, fad dieters, and those with severe GI disease.

Deficiency. Riboflavin deficiency results in a syndrome that includes glossitis, lesions at the corners of the mouth (cheilosis), and sore throat.

Toxicity. Riboflavin has no significant toxicities.

Niacin (Nicotinic Acid)

Niacin plays a key role in many metabolic reactions and is a component of nicotinamide adenine dinucleotide (NAD) and nicotinamide adenine dinucleotide phosphate (NADP), which participate in oxidation-reduction reactions.

Source. Niacin is found in lean meats, liver, poultry, and legumes.

Deficiency. Niacin deficiency results in a characteristic clinical syndrome called *pellagra*. Signs and symptoms include stomatitis with a red, swollen tongue, excessive salivation, enlarged salivary glands, gingivitis, papillary loss, dementia, diarrhea, and dermatitis. Niacin deficiency occurs most often in alcoholics, people living in poverty-stricken areas, those with GI problems, hyperthyroidism, pregnancy, fad dieters, and those with infections.

Toxicity. Niacin toxicity is characterized by cutaneous flushing, pruritus, and GI distress. Chronic use can lead to dry skin, xerostomia, hyperuricemia, peptic ulcer disease, blurred vision, nervousness, panic, and hyperglycemia.

Vitamin B$_6$ (Pyridoxine)

Vitamin B$_6$ also acts as a coenzyme in a number of metabolic reactions involving amino acid transformation.

Source. Vitamin B$_6$ is found in most foods including whole-grain cereals, meats, legumes, eggs, and some vegetables.

Clinical Use. Vitamin B$_6$ is used in conjunction with **isoniazid** for the treatment of tuberculosis. It can cancel the therapeutic and side-effects of **levodopa** when levodopa is used to treat Parkinson's disease. This is not the case when levodopa is combined with decarboxylase inhibitor. It is usually used in combination with other B vitamins to treat vitamin B deficiencies.

Deficiency. Vitamin B$_6$ deficiency is rare but it is characterized by oral lesions, glossitis, and stomatitis.

Toxicity. Vitamin B$_6$ has no significant toxicities.

Folic Acid

Folic acid acts physiologically as tetrahydrofolic acid, an acceptor for single carbon groups in many metabolic reactions including those involving DNA (deoxyribonucleic acid) and RNA (ribonucleic acid) synthesis.

Source. Sources of folic acid include liver, some fruits and vegetables, wheat germ, and yeasts.

Clinical Use. Folic acid is used to treat the hematologic effects of *pernicious anemia.* It is added to prenatal vitamins in an attempt to reduce neural tube defects in unborn children. It is also given in combination with other B vitamins to those who are deficient in them.

Deficiency. Folic acid deficiency is characterized by megaloblastic anemia and microcytic anemia. Other symptoms include weakness, weight loss, loss of skin pigmentation, and irritability. Oral symptoms include glossitis, angular cheilosis, and gingivitis. Folic acid deficiency is a result of inadequate diet, pregnancy, malabsorption syndromes, and chronic alcoholism.

Toxicity. Folic acid has no significant toxicities.

Vitamin B$_{12}$ (Cyanocobalamin)

Vitamin B$_{12}$ acts physiologically as a coenzyme in the metabolism of fats, carbohydrates, and protein.

Source. Sources of vitamin B$_{12}$ include liver, milk, cheeses, and eggs.

Clinical Use. Vitamin B$_{12}$ supplementation is used in people who are strict vegetarians. It has been used to treat trigeminal neuralgia, depression, and tiredness.

Deficiency. Inadequate absorption of vitamin B_{12} can result in pernicious anemia, which is caused by a lack of intrinsic factor in the GI tract that helps in the absorption of vitamin B_{12}. Signs and symptoms include weakness, numbness, and difficulty walking. The patient's skin may have a lemon-yellow hue. Oral manifestations include soreness and burning of the tongue, glossitis, and painful bright red lesions in the buccal and pharyngeal mucosa.

Toxicity. Vitamin B_{12} has no significant toxicities.

Pantothenic Acid

Pantothenic acid acts physiologically as part of coenzyme A, which is involved in various metabolic reactions including gluconeogenesis and the synthesis of fatty acids and sterols and steroid hormones.

Source. Sources include egg yolk, bran, yeast, and beef liver.

Clinical Use. Pantothenic acid has no significant pharmacodynamic effects.

Deficiency. Experimentally produced deficiency in humans is characterized by fatigue, headache, malaise, nausea, abdominal pain, and neuromuscular disorders.

Toxicity. Pantothenic acid has no significant toxic reactions.

Biotin

Biotin is a coenzyme that is required in several carboxylation reactions.

Source. Sources include liver, cow's milk, egg yolk, and yeast. It is also thought to be synthesized by intestinal bacteria.

Clinical Use. Biotin has no significant pharmacodynamic effects.

Deficiency. Biotin deficiency is extremely rare in humans and is characterized by dermatitis, loss of appetite, loss of hair, mental depression, nausea, and malaise.

Toxicity. Biotin has no significant toxicities.

Choline and Inositol

Choline and inositol are two B vitamins that have not been demonstrated to be necessary in the human diet. Choline serves as a precursor to acetylcholine and is involved in fat metabolism. There have been no demonstrated deficiencies or toxicities of either B vitamin in humans.

Dental Concerns

The dental hygienist can help to evaluate patients for vitamin deficiencies. Water-soluble vitamin deficiencies have many oral manifestations. The dental hygienist should ask the patient about his dietary intake or any health problems. The patient should be referred to his health-care provider for appropriate therapy.

SELECTED MINERALS

Though there are many different minerals available for daily vitamin supplementation, only calcium, iron, and zinc are discussed here.

Calcium

Calcium is essential for bone and teeth development and growth and is also necessary for the function of the nervous and muscular systems and cell membrane and capillary permeability. It is also needed for blood coagulation, cardiac function, membrane integritiy, renal function, and skeletal muscle contraction.

Source. Calcium is found in milk, cheese, yogurt, and cottage cheese. It is also found in sardines with bones, tofu, and shrimp. Orange juice can also be fortified with calcium.

Clinical Use. It is used to treat calcium deficiencies and osteoporosis. Calcium is used during cardiopulmonary resuscitation, and for the treatment of hyperkalemia and hypermagnesemia.

Deficiency. Deficiencies are noted in strict vegetarians and those with poor dietary intake of calcium. Signs and symptoms include tetany, paresthesia, muscle cramps, and convulsions if calcium blood levels fall.

Toxicity. Adverse reactions include GI upset, constipation, and hypercalcemia if large doses are given to patients with chronic renal failure.

Iron

The basic role of iron is the transport and uptake of oxygen and carbon dioxide from one tissue to another and is essential for protein metabolism. It accomplishes this task in the form of hemoglobin.

Source. Sources of iron include beef liver and heart, egg yolk, wheat germ, brewer's yeast, red meats, and dried beans. Breads, flours, and cereals are fortified with iron.

Clinical Use. Iron is used as a supplement in patients with anemia or during pregnancy and lactation.

Deficiency. Iron deficiency occurs during growth, menstruation, pregnancy and lactation, and during periods of inadequate dietary intake (preschool children, adolescents, the elderly). Symptoms include pallor, irritability, fatigue, decreased resistance to infection, and a sore mouth.

Toxicity. Acute toxicity (overdose) is characterized by intestinal bleeding, which can result in shock or death. Treatment includes gastric lavage, phosphate, or chelating agents if warranted. Common complaints of usual doses include GI symptoms (nausea and constipation).

Zinc

Zinc is a component of insulin. It is also required to transport carbon dioxide in the blood and eliminate it from the lungs, and it rids the body of lactic acid during exercise.

Source. Zinc is found in high quantities in seafood and meat. Cereals and legumes contain zinc but it is poorly absorbed from these foods.

Clinical Use. Zinc is used to treat zinc deficiencies.

Deficiency. Zinc deficiency can cause delayed wound healing, slowed growth, and sexual immaturity.

Toxicity. Acute ingestion of zinc can lead to nausea, vomiting, fever, and diarrhea. Excessive doses can cause lymphocytic and polymorphonuclear leukocytic function impairment in healthy adults.

Dental Concerns

The dental hygienist can help to evaluate patients for mineral deficiencies. The dental hygienist should ask the patient about dietary intake or any health problems. The patient should be referred to her health-care provider for appropriate therapy.

DRUG-INDUCED VITAMIN DEFICIENCIES

Certain drugs cause vitamin deficiencies and Table 11-2 reviews some of those deficiencies. The exact mechanism of action of these interactions is unknown, though they may be the result of an interference of intestinal absorption of the vitamin.

Table 11-2   Drug-Induced Vitamin Deficiencies

Vitamin	*Drug(s)*
Vitamin A	Cholestyramine
	Neomycin
Vitamin D	Anticonvulsants
	Cholestyramine
	Irritant cathartics
	Mineral oil
Vitamin K	Antibiotics
	Anticonvulsants
	Cholestyramine
	Coumarin/warfarin
	Mineral oil
	Salicylates

Table 11-2 (*cont.*)

Vitamin	Drug(s)
Vitamin C	Estrogen-containing OCs*
	Salicylates
	Tetracyclines
Folic acid	Anticonvulsants
	Cholestyramine
	Estrogen-containing OCs
	Pyrimethamine
	Salicylates
	Sulfasalazine
	Triamterene
	Trimethoprim
Folate	Methotrexate
Thiamine	Estrogen-containing OCs
Riboflavin	Estrogen-containing OCs
Niacin	Isoniazid
	Tetracycline
Pyridoxine	Levodopa
Vitamin B_6	Estrogen-containing OCs
	Hydralazine
	Isoniazid
Vitamin B_{12}	Cholestyramine
	Colchicine
	Estrogen-containing OCs
	Neomycin
	Chronic nitrous oxide
	Potassium chloride

*OCs = oral contraceptives.

Source: Cunningham RK, Smith CM, Interactions: Drug-allergy; drug-drug; drug-food. In Smith CM, Reynard AM (eds.), *Textbook of Pharmacology*, 1st ed. W. B. Saunders Company, Philadelphia, 1992.

Summary

Vitamins are categorized as either fat soluble or water soluble and are found in most food sources. Minerals are also present in food sources. Vitamins and minerals are essential for growth and development. Vitamin and mineral deficiencies are usually a result of inadequate dietary intake, medical illness, or medicines. Some medications and medical illnesses may prevent the absorption of either fat- or water-soluble vitamins. Vitamin toxicity may be due to medical illness, medications that increase vitamin absorption, or ingestion above and beyond recommended dietary intakes.

Many vitamin deficiencies and toxicities have oral manifestations with which the dental hygienist should become familiar. Dental hygienists can help patients by identifying these signs and symptoms and asking about dietary habits. Medication/health histories can help to identify patients at risk for drug-induced vitamin deficiencies and those with chronic illnesses that may predispose them to a vitamin deficiency.

Case Study: Paula Juaneza

Paula Juaneza is 32 years old and is new to your practice. She is a native of the Phillipine Islands, has been in the United States about 8 months, and speaks very little English. Her cousin, a naturalized citizen, brought her to the practice today for her first oral examination in about 2 years and is acting as her translator. During the medication/health history, you learn that Paula is quite concerned about some oral changes. Ms. Juaneza tells you that her gums have been swollen and bleeding and she is particularly concerned with the fact that her teeth are loose. Ms. Juaneza prides herself on her good oral self-care. During the oral examination, you and the dentist both observe swollen and bleeding gums as well as loose teeth. Upon further questioning, Ms. Juaneza tells you that she has not had any fresh fruit or vegetables since coming to the United States. Her ability to speak and understand English is minimal and she feels very uncomfortable shopping on her own. The rest of the family eats on the go and is not concerned with the fruit and vegetable supply at home.

1. What condition does Ms. Juaneza have?
2. What are some sources of vitamin C?
3. Are there any toxicities to vitamin C, and if so, what are they?
4. What are the clinical uses of vitamin C?
5. How does vitamin C work?
6. What could you recommend for this patient and why?
7. What should Ms. Juaneza be told about your recommendations?
8. Can any drugs cause a vitamin C deficiency? If so, what are they?

Case Study: Joan Henderson

Joan Henderson is a 66-year-old who was diagnosed with Parkinson's disease about 10 years ago. Her disease has progressed despite treatment with anticholinergic drugs and levodopa. Her physician was reading about some of the successes with vitamin E in people with Parkinson's disease. Mrs. Henderson tells you this during your routine medication/health history. Mrs. Henderson's medications now include vitamin E supplements and levodopa.

1. What is vitamin E and what is its mechanism of action?
2. What are some sources of vitamin E? Would it help Mrs. Henderson to increase her dietary intake of foods rich in vitamin E?
3. What are some causes of vitamin E deficiency?
4. Are there any toxicities of which Mrs. Henderson needs to be aware?
5. What vitamin supplement is usually necessary for patients taking levodopa?

Review Questions

1. What is the recommended dietary allowance and how is it determined?
2. Compare and contrast fat-soluble and water-soluble vitamins.
3. What are the toxicities and deficiencies of vitamin A?
4. Who is at risk for vitamin D deficiency and what are its signs and symptoms?
5. What are the sources of vitamin K and what are its signs and symptoms of deficiency?
6. What are the B vitamins and who is at risk for vitamin B deficiency?
7. What are the oral manifestations of vitamin B deficiency?
8. What are choline and inositol and what is their function?
9. What are sources of calcium and who is at risk for deficiency? Include signs and symptoms of deficiency.
10. What is zinc and what is its relevance to maintaining a healthy diet and body?

BIBLIOGRAPHY

Alhadeff LC, Gualtieri T, Lipton M: Toxic effects of water-soluble vitamins. *Nutr Rev* 42:33–40, 1984.

Allen LV Jr: Nutritional products. In *Handbook of Nonprescription Drugs,* 10th ed. American Pharmaceutical Association, Washington, DC, 1993.

Cunningham RK, Smith CM: Interactions: Drug-allergy; drug-drug; drug-food. In Smith CM, Reynard AM (eds.), *Textbook of Pharmacology,* 1st ed. W. B. Saunders Company, Philadelphia, 1992.

Food and Nutrition Board: *Recommended Dietary Allowances,* 10th ed. National Academy of Sciences, National Research Council, Washington, DC,1989.

Horvath PJ: Vitamins as therapeutic agents. In Smith CM, Reynard AM (eds.), *Textbook of Pharmacology,* 1st ed. W. B. Saunders Company, Philadelphia, 1992.

Marcus R, Coulston AM: Water-soluble vitamins. In Goodman Gilman A, Rall TW, Nies AS, Taylor P (eds.), *Goodman and Gilman's The Pharmacological Basis of Therapeutics,* 8th ed. Pergamon Press, New York, 1990.

Marcus R, Coulston AM: Fat-soluble vitamins. In Goodman Gilman A, Rall TW, Nies AS, Taylor P (eds.), *Goodman and Gilman's The Pharmacological Basis of Therapeutics,* 8th ed. Pergamon Press, New York, 1990.

Roe DA: Nutrient and drug interactions. *Nutr Rev* 42:141–154, 1984.

Roe DA: *Drug-Induced Nutritional Deficiencies,* 2nd ed. AVI, New York, 1985.

Smith C, Bidlack W: Dietary concerns associated with the use of medications. *J Am Diet Assoc* 84:901–914, 1984.

CHAPTER 12

Oral Conditions and Their Therapies

Key Words

Alveolar Osteitis
Candidiasis
Cheilosis
Gingivitis

Oral Lesions
Periodontitis
Xerostomia

LEARNING OBJECTIVES

After completion of this chapter and its learning activities, the student should be able to:

1. Describe actinic lip changes and angular cheilosis and their causes.
2. Describe acute necrotizing ulcerative gingivitis and its therapies.
3. List the different types of periodontitis including causes, signs and symptoms, and therapies.
4. Review the common oral lesions (recurrent aphthous stomatitis and herpes infection) including causes, signs and symptoms, and therapies.
5. Describe the causes and therapies of oral candidiasis.
6. Describe alveolar osteitis and its causes.
7. Describe root sensitivity and its therapies.
8. List the drugs that can cause xerostomia.
9. Discuss the treatments of xerostomia.

INTRODUCTION

Though dental hygienists do not directly treat oral conditions, they are among the first to note changes in a person's oral cavity. They may also be called upon to review therapies with patients and patients may ask them questions about their therapy. This chapter briefly reviews several different oral conditions and their therapies.

ACTINIC LIP CHANGES

Actinic lip changes are the result of long-term exposure to the sun's ultraviolet rays and can become irreversible. Application of a sunscreen/sunblock with a sun protective factor (SPF) of 15 prior to sun exposure and use repeatedly thereafter will help to minimize further changes. **5-fluorouracil** (5-FU) is indicated if keratotic changes have occurred and a topical steroid may be used to treat any possible skin irritations of 5-FU.

ANGULAR CHEILOSIS

Angular *cheilosis* may be a simple redness at the angles of the mouth or it can progress to fissures, erosions, ulcers, or crusting and may or may not be painful. Causes include *Candida albicans* (fungal infection), streptococci and staphylococci (bacterial infections), drugs (immunosuppressives, steroids, radiation therapy), or vitamin B deficiency. Treatment is based on the cause and includes antifungal treatment (Chapter 6) if it is *Candida albicans*, antibiotics if it is bacterial (Chapter 6), or supplementation with B-complex vitamins if the cause is vitamin B deficiency (Chapter 11).

ACUTE NECROTIZING ULCERATIVE GINGIVITIS

Acute necrotizing ulcerative *gingivitis* (ANUG) is also referred to as Vincent's stomatitis and trench mouth and is characterized by necrosis and ulceration of the gingiva with underlying inflammation and a distinctive odor. Patients present with sudden burning of their mouth and an inability to eat. The disease most commonly starts in the interdental papillae and can be localized or generalized. The lesions appear after a few days, at which time the papillae appear punched out and are covered by a white necrotic pseudomembrane.

Causes include bacterial (spirochetes) and environmental factors. It is seen most frequently in the United States in teenagers and young adults. Predisposing factors include anxiety, emotional stress, smoking, malnutrition, and poor oral hygiene. Good oral hygiene is the mainstay of therapy and hydrogen peroxide and saline mouth rinses are also useful.

Treatment begins with a complete debridement of plaque with careful scaling over one to two visits. The patient should begin a home treatment program consisting of meticulous plaque control. The patient can also rinse with a dilution of hydrogen peroxide and warm water for further relief after scaling at home. Other therapies should be symptomatic and include **aspirin** or **acetaminophen** for fever, or vitamin supplements if malnourished, or food supplements (which include vitamins) if unable to eat due to oral pain. Antibiotics, such as **penicillin** and **metronidazole,** are useful but are only recommended for those with signs of systemic infection (fever and severe malaise) or for those who have immunosuppressive illnesses.

PERIODONTITIS

Periodontitis is the most common type of periodontal disease which is characterized by tissue inflammation, loss of connective tissue, and a destruction of collagen fiber.

Most forms of this disease are related to plaque accumulation and retention. Successful treatment consists of complete plaque removal, including products of plaque, calculi, and plaque retention factors at appropriate intervals. The patient should continue treatment at home by maintaining personal plaque control.

The American Academy of Periodontology has recommended that periodontitis be categorized based on its etiology, clinical presentation, pathogenesis, progression, and response to therapy. These categories are as follows: adult periodontitis, early-onset periodontitis, periodontitis associated with systemic disease, acute necrotizing ulcerative periodontitis, and refractory periodontitis.

ADULT PERIODONTITIS

Adult periodontitis is a multibacterial disease of which the primary pathogen is *Porphyromonas gingivalis*. The disease is characterized by a slow progression of bone resorption. Disease severity is related to the amount of plaque and calculus present on the surfaces of the teeth. Its rate of progression is dependent on disease activity and the patient's level of resistance.

Adult periodontitis usually appears after age 30 and progresses slowly until teeth are lost as a result of extraction or exfoliation. The disease is further classified as slight, moderate, or advanced.

Treatment of adult periodontitis begins with the plaque and calculus removal from the root surfaces and educating the patient about the importance of personal plaque control. Though the disease is multibacterial, antibiotics are not usually indicated for treatment. The intent of treatment is to replace the infection with younger, less established plaque that is associated with health.

EARLY-ONSET PERIODONTITIS

Early-onset periodontitis can be further categorized: prepubertal, juvenile, and rapidly progressive. These diseases occur in patients younger than 30 years of age.

Prepubertal Periodontitis

This disease can be localized or generalized, can affect both primary and secondary teeth, and is rare. The disease is characterized by severe gingival inflammation, rapid bone loss, and early tooth loss. Patients loose deciduous teeth because of periodontal infection and permanent teeth become infected as they erupt. Antibioitic therapy slows down the progression of prepubertal periodontitis. Prepubertal periodontitis does not respond well to scaling and rooting.

Juvenile Periodontitis

This category of periodontitis is further classified as localized and generalized.

Localized Juvenile Periodontitis. Localized juvenile periodontitis is characterized by minimal gingival inflammation with rapid and severe vertical bone loss, deep pocket formation, and mobility and migration of incisors and first molars in patients under 20 years of age. *Actinobacillus actinomycetemcomitans* is the bacteria most often reported in the plaque associated with this disease. Treatment consists of mechanical debridement with scaling and root planing in conjunction with antibiotic therapy (usually tetracycline; Chapter 6).

Generalized Juvenile Periodontitis. Generalized juvenile periodontitis differs from the localized form in that there is a significant amount of clinical inflammation with heavy plaque and calculus buildup. Bacterial flora include *P. gingivalis, Eikenella corrodens,* and *A. actinomycetemcomitans.* Treatment consists of home plaque control, scaling and root planing, and antibiotic therapy.

Rapidly Progressive Periodontitis

This disease occurs in people between the ages of 20 and 30 and is characterized by severe gingival inflammation with varying degrees of plaque and calculus buildup. Bone and connective tissue loss occurs over a period of weeks or months. Treatment consists of eliminating local factors through good plaque control, scaling and root planing, possible periodontal surgery, and antibiotics. Antibiotics include **tetracycline,** metronidazole, **amoxicillin/clavulanic acid, ciprofloxacin,** and several antibiotic combinations (Chapter 6).

PERIODONTITIS ASSOCIATED WITH SYSTEMIC DISEASE

This classification is useful for the dental practitioner because it helps to emphasize underlying disease processes. Systemic illnesses such as diabetes increase the severity and rate of periodontal disease. Systemic illnesses can worsen periodontitis because they weaken the patient's resistance and ability to fight off infection. Increased personal, home plaque care, and frequent dental visits are required.

ACUTE NECROTIZING ULCERATIVE PERIODONTITIS

This disease is an extension of ANUG. The disease causes a severe progressive destruction of the gingiva and alveolar mucosa that spreads to deeper tissue. The gingiva are very red with extensive necrosis of the soft tissue. The disease is characterized by intense pain, distinctive mouth odor, punched-out tips of interdental papillae, and spontaneous bleeding. It is associated with immune deficiency diseases such as human immunodeficiency virus (HIV) and may also occur in malnutritional patients and those under extreme stress.

REFRACTORY PERIODONTITIS

Refractory periodontitis is unresponsive to appropriate treatment. The disease may occur at single or multiple sites that remain infected despite therapy.

ANTIBIOTIC THERAPY FOR PERIODONTAL DISEASE

Antibiotic therapy is indicated for patients who do not respond to debridement with scaling and root planing and good personal plaque control. It is also indicated when a bacterium has been identified. Several antibiotics are briefly reviewed. These antibiotics are discussed in detail in Chapter 6.

Metronidazole is bactericidal against spirochetes, *Bacteroides* species, and *P. gingivalis*. It is not effective against *A. actinomycetemcomitans* and is not used to treat juvenile periodontitis.

Penicillins are less effective against periodontal disease because of the high rate of resistance. Amoxicillin with clavulanic acid appears to be useful in the treatment of refractory periodontitis.

Tetracycline antibiotics concentrate in gingival fluid and are particularly useful in treating periodontal disease. They are helpful in the treatment of localized juvenile periodontitis because they are active against *A. actinomycetemcomitans*. The different types of tetracycline drugs and delivery systems are reviewed in Chapter 6.

NONSTEROIDAL ANTIINFLAMMATORY DRUGS FOR THE TREATMENT OF PERIODONTAL DISEASE

Recently, nonsteroidal antiinflammatory drugs (NSAIDs) have demonstrated potential benefits in inhibiting the progression of periodontal disease. NSAIDs, such as **ibuprofen,** have been shown to inhibit the inflammatory process of periodontal disease. Prostaglandins may play a role in periodontal disease and NSAIDs inhibit prostaglandin synthesis, which can affect the progression of gingival inflammation and alveolar bone loss.

ORAL LESIONS

Oral lesions include recurrent aphthous stomatitis (RAS) and herpes infection. They are often referred to as "canker sores" (RAS) and "cold sores" (herpes infection).

Recurrent Aphthous Stomatitis

This common condition affects many people and its cause is unknown. Aphthous ulcers can appear on any nonkeratinized surface in the mouth including the lips, buccal mucosa, tongue, floor of the mouth, or soft palate. The main goal of RAS treatment is to control discomfort and to promote healing. Analgesics and mouthwashes are used to control oral pain and discomfort. Topical protectants with or without steroids can provide symptomatic relief. Tetracycline suspension is often prescribed and the patient swishes and either swallows or expectorates, and it is sometimes mixed with viscous lidocaine 2% in a 1:1 mix. If the condition is severe, systemic steroids are begun with tapering doses in conjunction with topical steroids.

Herpes Infection

Primary herpes, also referred to as "cold sores" or "fever blisters," is caused by the herpes simplex type 1 virus. The lesions are painful, arise in the same location throughout the oral mucosa, are recurrent and cosmetically objectionable. The mature lesion often has a crust with an erythematous base and systemic symptoms can develop. Treatment includes aspirin or acetaminophen and/or a tepid bath for fever. Painful local symptoms can be treated with **diphenhydramine,** viscous **lidocaine,** or **kaolin,** or a combination of the three. Topical protectants also provide symptomatic relief and include **sodium carboxymethylcellulose** (Orabase) with or without benzocaine. **Acyclovir** (Chapter 6) can help to shorten the course of the disease and can be administered topically, orally, or intravenously. Prophylactic measures include applying a sunscreen/sunblock with an SPF of 15 or greater prior to sun exposure.

ORAL CANDIDIASIS

Oral *candidiasis* is caused by *Candida albicans* and occurs in both the oral and vaginal mucosa. It is often referred to as "thrush" when it occurs in the oral mucosa and is characterized by white "milk curd"–appearing plaques attached to the oral mucosa that can be wiped off. It occurs most frequently in pregnant women, infants, and immunocompromised patients. Treatment is with antifungal drugs and includes nystatin aqueous suspension or vaginal tablets, pastilles, or **clotrimazole** troches (Chapter 6). Other therapies include systemic **ketoconazole** or **fluconazole** (Chapter 6).

ALVEOLAR OSTEITIS

Alveolar osteitis, or "dry socket," is caused by loss or necrosis of a blood clot that exposes bone in the extraction socket. This exposed area is very painful and the patient may also have accompanying fever, lymphadenopathy, and a foul odor. Treatment includes debridement, packing, analgesics, antibiotics (if necessary), and supportive therapy.

ROOT SENSITIVITY

Root sensitivity can be precipitated by hot or cold and sweet or sour foods. It may be the result of occlusal trauma or roots that may have become exposed during periodontal surgery, extensive root planing, or an accumulation of plaque and its byproducts. Treatment includes occlusal adjustment if it is due to occlusal trauma or burnishing with glycerin and applications of sodium fluoride or stannous fluoride. Home therapy includes brushing with concentrated sodium chloride and 0.4% stannous fluoride, or a sodium fluoride gel may be applied in a bite guard.

XEROSTOMIA

Xerostomia or dry mouth is often drug induced, a result of aging, or it may be due to illness. Radiation therapy to the head and neck may also cause xerostomia because of its ability to affect the salivary glands and alter consistency and reduce volume of saliva. Table 12-1 lists drugs that are likely to cause dry mouth. Treatment includes consumption of plenty of water, ice chips, tart sugarless gum or candy, or artificial saliva; especially for patients undergoing radiation therapy. An example of an artifi-

Table 12-1   Drugs That Cause Xerostomia

Drug Class	Example
Anticholinergics	Benztropine (Cogentin)
Antihypertensives	Methyldopa (Aldomet)
	Clonidine (Catapress)
	Prazocin (Minipress)
Antipsychotics	Haloperidol (Haldol)
	Fluphenazine (Prolixin)
	Chlorpromazine (Thorazine)
	Thioridazine (Mellaril)
Tricyclic antidepressants	Amitriptylline (Elavil)
	Nortriptylline (Pamelor)
	Desipramine (Norpramin)
Antihistamines	Diphenhydramine (Benadryl)
	Chlorpheniramine (Chlor-Trimeton)
α-adrenergic agonists	Pseudoephedrine (Sudafed)
Benzodiazepines	Alprazolam (Xanax)
	Diazepam (Valium)
	Lorazepam (Ativan)
	Triazolam (Halcion)
Diuretics	Triameterene/hydrochlorothiazide (Dyazide)
	Hydrochlorothiazide (various)

cial saliva, product is XeroLube, which is composed of a variety of ingredients including cellulose, sorbital, sodium combinations, and phosphates.

Pilocarpine HCI (Salagen) is an oral cholinomimetic drug that is indicated for the treatment of xerostomia due to salivary gland hypofunction as a result of chemotherapy or radiation therapy to the head and neck. It acts predominantly on muscarinic receptors of the parasympathetic nervous system, which stimulates secretions of the exocrine glands.

Summary

Oral conditions and their therapies are an important part of dental care. The dental hygienist can help the patient by knowing what to look for during an oral examination and how to communicate that information to the dentist and the patient. Therapies vary for the different oral conditions and the dental hygienist should know about them and what to tell patients about their medication. Many oral conditions are a result of predisposing factors or poor oral health care. The dental hygienist can teach the patient how to minimize predisposing factors and how to improve oral hygiene.

Case Study: Blake Blackstone

Blake Blackstone is a 16-year-old high school junior who is new to your dental hygiene practice. She is in today for an oral examination. During the initial medication/ health history you note that Ms. Blackstone does not perform personal plaque prevention at home despite an understanding of periodontal disease. She just does-n't have the time for it. She manages to brush her teeth with a toothpaste that has a tartar-control element in it. During the oral examination both you and the dentist note minimal gingival inflammation but notice deep pocket formation and mobili-ty and migration of her first molars.

1. What is happening to Ms. Blackstone?
2. What is localized juvenile periodontitis and who does it affect?
3. Compare and contrast the different types of early-onset periodontitis.
4. How can juvenile periodontitis be treated?
5. What is the role of antibiotics in the treatment of localized juvenile periodontitis?
6. What should Ms. Blackstone be told about localized juvenile periodontitis and its treatment?

Case Study: Malcolm Smith

Malcolm Smith is 52 years old and has been a long-time patient of this dental prac-tice. His medication/health history is significant for prostate cancer, which has metas-tasized to his bones. He is receiving both oral and intravenous chemotherapy. His chief complaint today is a constant dry mouth that is not relieved by drinking water or juices or sucking on sugarless candy. He would like some help with this problem.

1. What are some of the causes of xerostomia?
2. Which drugs cause xerostomia?
3. How can xerostomia be treated?
4. What is Salagen and what is its role in the treatment of xerostomia?
5. How is Salagen different from other drugs used to treat xerostomia?

Review Questions

1. What is the best way to avoid actinic lip changes?
2. What is angular cheilosis and how is it treated?
3. What is acute necrotizing ulcerative gingivitis and how is it best treated?
4. Compare and contrast the different types of periodontitis.
5. Compare and contrast recurrent aphthous stomatitis and herpes infection.
6. What is alveolar osteitis and how is it treated?

BIBLIOGRAPHY

American Academy of Periodontology: *Proceedings of the World Workshop on Clinical Periodontology,* vol. 1. American Academy of Periodontology, Chicago, 1989, pp. 123–131.

Carranza FA (ed.): *Glickman's Clinical Periodontology,* 7th ed. W. B. Saunders Company, Philadelphia, 1990.

Fleser CR: Newly released therapeutic agents. *Dent Products Report,* January 60–61, January 1996.

Flynn AA: Oral health products: In *Handbook of Nonprescription Drugs,* 10th ed. American Pharmaceutical Association, Washington, DC, 1993.

Genco RJ: Systemic antimicrobials in the management of periodontal diseases. In *Periodontal Disease Management,* vol. 4. American Academy of Periodontology, Chicago, 1994, pp. 237–252.

Howell TH, Williams RC: Nonsteroidal antiinflammatory drugs as inhibitors of periodontal disease progression. *Crit Rev Oral Biol Med* 4:177–196, 1993.

Lynch MA, Brightman VJ, Greenberg MS (eds.): *Burket's Oral Medicine,* 9th ed. J. B. Lippincott Company, Philadelphia, 1994.

Newman MG, Kornman KS, Doherty FM: A 6-month multicenter evaluation of adjunctive tetracycline fiber therapy used in conjunction with scaling and root planing in maintenance patients: Clinical results. *J Periodontol* 65:685–691, 1994.

Taggart EJ: Gingival diseases. In Perry DA, Beemsterboer PL, Taggart EJ (eds.), *Periodontology for the Dental Hygienist,* 1st ed. W. B. Saunders Company, Philadelphia, 1996.

Taggart EJ: Periodontal diseases. In Perry DA, Beemsterboer PL, Taggart EJ (eds.), *Periodontology for the Dental Hygienist.* 1st ed. W. B. Saunders Company, Philadelphia, 1996.

Williams RC, Jeffcoat MK, Howell TH, Rolla A, Stubbs D, Teoh KW, et al: Altering the progression of human alveolar bone loss with nonsteroidal anti-inflammatory drugs. *J Periodontol* 60:485–490, 1989.

PART III

MEDICATIONS THAT DENTAL PATIENTS ARE TAKING

CHAPTER 13

Treatment of Cardiovascular Disorders

Key Terms

Angina pectoris
Arrhythmia
Cardiac Glycosides
Cardiovascular disease

Cholesterol
Coagulation
Congestive Heart Failure
Hypertension

LEARNING OBJECTIVES

After completion of this chapter and its learning activities, the student should be able to:

1. Discuss the dental concerns associated with cardiovascular disease.
2. Describe congestive heart failure as one of the most common categories of cardiovascular disease.
3. Describe the pharmacologic effects and adverse reactions of cardiac glycosides.
4. List other drugs used to treat congestive heart failure.
5. Define arrhythmia and list its causes.
6. Describe the four classifications of antiarrhythmics.
7. Define angina and review the classes of medication used to treat it.
8. Describe hypertension and the stepped-care approach to treating it.
9. List the different classes of antihypertensive medications including pharmacologic effects and adverse reactions.
10. Describe the factors that may place one at risk for hyperlipidemic disorders.
11. List the categories of drugs used to treat high cholesterol including pharmacologic effects and adverse reactions.
12. Briefly review the coagulation process.
13. Briefly review the drugs used to treat coagulopathies.
14. Discuss the dental concerns associated with the drugs used to treat cardiovascular disorders.

INTRODUCTION

Cardiovascular disease is among the leading causes of death in the United States and refers to disorders that primarily affect the heart and blood vessels. Several examples include congestive heart failure (CHF), hypertension, and angina. Despite it being the leading cause of death in the United States, many patients are living longer, more productive lives because of advances in medicine and better screening procedures for cardiovascular disease.

The dental hygienist is usually among the first in the dental clinic to determine whether or not a patient has a heart problem because of the reviewed medication/health history. A complete medication/health history will help to determine whether or not the patient's physician should be consulted before any dental treatment is given. A general knowledge of the diseases and their management will allow the dental hygienist to provide the patient with the best possible dental care. The intent of this chapter is to briefly discuss the different cardiovascular disorders and the medications used to treat them, including the mechanism of action, adverse reactions, and dental concerns. There is also a brief review of cholesterol and coagulation disorders and their treatments.

DENTAL CONCERNS ASSOCIATED WITH CARDIOVASCULAR DISEASE

As with medications, certain cardiovascular conditions may prohibit or restrict dental treatment. Absolute contraindications include uncontrolled arrhythmias, uncontrolled CHF, significant, uncontrolled hypertension, unstable or recent onset of angina, or an acute or recent myocardial infarction (MI) (within the past 3–6 months). In some instances dental procedures may be performed after consultation with the patient's physician.

Most patients with controlled cardiovascular disease can be treated in the dental office. One should consider the type and length of procedure, stress of the procedure, necessity, and any medications to be used prior to performing that procedure. Lastly, dental office personnel should consult with the dentist prior to performing any dental procedure on a patient with cardiovascular disease.

CONGESTIVE HEART FAILURE

The heart functions as a two-part pump with a right and left side that circulates blood throughout the body in order to help the body meet its oxygen requirements. Problems arise when the heart is unable to meet the body's oxygen requirements and starts to pump inefficiently. The heart muscle becomes stretched beyond its maximum effectiveness and can no longer pump out excess blood. The heart becomes enlarged and floppy. This inefficient pumping mechanism results in decreased cardiac output and circulation and is referred to as *congestive heart failure*.

When less blood is pumped to the rest of the body, many organs receive less blood flow and the blood backs up behind the part of the heart that is failing. Right-sided heart failure results in systemic congestion, which causes edema in the extremities (ankles or buttocks) and is evidenced by pitting of the legs or buttocks. Left-sided failure results in pulmonary edema and is characterized by dyspnea and orthopnea. Many patients have both right- and left-sided heart failure.

Cardiac Glycosides

The major drugs used to treat CHF are the *cardiac glycosides,* which are found in a number of plants (foxglove) and on the skin of the common toad. This group of drugs was first described by William Withering in 1785 for its use in the treatment of edema and other diseases. The glycosides are related chemically, have the same action in the body, and differ in terms of their route of administration, onset, and duration of action. They include **digitalis, digitoxin,** and **digoxin.** Digoxin (Lanoxin) is discussed here as it is the most commonly used cardiac glycoside.

Pharmacologic Effects. The major pharmacologic effect of digoxin is to increase the force and efficiency of contraction of the failing heart. The improved contractile force allows the heart to work more efficiently with subsequent increase in cardiac output. Heart size decreases and improved systemic circulation leads to improvement in tissue perfusion and a decrease in edema.

Improved cardiac output reduces heart rate, and digoxin also slows atrioventricular (AV) conduction, prolongs the refractory period of the AV node, and decreases the rate of the sinoatrial (SA) node. These effects are important in the treatment of arrhythmias.

Adverse Reactions. Digoxin has a very narrow margin of safety and blood levels are checked to monitor for possible toxicity. Changes in dose, metabolism, or absorption can produce toxic effects. Gastrointestinal effects (GI) include anorexia, nausea, vomiting, and copious salivation, which are usually the first signs of digoxin toxicity. They can occur at both therapeutic and toxic doses. Dose reduction can usually decrease this toxic effect. *Arrhythmias* and other conduction disturbances can occur with very high doses of digoxin. Neurologic adverse effects include headache, muscle weakness, facial pain, delirium, hallucinations, convulsions, and visual disturbances (green and yellow vision, halo around lights).

Drug Interactions. **Quinidine, verapamil, amiodarone**, and antibiotics that decrease gut flora and prevent bacterial inactivation of digoxin, as well as anticholinergics that decrease intestinal motility, can raise digoxin levels. Diuretics can cause hypokalemia and may potentiate an arrhythmia in a person taking digoxin. Sympathomimetic agents, including over-the-counter cough, cold, and allergy products, can enhance the chance of arrhythmias in patients taking digoxin.

Dental Concerns. Patients with CHF are of concern to the dental hygienist. Several medications used in dentistry may increase digoxin blood levels and increase the patient's risk of having an arrhythmia. The dental hygienist can take certain steps to minimize or avoid adverse reactions or drug interactions in these patients. They include watching for signs of toxicity including nausea, vomiting, copious salivation, and vision changes. Should these occur, the dental hygienist should notify the dentist and encourage the patient to see his physician immediately or go to the nearest emergency-care facility. Caution should be exercised if a local anesthetic with epinephrine is used because of the possible chance of arrhythmia (Chapter 4). **Tetra-cycline** and **erythromycin** should be avoided because of the possible increase in digoxin blood levels (Chapter 6). Lastly, the dental hygienist should monitor the patient's pulse. Abnormally slow rates and irregular rhythms could mean bradycardia or an arrhythmia. This information should be reported to the dentist for evaluation and the patient should be encouraged to contact his physician.

Other Drugs Used to Treat CHF

Though cardiac glycosides have been the main drugs used to treat CHF, diuretics, vasodilators, and angiotensin-converting enzyme inhibitors are also used. They are discussed in the section on hypertension in this chapter.

ARRHYTHMIAS

An *arrhythmia* is any sort of inappropriate electrical activity in the heart that can occur in both normal and diseased hearts. Symptoms range from mild palpitations to cardiac arrest, and diagnosis is made by evaluating signs and symptoms presented by the patient and confirmed by an electrocardiogram (EKG).

In a normal heart, the sinoatrial (SA) node serves as the pacemaker that regulates heart rate. The normal conduction route of the heart begins in the SA node and travels to the atrioventricular (AV) node down the bundle of His into the right and left bundle branches until it reaches the Purkinje fibers (Figure 13-1). This conduction route produces rhythmic contractions of various parts of the heart.

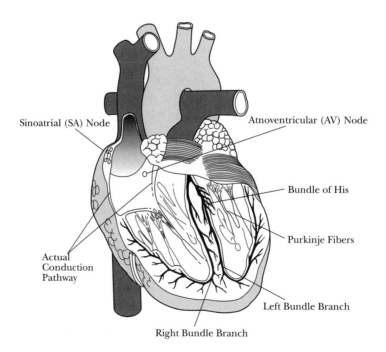

Figure 13-1   *Normal conduction route of the heart*

Arrhythmias most often occur when there is a defect in the AV node that causes it to fire abnormal impulses, or a defect in conduction, or both. The automatic firing of the AV node is under the influence of sodium, potassium, and calcium, which all play a significant role in cardiac action potential or nerve impulse. Cardiac disease or injury can alter normal cardiac rhythm.

Classification of Antiarrhythmic Drugs

There are four classes of drugs used to treat arrhythmias and they are reviewed in Table 13-1. Many of these antiarrhythmic drugs are used to treat other cardiovascular diseases and other illnesses as well. Digoxin is used to treat arrhythmias and is not given a class number.

Class I drugs have actions similar to local anesthetics and work by interfering with the influx of sodium into the nerve cell membrane. This prevents depolarization and transmission of the nerve impulse. This group is further divided in I-A, I-B, and I-C based on their effect on the myocardial action potential. Class I-A drugs prolong the action potential, Class I-B drugs shorten the action potential, and Class I-C drugs slow conduction without affecting the action potential.

Class II drugs are the β blockers and they decrease the effects of sympathetic stimulation and of endogenous catecholamines like epinephrine and norepinephrine.

Table 13-1   Classification of Antiarrhythmic Drugs

Class	*Mechanism of Action*
Class I	
I-A Disopyramide (Norpace)	Sodium channel blockers
Procainamide (Pronestyl)	
Quinidine (Quinaglute)	
I-B Lidocaine (Xylocaine)	Sodium channel blockers
Tocainide (Tonocard)	
Mexiletine (Mexitil)	
I-C Flecainide (Tambocor)	Sodium channel blockerr
Encainide (Enkaid)	
Propafenone (Rythmol)	
Class II	
Propranolol (Inderal)	β blocker
Class III	
Amiodarone (Cordarone)	Adrenergic neuronal blockers
Bretylium (Bretylol)	
Class IV	
Verapamil (Calan)	Calcium channel blockers
Diltiazem (Cardizem)	

Sources: Tisdale JE, Webb CR, Are antiarrhythmic drugs obsolete? *Clin Pharm* 49:714–726, 1992.

Class III drugs are neuronal blockers and work by decreasing the release of nor-epinephrine from adrenergic nerve endings and increasing the refractory period of the ventricles.

Class IV drugs are the calcium channel blockers that block the influx of calcium into the cardiac muscle cells and smooth muscle cells of blood vessels. They decrease the rate of firing of the SA and AV nodes, which slows down heart rate and causes vasodilation.

Dental Concerns

The medication/health history will help the dental hygienist to determine whether or not a patient has or has had arrhythmias. The patient should be questioned about the specific use of a medication since different cardiovascular medications can be used to treat arrhythmias or other types of cardiovascular disease. As stated previously, patients with controlled arrhythmias can undergo dental procedures. The patient's pulse should be checked for normal rate and rhythm. All findings should be reported to the dentist and documented in the patient's dental record.

ANGINA

Angina pectoris is a cardiovascular disease characterized by pain and discomfort in the chest and is caused by a lack of oxygen to the cardiac muscle and an imbalance between myocardial oxygen supply and demand. Pain can also radiate to the lower jaw, neck, and back; lower jaw pain can initially be confused with a toothache. Angina attacks are usually precipitated by anything that increases myocardial oxygen demand such as exercise, stress, excitement, or digestion of a heavy meal. This type of angina is referred to as stable or static angina because it is predictable. A second type of angina is termed variant or spastic because it can occur at any time and is caused by coronary artery spasm.

Pharmacotherapy of Angina

At one time, the nitrates and nitrites were the most commonly used drugs in the treatment of angina. Today, one can choose from not only nitrates and nitrites but β blockers and calcium channel blockers (Table 13-2). These drugs work primarily by reducing the workload on the heart, which decreases myocardial oxygen requirements.

Nitrates and Nitrites. **Nitroglycerin** is the most frequently used drug of this class for the management and prevention of angina induced by stress or exercise. It works by relaxing vascular smooth muscle throughout the body, which causes a decrease in blood pressure and cardiac work. This reduced workload reduces oxygen demand on the heart.

DOSE FORMS. Nitroglycerin can be used sublingually or by spray to treat an acute attack, or orally or topically for prophylaxis of angina attacks. Sublingual tablets cause a burning sensation when placed under the tongue. If the patient does not experience a burning sensation, it could mean that the tablets are no longer effective and they should be replaced. Ointments (topical) should be applied with

Table 13-2　Selected Drugs in the Treatment of Angina

Drug	*Dose Form*	*Onset of Action*	*Duration of Action*
Nitrites			
Amyl nitrite	Ampule for inhalation	30–60 sec	10 min
Short-Acting Nitrates			
Nitroglycerin (NTG, Nitrostat)	Sublingual	1–3 min	15–60 min
Isosorbide dinitrate (Isordil)	Sublingual	2–5 min	2–4 hours
Long-Acting Nitrates			
Isosorbide dinitrate (Isordil)	Oral	30 min	3–6 hours
Isosorbide mononitrate (Ismo)	Oral		
Nitroglycerin (Nitro-Bid)	Sustained release, oral tablets	30–60 min	3–8 hours
Nitroglycerin (Nitro-Bid, Nitrol)	Ointment	15–45 min	2–10 hours
Nitroglycerin (Nitro-Dur, Transderm Nitro)	Transdermal patches	30–60 min	24 hours
Pentaerythritol (Peritrate)	Oral	30 min	10 hours
β Blockers			
Propranolol (Inderal)	Oral	30 min	6–8 hours
Calcium Channel Blockers			
Verapamil (Calan, Isoptin)	Oral	30 min	4 hours
Nifedipine (Procardia, Adalat)	Oral	15 min	4–8 hours
Diltiazem (Cardizem)	Oral	30 min	6–8 hours
Nicardipine (Cardene)	Oral	15 min–1 h	6–8 hours
Amlodipine (Norvasc)	Oral	5–10 hours	> 24 hours

Sources: Yedinak KC, Use of calcium channel antagonists for cardiovascular disease. *Am Pharm* N533:49–64, 1993; Yedinak KC, Selection and use of beta-blockers for patients with cardiovascular disease. *Am Pharm* N534:28–36, 1994.

the applicator provided. Patients should be encouraged to carry their nitroglycerin with them at all times, especially to a dental appointment. The nitroglycerin should be within immediate reach of the patient during dental treatment.

STORAGE.　Sublingual nitroglycerin breaks down easily and should be stored in its original container away from heat and moisture. The tablets remain active until the expiration date on the bottle as long as the bottle remains unopened. Once the bottle is opened the patient should discard the remaining tablets after 3 months from the opening date or sooner if indicated by the expiration date.

ADVERSE REACTIONS.　Adverse reactions are many and include throbbing headache, facial flushing, dizziness, hypotension, and gastrointestinal (GI) upset. Hypotension is a result of vascular relaxation and is enhanced by hot weather and alcohol. Most headaches respond to **acetaminophen** or **aspirin.** Most patients develop tolerance to these adverse reactions over time.

TOLERANCE.　Patients develop tolerance to the effects of nitrates and nitrites with repeated administration especially if the medication is used too often. This also includes daily doses for prophylaxis of angina. It has been recommended that patients use intermittent therapy to avoid tolerance, including every other day dosing or drug-free periods. The most commonly recommended drug-free period is to have the patient take the drug upon arising in the morning and the next dose 7 hours later.

Beta Blockers. Beta blockers decrease heart rate, reduce blood pressure, and decrease cardiac contractility, which leads to a decrease in the amount of cardiac work and a decrease in myocardial oxygen demand. These drugs are effective in reducing both exercise- and stress-induced angina and are used for long-term treatment. Although four β blockers are used (**atenolol, metoprolol, nadolol,** and **propranolol**), propranolol is the most commonly used drug. Adverse reactions include bradycardia, congestive heart failure, headache, dry mouth, blurred vision, sedation, and unpleasant dreams.

Calcium Channel Blockers. The calcium channel blockers are the newest drugs used to treat angina. These drugs work by decreasing the influx of calcium ions into the cardiac and vascular smooth muscle. Vasodilation occurs in the vascular smooth muscle, which decreases venous return, thereby causing less cardiac work and myocardial oxygen demand. Calcium channel blockers also dilate larger coronary arteries and decrease coronary spasm. Examples include **verapamil, diltiazem, nifedipine, nicardipine, amlodipine,** and **bepridil.** Adverse reactions include dizziness, weakness, constipation, dysgeusia, gingival hyperplasia, and hypotension. Patients taking these drugs should be instructed on the importance of oral hygiene and should have frequent dental appointments to help avoid or minimize gingival hyperplasia.

Dental Concerns

Dental appointments and procedures may precipitate angina attacks in some patients. Dental personnel should anticipate this and help to prevent them, possibly by prescribing a sedative-hypnotic (Chapter 9) prior to the appointment to help reduce patient anxiety. The patient could self-administer a sublingual nitroglycerin tablet prior to the procedure to prevent an angina attack. The patient should rise slowly from the dental chair to help minimize hypotension.

HYPERTENSION

Hypertension is defined as a systolic blood pressure (SBP) of 140 mm Hg or greater and/or a diastolic blood pressure (DBP) of 90 mm Hg or greater and is classified as either essential, secondary, or malignant. Essential hypertension is due to unknown etiology and affects 90% of diagnosed hypertensives. Secondary hypertension occurs in about 10% of diagnosed hypertensives and is due to an identifiable condition such as renal disease or CHF. Malignant hypertension occurs in about 5% of patients with essential or secondary hypertension.

According to data from the National Health and Nutrition Examination Survey III, hypertension affects as many as 50 million Americans (Joint National Committee on Detection, Evaluation, and Treatment of High Blood Pressure, 1993). The prevalence of high blood pressure increases with age, is greater in African-Americans than Caucasians, and is greater in less educated people of both races. High blood pressure prevalence is greater for men than women during young adulthood and middle age. Women have a higher prevalence than men once they reach menopause. African-Americans and Caucasians living in the southeastern United States have a higher rate of high blood pressure than those living in other parts of the country (Roccella and Lenfant, 1989).

Hypertension produces few, if any, symptoms and can lead to target organ disease if left untreated. Nonfatal and fatal cerebrovascular accidents (stroke), cardiovascular disease, and renal disease increase progressively with higher levels of SBP and/or DBP (JNC, 1993). Fortunately, there have been many advances in the treatment of hypertension that reduce both morbidity and mortality. The next section reviews lifestyle modifications and classes of drugs used to treat hypertension including pharmacologic effects, adverse reactions, selected drug interactions, and dental concerns.

Treatment of Hypertension

Hypertension is treated with a combination of both lifestyle modifications and drug therapy in an effort to maintain an SBP below 140 mm Hg and a DBP below 90 mm Hg. Figure 13-2 reviews this "stepped-care" approach to treating hypertension. Medications are chosen based on the patient, age, sex, adverse reaction profile of the drug, any known cardiovascular risk factors, and other illnesses.

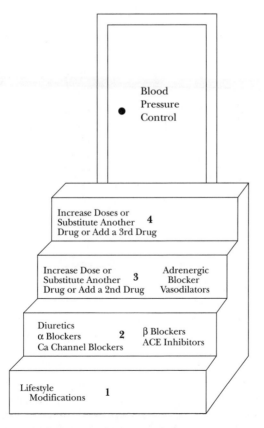

Figure 13-2   *"Stepped-care" approach to treating hypertension*

Lifestyle Modifications. Lifestyle modifications include weight reduction, exercise, moderate dietary sodium and alcohol intake, and tobacco avoidance. Other dietary changes include low-fat and low-cholesterol diets and maintaining adequate potassium, calcium, and magnesium dietary intake. Patients should be encouraged to modify their lifestyle. This may not only reduce their blood pressure but may also reduce other risk factors for cardiovascular disease.

Diuretics. Diuretics are among the most commonly used drugs to treat hypertension and include thiazides and thiazide-like diuretics, loop diuretics, and potassium-sparing diuretics. Table 13-3 reviews the doses and adverse reactions of selected diuretics.

THIAZIDE DIURETICS. These are the most widely used diuretics. They may be used alone or in combination with other antihypertensive drugs. The major pharmacologic effect of these drugs is diuresis produced by the inhibition of the reabsorption of sodium in the distal convoluted tubules (DCT) of the kidneys. Potassium loss also occurs because of the increased amount of sodium in the DCT.

LOOP DIURETICS. These are the most potent diuretics and work by preventing sodium and chloride reabsorption in the loop of Henle at the base of the kidney. They are used during emergencies when rapid diuresis is necessary and are also used in patients who do not respond to thiazide diuretics.

Table 13-3   Selected Diuretics in the Treatment of Hypertension

Drug	*Dose (mg/day)*	*Adverse Reactions*
Thiazide Diuretics		
Chlorthalidone (Hygroton)	12.5–50	Hypokalemia
Hydrochlorothiazide (Esidrix, HydroDiuril, others)	12.5–50	Hypomagnesemia, hyperuricemia, Hypercalcemia,
Indapamide (Lozol)	2.5–5	Hypomagnesemia, hyperuricemia, Hypercalcemia, Hyperglycemia, Hypercholesterolemia, Hypertriglyceridemia, Sexual dysfunction, Weakness
Loop Diuretics		
Bumetanide (Bumex)	0.5–5	Same as thiazides except that they do not cause hypercalcemia
Furosemide (Lasix)	20–320	
Potassium Sparing		
Amiloride (Midamor)	5–10	Hyperkalemia
Spironolactone (Aldactone)	25–100	Gynecomastia, mastodynia, menstrual irregularities, diminished libido in males
Triamterene (Dyrenium)	50–150	

Sources: Joint National Committee on Detection, Evaluation, and Treatment of High Blood Pressure, The fifth report of the Joint National Committee on detection, evaluation, and treatment of high blood pressure (JNC V). *Arch Intern Med.* 153:154–183, 1993.

POTASSIUM-SPARING DIURETICS. These medications work by one of two mechanisms of action. **Spironolactone** competitively antagonizes aldosterone, which results in sodium excretion and loss of fluid volume through diuresis. **Triamterene** promotes sodium excretion in the collecting tubules of the kidneys. With both drugs, potassium is not exchanged for sodium. Sodium is not reabsorbed and stays in the tubules along with water.

Adrenergic Antagonists. This group of drugs works by blocking α and β receptors, which reduces sympathetic activity to the heart and/or blood vessels, thereby reducing cardiac output and/or peripheral resistance. Table 13-4 reviews the adrenergic blockers currently available in the United States.

Beta receptors have been divided into β_1 and β_2 receptor subtypes. Beta$_1$ receptors are primarily located in cardiac muscle, and stimulation results in increased heart rate, cardiac contractility, and AV conduction. Beta$_2$ receptors are located primarily in the bronchial and vascular smooth muscle, and stimulation results in vasodilation of skeletal muscle and bronchodilation of pulmonary muscle.

Table 13-4   Adrenergic Blockers in the Treatment of Hypertension

Drug	Dose (mg/day)	Adverse Reactions
β Blockers		
Acebutolol (Sectral)	200–1200	Bronchospasm, fatigue, insomnia,
Atenolol (Tenormin, others)	25–100	mask symptoms of hypoglycemia,
Betaxolol (Kerlone)	5–40	hypertriglyceridemia, decrease
Bisoprolol (Zebeta)	5–20	HDL cholesterol, strange dreams,
Carteolol (Cartrol)	2.5–10	exacerbation of CHF, depression,
Metoprolol (Lopressor)	50–200	may aggravate peripheral vascular
Metoprolol LA (Toprol XL)	50–200	insufficiency
Nadolol (Corgard)	20–240	
Penbutolol (Levatol)	20–80	
Pindolol (Visken, others)	10–60	
Propranol (Inderal, others)	40–240	
Propranolol LA (Inderal LA, others)	60–240	
Timolol (Blocarden, others)	20–40	
α Blockers		
Doxazosin (Cardura)	1–16	Orthostatic hypotension, syncope,
Prazosin (Minipress)	1–20	weakness, palpitations, headache
Terazosin (Hytrin)	1–20	
α and β Blockers		
Labetalol (Normodyne, Trandate)	200–1200	Bronchospasm, may aggravate peripheral vascular insufficiency, orthostatic hypotension

Sources: Joint National Committee on Detection, Evaluation, and Treatment of High Blood Pressure, The fifth report of the Joint National Committee on Detection, Evaluation, and Treatment of High Blood Pressure (JNC V). *Arch Intern Med* 153:154–183, 1993. Yedinak KC, Use of calcium channel antagonists for cardiovascular disease. *Am Pharm* NS33:49–64, 1993.

The α receptor has also been divided into α_1 and α_2 receptor subtypes. Alpha$_1$ receptors are located on postsynaptic receptor tissues, and stimulation results in vasoconstriction and increased peripheral vascular resistance. Alpha$_2$ receptors are located on presynaptic receptor tissues, and stimulation results in a feedback inhibition of norepinephrine release.

BETA-ADRENERGIC BLOCKERS. These drugs are classified as either β_1 specific or β_1/β_2 nonspecific. Examples include **propranolol, timolol, atenolol,** and **pindolol.** Some advantages of β_1-specific blockers (**metoprolol**) include a lower propensity for bronchoconstriction, a lesser degree of adverse metabolic effects in patients with diabetes, a reduced capacity for the exacerbation of intermittent claudication and bronchial asthma.

These medications exert their pharmacologic effect by decreasing output, which lowers blood pressure. Other effects include lowering of plasma renin levels, reduction in plasma volume, decrease in sympathetic outflow from the central nervous system (CNS), and decrease in peripheral vascular resistance. They are used either alone or in combination with other antihypertensives.

ALPHA-ADRENERGIC BLOCKERS. These drugs exert their pharmacologic effect by blocking peripheral α_1 receptors, which lowers blood pressure. Examples include **prazosin, terazosin,** and **doxazosin.** Prazosin is sometimes used in combination with diuretics because it can cause fluid retention. These drugs are used in patients with moderate to severe hypertension.

ALPHA- AND β-ADRENERGIC BLOCKERS. **Labetalol** is a nonspecific β blocker with α-blocking activity. It is used alone or in combination with diuretics.

Angiotensin-Converting Enzyme (ACE) Inhibitors. The ACE inhibitors are another group of antihypertensive drugs that have come to the forefront in both the initial management of mild hypertension and the treatment of moderate to severe hypertension. Examples include **captopril, enalapril,** and **lisinopril** and they are reviewed in Table 13-5.

ACE inhibitors work by blocking the conversion of angiotensin I to angiotensin II (Figure 13-3). This results in vasodilation, decreased aldosterone formation, an increase in bradykinin, and an increase in vasodilatory prostaglandins. These medications are potassium sparing and may cause hyperkalemia in patients receiving potassium-sparing diuretics or those taking potassium supplements.

Angiotensin II Receptor Antagonists. This is the newest class of drugs in the treatment of hypertension and **losartan** (Cozaar) is the only drug available for use in the United States. It is reviewed in Table 13-5.

Losartan works by preventing the binding of angiotensin II to the angiotensin I receptor (Figure 13-3). This causes a relaxation of vascular smooth muscle, promotes vasodilation, and increases renal salt and water excretion. It also reduces plasma volume and decreases cellular hypertrophy. Adverse reactions include dizziness, edema, orthostatic hypotension, headache, fatigue, and cough.

Calcium Channel Blockers. The calcium channel blockers are used in the second step of the "stepped-care" approach to treating hypertension. Examples include **dilti-**

Table 13-5 ACE Inhibitors and Angiotensin II Receptor Antagonists

Drug	Dose (mg/day)	Adverse Reactions
ACE Inhibitors		
Benazepril (Lotensin)	10–40	Cough, rash
Captopril (Capoten)	12.5–150	
Enalapril (Vasotec)	2.5–40	Angioedema,
Fosinopril (Monopril)	10–40	Hyperkalemia
Lisonopril (Prinivil, Zestril)	5–40	
Quinapril (Accupril)	5–80	
Ramipril (Altace)	1.25–20	
Angiotensin II Receptor Antagonists		
Losartan (Cozaar)	25–100	Dizziness

Sources: Joint National Committee on Detection, Evaluation, and Treatment of High Blood Pressure, The fifth report of the Joint National Committee on Detection, Evaluation, and Treatment of High Blood Pressure (JNC V). *Arch Intern Med* 153:154–183, 1993, Weber MA, Byyny RL, Pratt JH, et al., Blood pressure effects of the angiotensin II receptor blocker, losartan. *Arch Intern Med* 155:405–411, 1995.

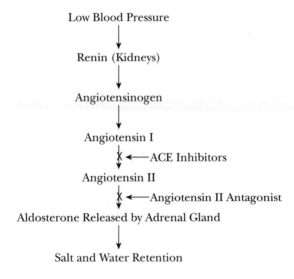

Figure 13-3 *Renin-angiotensin system*

azem, verapamil, and **nifedipine** (see Table 13-6). They may be used alone or in combination with other antihypertensive agents.

Calcium channel blockers work by blocking the inward movement of calcium ions across cell membranes. This causes smooth muscle relaxation and coronary vasodilation. The calcium channel blockers also cause systemic vasodilation, which

Table 13-6   Calcium Channel Blockers Used in the Treatment of Hypertension

Drug	Dose (mg/day)	Adverse Reactions
Conventional		
Amlodipine (Norvasc)	2.5–10	Constipation (Verapamil only),
Diltiazem (Cardizem, Dilacor)	90–360	Headache,
Felodipine (Plendil)	5–20	Dizziness,
Isradipine (DynaCirc)	2.5–10	Peripheral edema,
Nicardipine (Cardene)	60–120	Gingival hyperplasia,
Nifedipine (Procardia, Adalat)	30–120	Tachycardia (Amlodipine, Felodipine,
Verapamil (Calan, Isoptin)	80–480	Isradipine, Nicardipine, and Nifedipine),
		Heart block (ditiazem and verapamil only),
		Bradycardia (diltiazem and verapamil only)
Controlled Release		
Diltiazem		
Cardizem SR	240–360	Same as conventional dose forms
Cardizem CD	240–360	
Dilacor XR	240–360	
Felodipine (Plendil ER)	5–10	
Nicardipine (Cardene SR)	90–120	
Nifedipine		
Procardia XL	60–90	
Adalat CC	30–60	
Verapamil		
Calan SR	240–360	
Isoptin SR	240–360	
Verelan	240–360	

Sources: Joint National Committee on Detection, Evaluation, and Treatment of High Blood Pressure, The fifth report of the Joint National Committee on Detection, Evaluation, and Treatment of High Blood Pressure (JNC V). *Arch Intern Med* 153:154–183, 1993; Yedinak KC, Use of calcium channel antagonists for cardiovascular disease. *Am Pharm* N533:49–64, 1993.

reduces afterload on the heart and reduces blood pressure. The adverse reactions associated with calcium channel blockers are reviewed in Table 13-6.

As with most antihypertensives, calcium channel blockers can cause xerostomia and dysgeusia. There have also been reports of gingival hyperplasia with nifedipine, diltiazem, **felodipine,** and verapamil (Barak et al., 1987; Brown et al., 1991; Frattore et al, 1991; Todd and Faulds, 1992).

Gingival hyperplasia can occur within 1 month to several months after beginning calcium channel blocker therapy. The hyperplasia begins as nodular and firm tissue and progresses to red gingiva that bleed easily upon probing. It begins in the anterior labial papillae and can include the lingual and palatal gingiva and eventually extend onto crown surfaces. Patients should be encouraged to maintain meticulous oral hygiene and make frequent visits to the dental office for checkups. Gingival hyperplasia reverts to normal tissue upon discontinuation of the drug and usually does not reappear. It may take several months for the gingival hyperplasia to clear up once the drug has been discontinued.

Centrally Acting α_2-Agonists. These drugs include **clonidine** and **methyldopa,** which are also reviewed in Chapter 3. They lower blood pressure by the depression of sympathetic outflow from the CNS and are used infrequently.

> CLONIDINE. Clonidine works on the cardiovascular regulatory center in the brain and decreases sympathetic outflow. Adverse reactions include drowsiness, sedation, dry mouth, fatigue, and orthostatic hypotension.

> METHYLDOPA. Methyldopa works by stimulating central α_2 receptors that inhibit efferent sympathetic activity. Adverse reactions include drowsiness, sedation, depression, and fatigue.

Peripheral-Acting Adrenergic Antagonist. **Reserpine** inhibits catecholamine release from neuronal storage sites, which results in a lowering of blood pressure. Adverse reactions include lethargy, nasal congestion, and depression. Reserpine is also reviewed in Chapter 3.

Direct Vasodilators. This group of drugs includes **hydralazine** which works by causing direct vasodilation of arterioles. Adverse reactions include headache, tachycardia, and fluid retention.

Dental Concerns Associated with Antihypertensive Drugs

Antihypertensive drugs can cause a number of adverse reactions that can affect oral health and hygiene. They can also interact with some of the drugs used in the dental process. The dental hygienist should know about these drugs and how they can impact on the dental process. She should be able to effectively counsel the patient on these issues. The next sections focus on these adverse reactions and drug interactions.

Orthostatic Hypotension. Antihypertensive drugs cause orthostatic hypotension, which can be triggered after lying back in the dental chair. The dental hygienist should raise the chair slowly and let the patient wait a few minutes before rising *slowly* from the chair. The patient's blood pressure should be taken at the beginning of each appointment to determine whether or not to proceed with the dental procedure.

Xerostomia. Many patients complain of the xerostomia associated with antihypertensive drugs. This can best be combated by explaining to the patient that it may occur and what to do if it should happen. Patients should be instructed to drink plenty of water and suck on tart sugarless gum or candy. Caffeine-containing beverages exacerbate xerostomia and should be avoided. Patients should also practice good oral hygiene and come in for regularly scheduled cleanings. Artificial saliva is available for those with serious xerostomia.

Gingival Hyperplasia. Gingival hyperplasia is associated with several of the calcium channel blockers. Patients should be instructed to perform meticulous oral hygiene and return for frequent cleanings.

CNS Sedation. Several of the antihypertensive drugs cause sedation and this may be a concern if an opioid analgesic or a benzodiazepine is prescribed. Patients should be instructed on the increased likelihood of sedation and should refrain from driving. They should also avoid anything that requires thought or concentration such as operating heavy machinery or anything that requires thought or concentration.

Gastrointestinal Effects. Several of the antihypertensive drugs can cause GI irritation. The addition of nonsteroidal antiinflammatory drugs may increase GI discomfort and the patient should be warned. Patients should be instructed to take their medication with food or milk to help avoid or minimize GI irritation.

Constipation. Constipation is an adverse reaction of some of the antihypertensive drugs, which may be aggravated by the addition of an opioid analgesic. Patients should be instructed to eat plenty of fruits, vegetables, and other foods rich in fiber. In some instances, patients may require a bulk laxative or stool softener.

HYPERCHOLESTEROLEMIA (HIGH CHOLESTEROL)

Elevation of plasma lipid levels above accepted normal values are a significant risk factor in the development of coronary artery disease, stroke, and hypertension. The important dietary lipids include fatty acids, triglyccrides, and *cholesterol* and are essential for the formation of cell membranes, nerve tissues, and lipoprotein. Excessive amounts of lipids, over time, permit the formation of fatty deposits or plaques (atherosclerosis) in arterial blood vessels. Both cholesterol and triglycerides play an important role in plaque formation. Cholesterol can be further divided into high-density lipoproteins (HDL), which are considered to be good, and low-density lipoproteins (LDL), which have a high cholesterol content and are not considered to be good for the body.

Pharmacotherapy of Hypercholesterolemia

Reports indicate that lowering elevated serum cholesterol concentrations decreases mortality from coronary artery disease and may cause regression of atherosclerosis (Kane et al., 1990). Patients with high cholesterol should first be treated with a low-cholesterol, low-fat diet. If this fails, dietary or lifestyle modifications should be combined with drug therapy. The overall goal of diet and drugs is to lower cholesterol below 200 mg/dl and increase the proportion of HDL relative to LDL.

A number of drugs are available to treat hypercholesterolemia and include bile acid sequestrants, nicotinic acid, **gemfibrozil, probucol,** and the HMG CoA reductase inhibitors. Table 13-7 reviews these drugs and their adverse reactions.

Bile Acid Sequestrants. These drugs (**cholestyramine** [Questran] and **colestipol** [Colestid]) bind with bile salts in the small intestine and the bound bile acids become insoluble. The bile salts are normally used to make new cholesterol and can no longer do this once they become insoluble.

Niacin. **Niacin** decreases triglycerides, total serum cholesterol and LDL cholesterol, and increases HDL cholesterol. Niacin also causes flushing and dry skin. The

Table 13-7 Drugs Used in the Treatment of High Cholesterol

Drug	Dose	Adverse Reactions
Bile Acid Sequestrants		
Cholestyramine (Questran)	16 gm bid to tid	Bloating, constipation, epigastric pain, flatulence, nausea, do not taste good
Colestipol (Colestid)	5 gm qd to tid in 2–6 fl oz water	
B Vitamin		
Niacin	1–2 gm bid to tid with or after meals	Hepatoxicity, flushing, itching, headache
Fibric Acid Derivative		
Gemfibrozil (Lopid)	1200 mg per day in 2 divided doses, 30 minutes before morning and evening meals	GI complaints
Antioxidant		
Probucol (Lorelco)	500 mg bid, 30 minutes before morning and evening meals	GI complaints, prolonged QT intervals
HMG CoA Reductase Inhibitors		
Fluvastatin (Lescol)	20–40 mg qd, at bedtime	Elevated transaminase levels, myopathy, dyspnea, flatulence, constipation, headache
Lovastatin (Mevacor)	20–40 mg qd to bid	
Pravastatin (Pravachol)	10–20 mg qd to bid	
Simvastatin (Zocor)	10–20 mg once day, usually in the evening	

Source: McKenney JM, New guidelines for managing hypercholesterolemia. *Am Pharm* N533:3–11, 1993.

prostaglandin-mediated flushing can be avoided by pretreating with aspirin or a nonsteroidal antiinflammatory drug.

Gemfibrozil. Gemfibrozil (Lopid) lowers plasma triglycerides and very low-density lipoprotein (VLDL) cholesterol and can increase HDL cholesterol.

Probucol (Lorelco). This drug generally lowers total cholesterol and LDL cholesterol and it also lowers HDL cholesterol. Probucol may prolong the QT interval and is not used very often.

HMG-CoA Reductase Inhibitors. This is the newest class of drugs used to treat hypercholesterolemia and includes **lovastatin** (Mevacor), **pravastatin** (Pravachol), **simvastatin** (Zocor), and **fluvastatin** (Lescol). These drugs lower HDL by interfering with its synthesis in the liver and they also lower LDL.

Dental Concerns

Patients with high cholesterol are at significant risk for coronary artery disease and stroke. The dental practitioner should always record the patient's blood pressure and pulse in the patient's dental record. Several cholesterol-lowering drugs have GI side effects that may be further aggravated by the addition of a nonsteroidal antiinflammatory drug. Patients should be made aware of this and should beencouraged to take their medicine with food or milk to help avoid or minimize GI upset.

Coagulation Process

Coagulation is the normal process that occurs when a blood vessel is severed or injured. This protective process is called hemostasis and is designed to prevent blood loss after injury to the blood vessel. On occasion the clotting mechanism can become overactive and a clot may form. This thrombus can completely occlude or partially impair blood flow to local tissue and cause an infarct or necrosis. If the thrombus dislodges (embolus), it enters the bloodstream and can travel to other tissues and organs and cause occlusion.

Anticoagulant drugs are administered to prevent clot formation. Figure 13-4 is a simplified overview of the clotting process. Thromboplastin, fibrin, and thrombin are all formed as a result of the clotting process and are necessary for the development of a clot.

Anticoagulant Pharmacotherapy

This section reviews the two more common drugs used to treat coagulation disorders.

Heparin. **Heparin** is one of the most commonly used anticoagulants and must be given by injection. It is used in hospitals and skilled-care facilities. Heparin works by inhibiting thrombin activity so that fibrinogen cannot be converted to fibrin. Its

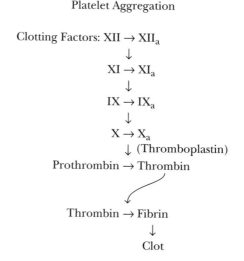

$$\text{Platelet Aggregation}$$

$$\text{Clotting Factors: XII} \rightarrow \text{XII}_a$$
$$\downarrow$$
$$\text{XI} \rightarrow \text{XI}_a$$
$$\downarrow$$
$$\text{IX} \rightarrow \text{IX}_a$$
$$\downarrow$$
$$\text{X} \rightarrow \text{X}_a$$
$$\downarrow \text{(Thromboplastin)}$$
$$\text{Prothrombin} \rightarrow \text{Thrombin}$$

$$\text{Thrombin} \rightarrow \text{Fibrin}$$
$$\downarrow$$
$$\text{Clot}$$

Figure 13-4   *Clot formation*

major adverse reaction is hemorrhage. Too high levels of heparin result in mucosal and GI bleeding, which drops both hematocrit and blood pressure. Other adverse reactions include hypersensitivity, hair loss, osteoporosis, and thrombocytopenia.

Warfarin (Coumadin). Oral anticoagulants are very different from heparin because they can be administered by mouth. **Warfarin** resembles vitamin K in its structure and acts as a vitamin K antimetabolite, interfering with a number of clotting factors including thrombin. The onset of action is delayed and may take up to 12–36 hours.

The most common adverse reaction associated with warfarin is hemorrhage. Other adverse reactions include nausea, diarrhea, urticaria, and hair loss. Warfarin interacts with aspirin and other nonsteroidal antiinflammatory drugs (Chapter 7). Antibiotics can potentiate the effects of warfarin because they can inhibit the synthesis of vitamin K, which is reviewed in Chapter 11. Warfarin metabolism is increased by **phenobarbital** and chronic alcohol ingestion. Warfarin metabolism is inhibited by acute alcohol intoxication, **cimetidine, disulfiram,** and **metronidazole.**

There are many dental concerns associated with patients taking warfarin. Patients should be encouraged to bring in their latest prothrombin time (PT) to each dental visit or they should have their PT measured just prior to the visit. PTs greater than two times normal may require a reduction in the warfarin dose. This should be discussed with the patient's physician prior to any procedure or dose reduction. If the dose is reduced, the dental procedure should be scheduled for up to several days after the reduction because of the latent time to onset and recovery of PT times. All dose changes should be discussed with the patient's physician.

Aspirin and nonsteroidal antiinflammatory drugs are contraindicated in these patients because of the increased risk of bleeding. Patients can take acetaminophen or opioid analgesics without aspirin.

Other Anticoagulants. There are several drugs that patients may be taking on a regular basis that are used as anticoagulants. They include **aspirin, ticlopidine** (Ticlid), and **dipyridamole** (Persantine). Aspirin (reviewed in Chapter 7) inhibits platelet aggregation, which prolongs bleeding time. It is used to decrease the incidence of heart attack and/or stroke in patients with previous heart attacks or strokes. Ticlopidine irreversibly inhibits ADP-induced platelet aggregation and is used in patients who cannot tolerate aspirin. Its adverse reactions and dental concerns are similar to aspirin. Dipyridamole also prevents platelet aggregation and is often used in combination with aspirin or warfarin.

Summary

Patients with cardiovascular disease, hypercholesterolemia, and coagulation disorders make up a large percentage of any dental practice. Medications and the illnesses themselves can affect the dental process and treatment. Detailed medication/health histories will help to determine patients' diseases and medications. The dental hygienist should have a general knowledge of the diseases and medications discussed in this chapter. Many of the drugs have adverse reactions, including oral effects, which can influence oral health care. The dental hygienist plays an important role in teaching patients how to manage or avoid these adverse reactions.

Case Study: Nina Papadopulos

Nina Papadopulos is 56 years old and has been coming to your practice for close to 15 years. She has no significant medical/health problems. She takes no prescription medications and only takes acetaminophen when she has a headache. During the maintenance medication/health history she tells you that her sister has been "nagging" her about her diet and insists Mrs. Papadopulos have her cholesterol checked. Mrs. Papadopulos went to the doctor last week and had this done. Her cholesterol was about 200 and her physician just advised her to watch her diet. Unfortunately, Mrs. Papadopulos feels that her sister is driving her crazy about "these numbers" and possible medication. Mrs. Papadopulos's cousin was placed on lovastatin for high cholesterol.

1. What is high cholesterol and what are some contributing factors?
2. What are the different nonpharmacologic methods of lowering cholesterol?
3. What is lovastatin and what is its role in treating high cholesterol?
4. What are the adverse reactions associated with lovastatin?
5. Compare and contrast the different medications used to treat high cholesterol. Include mechanisms of action and adverse reactions.
6. Do any of the cholesterol-lowering medications have any oral adverse reactions? If so, what are they and how should they be managed?

Case Study: Jack Blackstone

Jack Blackstone is 80 years old and had recently suffered a series of small strokes. His physician placed him on coumadin therapy. Mr. Blackstone has come to your practice for his scheduled maintenance visit. He is otherwise healthy (suffered very little residual effects from the stroke) and only takes occasional acetaminophen in addition to his coumadin. Mr. Blackstone needs to have a cavity filled and will return in 1 week. Mr. Blackstone is concerned because he often requires a dose or two of ibuprofen after this type of procedure.

1. What is the concern with coumadin and procedures that may cause bleeding?
2. What is coumadin and how does it work?
3. What are the adverse reactions associated with coumadin and other anticoagulant drugs?
4. What are the dental concerns associated with coumadin?

5. What would you tell Mr. Blackstone about them?
6. Why would Mr. Blackstone be concerned about taking ibuprofen while he is taking coumadin?
7. What should he take for pain relief?

Review Questions

1. What are some of the major cardiovascular contraindications to dental treatment?
2. What are the pharmacologic and adverse reactions associated with digoxin?
3. Describe the dental concerns associated with digoxin. What would you tell your patient about them?
4. Compare and contrast the different classes or groups of antiarrhythmics.
5. Compare and contrast the nitrates and nitrites.
6. What are the dental concerns associated with nitrates and nitrites? What would you tell your patient about them?
7. What are ACE inhibitors and what is their role in the treatment of cardiovascular disease?
8. What is the role of adrenergic antagonists in the treatment of cardiovascular disease and what are the adverse reactions of α and β blockers?

BIBLIOGRAPHY

Anon: Choice of cholesterol-lowering drugs. *Med Lett* 33:1–4, 1991.
Baker DW, Konstam MA, Bottorff M, Pitt B: Management of heart failure: I. Pharmacologic treatment. *JAMA* 272:1361–1366, 1994.
Barak S, Engelberg IS, Hiss J: Gingival hyperplasia caused by nifedipine. Histopathologic findings. *J Periodontol* 58:639–642, 1987.
Bettigole RE: Drugs acting on the blood and blood-forming organs. In Smith CM, Reynard AM (eds.), *Textbook of Pharmacology*, 1st ed. W. B. Saunders Company, Philadelphia, 1992.
Brown RS, Beaver WT, Bottomley WK: On the mechanism of drug-induced gingival hyperplasia. *J Oral Pathol Med* 20:201–209, 1991.
Dracup K, Baker DW, Dunbar SB, et al.: Management of heart failure: II. Counseling, education, and lifestyle modifications. *JAMA* 272:1442–1446, 1994.
Frattore L, Stablein M, Bredfeldt G, et al.: Gingival hyperplasia: A side-effect of nifedipine and diltiazem. *Special Care in Dentistry* 11:107–108, 1991.
Higgins DM, Smith CM: Drugs used in the treatment of angina pectoris. In Smith CM, Reynard AM (eds.), *Textbook of Pharmacology*, 1st ed. W. B. Saunders Company, Philadelphia, 1992.
Joint National Committee on Detection, Evaluation, and Treatment of High Blood Pressure: The fifth report of the Joint National Committee on Detection, Evaluation, and Treatment of High Blood Pressure (JNC V). *Arch Intern Med* 153:154–183, 1993.
Kane JP, et al.: Regression of Coronary atherosclerosis during treatment of familial hypercholesterolemia with combined drug regimens. *JAMA* 264:3007–3012, 1990.

Lathers CM: Treatment of congestive heart failure—digitalis glycosides. In Smith CM, Reynard AM (eds.), *Textbook of Pharmacology*, 1st ed. W. B. Saunders Company, Philadelphia, 1992.

Lathers CM, O'Rourke DK: Antiarrhythmic agents. In Smith CM, Reynard AM (eds.), *Textbook of Pharmacology*, 1st ed. W. B. Saunders Company, Philadelphia, 1992.

McKenney JM: New guidelines for managing hypercholesterolemia. *Am Pharm* NS33:3–11, 1993.

Roccella EJ, Lenfant C: Regional and racial differences among stroke victims in the United States. *Clin Cardiol* 12:IV18–IV22, 1989.

Summary of the second report of the National Cholesterol Education Program: Adult Treatment Panel II: Expert Panel on Detection, Evaluation, and Treatment of High Blood Cholesterol in Adults. *JAMA* 269:3015–3023, 1993.

Tisdale JE, Webb CR: Are antiarrhythmic drugs obsolete? *Clin Pharm* 49:714–726, 1992.

Todd PA, Faulds D: Felodipine. A review of the pharmacology and therapeutic use of the extended release formulation in cardiovascular disorders. *Drugs* 44:251–277, 1992.

Weber MA, Byyny RL, Pratt JH, et al.: Blood pressure effects of the angiotensin II receptor blocker, losartan. *Arch Intern Med* 155:405–411, 1995.

Yedinak KC: Use of calcium channel antagonists for cardiovascular disease. *Am Pharm* NS33:49–64, 1993.

Yedinak KC: Selection and use of beta-blockers for patients with cardiovascular disease. *Am Pharm* NS34:28–36, 1994.

CHAPTER *14*

Treatment of Gastrointestinal Disorders

Key Terms

Antacids
Constipation
Diarrhea
Emesis
Gastroesophageal Reflux Disease

Helicobacter pylori
H$_2$-Receptor Antagonists
Peptic Ulcer Disease
Proton Pump Inhibitors
Sucralfate

LEARNING OBJECTIVES

After completion of this chapter and its learning activities, the student should be able to:

1. Briefly discuss the prevalence of peptic ucler disease.
2. Discuss signs and symptoms of peptic ulcer disease.
3. Discuss the role of antacids in the treatment of peptic ulcer disease.
4. Discuss the role of H$_2$-receptor antagonists in the treatment of peptic ulcer disease.
5. Discuss the role of proton pump inhibitors in the treatment of peptic ulcer disease.
6. Discuss the role of antibiotics in the treatment of peptic ulcer disease.
7. Briefly describe gastroesophageal reflux disease and its therapies.
8. List the medications used to treat diarrhea.
9. List the different types of laxatives and know the advantages and disadvantages of each.
10. Define antiemetics and give examples.

INTRODUCTION

The gastrointestinal (GI) system is responsible for the digestion and absorption of nutrients and the absorption of drugs. This chapter reviews medications used to treat peptic ulcer disease, gastroesophageal reflux disease, and drugs that affect GI motility, including antidiarrheals, and laxatives. Several of these medications can affect the dental process. The dental hygienist should know about these medications, their effect on oral hygiene, and their effects on dental treatment.

PEPTIC ULCER DISEASE

Peptic ulcer disease (PUD) is one of the leading causes of significant morbidity and mortality in the United States. The annual incidence of PUD is 1% and the lifetime prevalence for duodenal ulcers is 10% for men and 5% for women (Soll, 1990). Billions of dollars are spent each year on the diagnosis and treatment of PUD, and this number is further increased when adding in the direct cost of medication and the indirect cost of time lost from work and social activities (Jensen, 1986).

Persons presenting with PUD complain of an aching or boring epigastric pain that is relieved by food or antacids. The pain may radiate to the back or chest and can wake the person up from a sound sleep.

Dental Concerns

Nonsteroidal antiinflammatory drugs (NSAIDs) are a known risk factor for developing a drug-induced ulcer. It is estimated that the risk for developing PUD is 2–11% for those taking NSAIDs compared to 1–2% for the general population (Soll, 1990). The dental hygienist should question the patient carefully about a history of PUD and both prescription and nonprescription use of NSAIDs. NSAIDs should be avoided in these patients.

Pharmacotherapy of Peptic Ulcer Disease

Currently, antacids, H_2-receptor antagonists, **sucralfate,** and proton pump inhibitors are available for the acute treatment of peptic ulcer disease. Acute treatment ranges from 4–6 weeks with proton pump inhibitors to 6–8 weeks with the other treatments. A combination of antibiotics with H_2-receptor antagonists or a proton pump inhibitor is available for the treatment of PUD as a result of *Helicobacter pylori* infection. Sucralfate and H_2-receptor antagonists are used for long-term maintenance therapy of PUD. **Misoprostol,** a synthetic analog of the prostaglandin PGE_2, is available for the prevention of nonsteroidal antiinflammatory drug–induced ulcers.

Antacids. Until 1977 when the H_2-receptor antagonist **cimetidine** came on the market, *antacids* were first-line therapy for PUD. Antacids are still used to treat PUD though usually in conjunction with an H_2-receptor antagonist. Antacids work by partially neutralizing hydrochloric acid in the stomach, thereby raising stomach pH to 3 or 4. This can decrease the erosive effect of acid and reduce pepsin production. There are several antacids available to treat PUD and they are listed in Table 14-1.

ALUMINUM AND MAGNESIUM. **Aluminum hydroxide, magnesium hydroxide,** and **aluminum-magnesium hydroxide gels** are nonsystemic antacids. Aluminum salts cause constipation and magnesium salts cause diarrhea. Both have poor neu-

Table 14-1   Treatment of Peptic Ulcer Disease

Generic Name	Brand Name	Acute Dosing	Maintenance Dose
Antacids			
Magnesium, aluminum hydroxide	Maalox, Mylanta, others	Various doses 1 and 3 hours after meals and at bedtime	
Sucralfate	Sucralfate	2 gm bid or 1 gm qid on an empty stomach	1 gm bid on an emty stomach
H₂-Receptor Antagonists			
Cimetidine	Tagamet	400 mg bid	400 mg/day hs
Famotidine	Pepcid	20 mg bid	20 mg/day hs
Nizatidine	Axid	150 mg bid	150 mg/day hs
Ranitidine	Zantac	150 mg bid	150 mg/day hs
Proton Pump Inhibitors			
Omeprazole	Prilosec	20 mg qd	
Lansoprazole	Prevacid	30 mg qd	
Selected Medication for the Treatment of *H. pylori*			
Bismuth subsalicylate	Pepto-Bismol	Two 262-mg tablets qid × 2 weeks	
Metronidazole	Flagl	250 mg tid–qid × 2 weeks	
Tetracycline or amoxicillin	Various	250–500 mg qid × 2 weeks	
Plus H₂-receptor antagonist	Various	Full dose (acute) at bedtime × 4–6 weeks	

Sources: Graham DY, Lew GM, Klein PD, et al., Effect of treatment of *Helicobacter pylori* infection on the long-term recurrence of gastric or duodenal ulcers. *Ann Intern Med* 116:705–708, 1992; Hentschel E, Brandstatter G, Dragosics B, et al., Effect of ranitidine and amoxicillin plus metronidazole on the eradication of *Helicobacter pylori* and the recurrence of duodenal ulcer, *New Engl J Med* 328:308–312, 1993; NIH Consensus Development Panel on *Helicobacter pylori* in peptic ulcer disease. *JAMA* 272: 65–69, 1994; Pinson JB, Weart CW, Antacid products. In *Handbnook of Nonprescription Drugs*, 10th ed. American Pharmaceutical Association, Washington, DC, 1993, pp. 147–179.

tralizing capabilities when used alone. These agents are used in combination in order to obtain a reasonable effect and to minimize adverse reactions. Antacids can inhibit the GI absorption of **tetracycline, digoxin, iron, chlorpromazine,** and **indomethacin** and increase the GI absorption of **levodopa.**

Disadvantages of aluminum and magnesium antacids include the need for large and frequent doses and storage in large, bulky containers, which are leading causes of noncompliance.

CALCIUM CARBONATE. **Calcium carbonate** is nonsystemic antacid that is effective in neutralizing acid production. However, it can cause acid rebound, kidney stone formation, and constipation. Calcium carbonate antacids are available as

Tums or any number of generic equivalents and are primarily used to treat the symptoms of heartburn.

SODIUM BICARBONATE. **Sodium bicarbonate** (baking soda) is a systemically absorbed antacid that rapidly neutralizes gastric acids. However, it can cause severe alkalosis because of its systemic absorption. It also contains sodium and should be avoided in patients on sodium-restricted diets or cardiovascular patients.

Sucralfate. **Sucralfate** (Table 14-1) is an aluminum hydroxide complex of sucrose that binds selectively to ulcerated tissue. This produces a coating that is impenetrable to hydrochloric acid, pepsin, and bile salts. Adverse reactions are minor and include constipation, diarrhea, and nausea. **Sucralfate** has been reported to decrease the absorption of phenytoin and the quinolones. It is as effective as H_2-receptor antagonists in healing duodenal ulcers.

H_2-Receptor Antagonists. Because of their safety, efficacy, and tolerability, the *H_2-receptor antagonists* (Table 14-1) have become the mainstay of therapy for PUD. They are associated with a healing rate of 78% at 4 weeks and 92% at 8 weeks of therapy in patients with duodenal ulcers. The healing rate is 88% at 8 weeks for patients with gastric ulcers (Feldman and Burton, 1990).

MECHANISM OF ACTION. H_2-receptor antagonists block the binding of histamine, thereby decreasing gastric acid production.

ADVERSE REACTIONS. H_2-receptor antagonists are generally well tolerated. The more common adverse reactions include headache, lethargy, confusion, depression, and hallucinations. They occur more frequently with cimetidine. Cimetidine also has antiandrogenic activity, which may result in gynecomastia and impotence. Famotidine has been associated with dry mouth and taste changes. Granulocytopenia, thrombocytopenia, and neutropenia are hematologic adverse reactions associated with cimetidine. Reversible hepatic and abnormal liver function tests have been reported with all four H_2-receptor antagonists.

DRUG INTERACTIONS. Cimetidine, famotidine, and ranitidine are metabolized primarily by the liver and undergo first-pass metabolism. Cimetidine, and ranitidine to a lesser extent, inhibit the P450 oxidase system in the liver. As a result, cimetidine can decrease the clearance and increase the serum levels of such drugs as warfarin, lidocaine, metronidazole, phenytoin, carbamazepine, and diazepam. Neither famotidine nor nizatidine inhibit the P450 system. Nizatidine undergoes renal excretion. The doses of all three drugs should be decreased in patients with moderate to severe renal failure and liver disease, the elderly, and children.

Concurrent administration of antacids can decrease the absorption of cimetidine, ranitidine, and famotidine. Antacids should not be taken 2 hours before or 2 hours after an H_2-receptor antagonist. H_2-receptor antagonists should be taken with meals to prolong their effect. All H_2-receptor antagonists except famotidine have been shown to inhibit alcohol dehydrogenase and can increase the effects of alcohol.

DENTAL CONCERNS. It is most important to carefully question patients about their use of both prescription and nonprescription H_2-receptor antagonists. Both famotidine (Pepcid AC), cimetidine (Tagamet HB), ranitidine (Zantac 75) and anizatidine (Axid AR) are now available as over-the-counter preparations for the treatment of heartburn and GI upset. Patients often forget that over-the-counter medications have the same adverse reactions and drug interactions as prescription products. The dental practitioner should use caution when lidocaine or diazepam are prescribed for a dental procedure and should use the lowest dose possible to avoid toxicity. The patient should be further advised about the sedating and amnestic effects of diazepam.

Proton Pump Inhibitors. **Proton pump inhibitors** are the newest class of medications to treat PUD (Table 14-1).

MECHANISM OF ACTION. Proton pump inhibitors irreversibly bind to the proton pump, which results in 90% or greater reduction in gastric acid secretion over 24 hours. They are indicated for the treatment of active duodenal ulcers, erosive esophagitis and the control of symptomatic gastroesophageal reflux disease (GERD) that is poorly responsive to customary medical treatment.

ADVERSE REACTIONS. Adverse reactions include abdominal pain and headache. Oral adverse reactions include esophageal candidiasis, mucosal atrophy of the tongue, and dry mouth. In rats, **omeprazole** has been noted to produce gastric carcinoid tumors. This is probably due to achlorhydria and hypergastremia. This effect has not been observed with short-term use in humans. Also several long-term studies for the treatment of GERD have been completed and there has been no evidence of gastric carcinoid tumors in humans (personal communication, Astra Merck, 1995).

DENTAL CONCERNS. A careful examination should be performed of the oral cavity of patients taking proton pump inhibitors for the presence of candidiasis, mucosal atrophy, and dry mouth. Instruct all patients on methods to avoid or minimize dry mouth. They include chewing sugarless gum, sucking on tart, sour sugarless candy, and drinking plenty of water. Patients should avoid all caffeine-containing beverages and fruit juices. Caffeine can exacerbate dry mouth and fruit juices can increase the likelihood of dental caries. Also, stress the importance of good oral hygiene and regular dental examinations. The dental practitioner should keep in mind that these medications are still new and the incidence of reported oral adverse reactions may be low. Question your patient carefully about any problems with oral adverse reactions.

Antiinfective Therapy. An area of growing research in PUD is the role of the gram-negative bacillus *Helicobacter pylori*. The organism is found in 95% of patients with duodenal ulcers and 75% percent of patients with gastric ulcers, although its relationship to the development of PUD is unknown (Blaser, 1987; Dooley and Cohen, 1988). The prevalence of colonization increases with age and is more common in socioeconomically deprived patients and patients living in custodial institutions.

Several studies have shown the eradication of this organism with a combination of bismuth and one or two antibiotics (NIH Consensus Development Panel, 1994; Graham et al., 1992; Hentschel et al., 1993). H_2-receptor antagonists or omeprazole are prescribed in conjunction with **bismuth** and antibiotics to help alleviate ulcer pain

(Table 14-1). This therapy should be considered in patients with evidence of *H. pylori* infection, especially if they have recurrent or persistent symptoms despite an appropriate course of traditional antiulcer therapy.

Prostaglandins. Misoprostol (Cytotec) is a synthetic analog of prostaglandin PGE_2 that stimulates gastric mucosal defenses, thereby decreasing gastric acid production. It is indicated for the prevention of NSAID-induced gastric ulcers. Its adverse reactions include GI discomfort and diarrhea. It is FDA (Food and Drug Administration) category X because of its ability to stimulate uterine contractions.

GASTROESOPHAGEAL REFLUX DISEASE

Gastroesophageal reflux disease (GERD) is a multifactorial process that involves lower esophageal sphincter (LES) incompetence, abnormal esophageal clearance, delayed gastric emptying, and the irritating effects of gastric contents. Almost 40% of Americans experience heartburn—the most common symptom of reflux—at least once a month, and up to 91% of patients with GERD experience nocturnal heartburn (Spechler, 1992; Demeester et al., 1976). GERD patients with nocturnal heartburn are more at risk for developing esophagitis and strictures from long term acid exposure.

Treatment

Lifestyle modifications along with medication appear to be the best defense in treating GERD. Lifestyle changes include elevating the head of the bed and avoiding alcohol, tobacco, and fatty foods. Therapies include antacids, H_2-receptor antagonists, and proton pump inhibitors and are reviewed in the peptic ulcer disease section. These medications neutralize or suppress acid production, which reduces acidity and the erosive quality of the refluxate.

Prokinetic agents are designed to address the upper GI tract and offer a more direct approach to treating the underlying physiologic causes of reflux.

Metoclopramide (Reglan). **Metoclopramide** stimulates the motility of the upper GI tract without stimulating secretions. It relaxes the pyloric sphincter and increases peristalsis in the duodenum, which results in an accelerated gastric emptying time. The medication is also used as an antiemetic. It blocks dopamine receptors and can cause Parkinson-like reactions. Other adverse reactions include sedation, restlessness, drowsiness, and fatigue. Added CNS depression can occur when other CNS depressants are used with this medication.

Cisapride (Propulsid). **Cisapride** is the newest medication in the treatment of GERD. Cisapride works by selectively stimulating the motor components of the GI tract. This action stimulates coordinated smooth muscle contraction, increases LES tone, improves esophageal peristalsis, and promotes gastric emptying; it has no effect on gastric secretion. Cisapride enhances the release of acetylcholine in the GI tract and it does not block dopamine receptors. Adverse reactions include headache, diarrhea, abdominal pain, nausea, rhinitis, and constipation. Because this drug accelerates gastric emptying time it may affect the absorption of other drugs.

Dental Concerns

Patients with GERD may experience reflux while lying back in the examination chair. It may be beneficial to elevate the head of the chair. Older medications such as metoclopramide may cause such Parkinson-like symptoms as dry mouth, which can adversely affect oral hygiene. Review the different ways of helping to avoid or minimize dry mouth with your patients as discussed previously. Patients may also experience muscle stiffness, acute dystonia, and other extrapyramidal symptoms associated with dopamine blockade. Extrapyramidal symptoms may make it impossible for the patient to practice good oral hygiene or sit for a dental examination.

CONSTIPATION

Constipation is a decrease in frequency of fecal elimination and is characterized by the passage of hard, dry stools. It is difficult to determine whether or not a person is constipated because normal frequency varies from 3 times per day to 3 times per week. Several conditions such as poor bowel habits, inadequate dietary fiber intake, inadequate fluid intake, narcotic drugs, anticholinergic drugs, and emotional stress can cause constipation. In addition, there can be underlying medical and pathophysiologic causes.

Pharmacologic Treatment

Several classes of medications are available to treat constipation and should only be used on a short-term basis. The different types of laxatives are reviewed in Table 14-2.

Bulk Laxatives. Inert, nonabsorbable substances, bulk laxatives that absorb and retain water, increase fecal mass, and increase rate of defecation. They are safe and approximate most closely the physiologic function of defecation.

Stool Softeners and Lubricants. Stool softeners wet and soften the stool by absorbing water in the intestine. Lubricants, such as mineral oil, were used frequently but are no longer recommended. Long-term use of lubricants can interfere with the absorption of the fat-soluble vitamins A, D, E, and K.

Saline Laxatives. Saline laxatives are potent, relatively nonabsorbable inorganic salts. They work by osmotically pulling water into the bowel and causing loose, watery stools within 1–3 hours. They are primarily used to evacuate the bowel for endoscopic examination and in preparation of bowel surgery.

Hyperosmotic Laxatives. The most common hyperosmotic laxative is the **glycerin** suppository. The laxative effect of glycerin is due to the combination of glycerin's osmotic effect with the local irritant effect of sodium stearate, which may cause rectal irritation.

Stimulant Laxatives. Stimulant laxatives work by increasing the propulsive peristaltic activity of the intestine by local irritation of the mucosa. Stimulants are usually used before radiologic examination of the GI tract and before bowel surgery. This type of laxative should not be used for simple constipation.

Table 14-2   Medications That Alter Gastrointestinal Function

Treatments	Drug Class	Drug Name
Laxatives	Bulk	Psyllium seed (Metamucil)
	Stool Softener	Dioctyl sodium sulfosuccinate (Colace)
	Lubricant	Mineral oil
	Saline	Magnesium citrate
	Hyperosmotic	Glycerin
	Stimulants	Senna (Senekot)
		Bisacodyl (Dulcolax)
Antidiarrheals	Opioids	Diphenoxylate (Lomotil)
		Loperamide (Imodium)
		Paregoric
	Absorbents	Kaolin + pectin (Kaopectate)
Antiemetics	Anticholinergic	Cyclizine (Marezine)
		Dimenhydrinate (Dramamine)
		Hydroxyzine (Atarax)
		Meclizine (Bonine)
		Scopolamine (Transderm-Scop)
		Trimethobenzamide (Tigan)
	Phenothiazines	Prochlorperazine (Compazine)
	Cannabinoids	Dronabinol (Marinol)
		Nabilone (Cesamet)

Sources: Curry CE Jr., Tatum-Butler D, Laxative products. In *Handbook of Prescription Drugs*, 10th ed. American Pharmaceutical Association, Washington, DC, 1993; Goodman Gilman A, Rall TW, Nies AS, Taylor P (eds.), *Goodman and Gilman's The Pharmacological Basis of Therapeutics*. Pergamon Press, New York, 1990; Longe RL, Antidiarrheal products. In *Handbook of Nonprescription Drugs*, 10th ed. American Pharmaceutical Association, Washington, DC, 1993.

DIARRHEA

Diarrhea is a symptom of increased GI motility and can either be acute or chronic. Acute diarrhea can occur very quickly and can be the result of infection, drugs, diet, or toxins. Chronic diarrhea may be the result of organ pathology. Both can lead to dehydration and electrolyte imbalance.

Pharmacologic Treatment of Diarrhea

Antidiarrheals are used to minimize fluid loss and electrolyte imbalances. The opioids (Table 14-2) are among the most effective antidiarrheals used today. They decrease the intestinal motility by acting on the smooth muscle of the small intestine thereby causing localized spasms that break up normal propelling activity of peristalsis.

Absorbents are designed to absorb the causative bacteria, virus, or toxin. Most of these agents are available without a prescription and the most common is **kaolin** and **pectin** (Kaopectate).

Dental Concerns

Dry mouth is a common adverse reaction of antidiarrheal medications. Review with the patient the steps necessary to avoid or minimize dry mouth. They have been discussed Chapter 3. Stress the importance of good oral hygiene and regular dental examinations.

Opioid antidiarrheal medications are also sedating. Use caution if an opioid analgesic, antianxiety agent, or any other medication that may cause sedation is prescribed. Counsel the patient about the likelihood of increased sedation and the potential for other central nervous system effects such as confusion, hallucinations, and fatigue. Encourage the patient to have someone drive her to and from her appointment. The patient should also be instructed not to perform any tasks that require thought or concentration (e.g., driving a car, operating heavy machinery, watching the children).

EMESIS

Vomiting may be the result of a bacterial or viral infection, motion sickness, drugs, radiation therapy, or pregnancy. In certain instances the treatment may depend on the cause of vomiting.

Pharmacologic Treatment

There are several different classes of drugs used to treat *emesis* and they are discussed next. These drugs are listed in Table 14-2.

Anticholinergic. Commonly used to treat nausea and vomiting due to motion sickness, examples of anticholinergic agents include **dimenhydrinate, meclizine,** and **scopolamine.** Scopolamine is available as a transdermal patch that is placed behind the ear and releases medication over a 3 day period. Adverse reactions include sedation, dry mouth, blurred vision, constipation, and urinary retention.

Trimethobenzamide is also an anticholinergic agent though its mechanism of action is different. It works by suppressing the chemoreceptor trigger zone. Its adverse reactions include sedation, headache, dry mouth, and agitation. The suppository dose form contains **benzocaine** and should be avoided in patients who are allergic to ester local anesthetics.

Antipsychotics. Phenothiazines are used to control severe nausea and vomiting and are available in oral and suppository dose forms. The adverse reactions of this class of medication are reviewed in Chapter 21. **Promethazine** has been used in dentistry to treat nausea and vomiting associated with surgery and anesthesia.

Cannabinoids. Cannabinoid antiemetics, **dronabinol** and **nabilone,** are used to treat nausea and vomiting associated with cancer chemotherapy in patients who have failed to respond to traditional antiemetic therapies. These agents are derived from the *Cannabis sativa L.* (marijuana) plant and produce similar effects. They are abusable and tolerance and dependence can result. Close supervision is required and adverse reactions include sedation, drowsiness, dizziness, perceptual difficulties, and confused thoughts.

Dental Concerns

Dry mouth is a common adverse reaction of many antiemetics. Review with the patient the steps necessary to avoid or minimize dry mouth. They are discussed in Chapter 3. Stress the importance of good oral hygiene and regular dental examinations.

Antiemetic medications can also be sedating. Use caution if an opioid analgesic, antianxiety agent, or any other medication that may cause sedation is prescribed. Again, counsel the patient about the likelihood of increased sedation and the potential for other central nervous system effects such as confusion, hallucinations, and fatigue. Encourage the patient to have someone drive him to and from his appointment. The patient should also be instructed not to perform any tasks that require thought or concentration (e.g., driving a car, operating heavy machinery, watching the children) if these medications are combined.

Summary

Peptic ulcer disease occurs within a large segment of the U.S. population. Causes are many and include medications. Nonsteroidal antiinflammatory drugs are one of the main causes of drug-induced peptic ulcer disease. The dental practitioner should carefully question patients about a history of peptic ulcer disease. NSAIDs should be avoided in patients with ulcers. However, NSAIDs can be taken if the patient is currently taking misoprostol which is a prostaglandin used to treat drug-induced peptic ulcer disease.

H_2-receptor antagonists, sucralfate, proton pump inhibitors, and antacids are used to treat peptic ulcer disease. Antibiotics are also being used to treat peptic ulcer disease due to *Helicobacter pylori* infection. Several of these medications have oral adverse reactions and some medications interact with sedating drugs prescribed from a dental office. The effects of these adverse reactions and drug interactions should be reviewed with the patient.

Gastroesophageal reflux disease occurs in a great number of patients. Lying back in a dental chair will often cause the patient to experience symptoms associated with GERD. Patients should sit in an upright position to help avoid this possibility. Medications used to treat GERD include H_2-receptor antagonists, proton pump inhibitors, sucralfate, antacids, metoclopramide, and cisapride. Several of these drugs have oral adverse reactions and drug interactions that should be reviewed with the patient.

There are many medications available to treat disorders such as constipation, diarrhea, and emesis. Many of the drugs used to treat these disorders cause dry mouth, sedation, confusion, and other CNS adverse reactions. The dental practitioner should address these adverse reactions with the patient and review the treatment of dry mouth. Caution should be used if CNS depressant drugs are prescribed.

Gastrointestinal disorders are common disorders for which many people take medications. These disorders and the medications used to treat them can interfere with dental treatment and oral hygiene. The dental hygienist should know about them and how to effectively counsel patients about them.

Case Study: Linda Thompson

Linda Thompson is 45-year-old executive with a local advertising agency and is new to your practice. Upon completion of her medication health history you learn that she is on omeprazole 20 mg for a duodenal ulcer that just won't heal. Her job is rather stressful and she is continually working late to meet deadlines. As a result, Ms. Thompson drinks approximately 10 cups of coffee a day, which is down from her normal 15–20 cups per day. Unfortunately, she frequents fast-food places for lunch and snacks. She tries to keep dinner with her family somewhat healthy. Ms. Thompson's other medications include nonprescription ibuprofen for headaches and other aches and pains and she has recently purchased Pepcid AC for heartburn. She takes at least 600–1200 mg of ibuprofen every 2–3 days.

1. What is the prevalence of PUD in the United States and why is this of great importance?
2. What is omeprazole and what is its role in the treatment of peptic ulcer disease?
3. What are the adverse reactions associated with omeprazole?
4. Are there any dental concerns associated with omeprazole? What should Ms. Thompson be told about them?
5. What is the role of NSAIDs in peptic ulcer disease?
6. What medication is appropriate to treat or prevent NSAID-induced PUD? How does this medication work?
7. What is Pepcid AC and what are some of its dental concerns?
8. What would a dental practitioner tell Ms. Thompson about Pepcid AC and other over-the-counter drugs H_2-receptor antagonists?

Case Study: Al Salvatori

Al Salvatori is a 56-year-old who has been coming to your practice for several years. He is slightly overweight and except for some problems with an occasional ulcer flair up and heartburn he is healthy. He is currently taking antacids to treat his heartburn and "ulcer" symptoms. Prior to starting your examination you review his health over the past 6 months. Mr. Salvatori tells you that he is on a new medication for his GI problems. It seems that he is also having problems with intense heartburn, especially at night. His provider diagnosed him with GERD and placed Mr. Salvatori on a new medication called cisapride 10 mg before meals and at bedtime.

1. What is the pathophysiology of GERD?
2. What are some of the risk factors of GERD?

3. What is the role of antacids, H_2-receptor antagonists, and proton pump inhibitors in the treatment of GERD?
4. What are prokinetic agents and what is the role of older drugs in the treatment of GERD?
5. What is cisapride? Include mechanism of action, adverse reactions, and any dental concerns.
6. What are the dental concerns associated with the medications used to treat GERD?
7. What are some dental concerns of GERD?
8. What would the dental practitioner tell Mr. Salvatori about these dental concerns?

Review Questions

1. What is the role of antacids in the treatment of PUD?
2. Compare and contrast the different antacids.
3. Are there any dental concerns associated with antacids? What would the dental practitioner tell the patient about them?
4. What is the role of sucralfate in the treatment of PUD?
5. What is the rationale for using antibiotics to treat PUD?
6. What are the different types of antiemetics and how do they work? What are the dental concerns associated with antiemetics?
7. What are the different types of laxatives? Give the advantages and disadvantages of each.
8. What are the different types of antidiarrheals. What are the dental concerns associated with antidiarrheals?

BIBLIOGRAPHY

Blaser MJ: *Campylobacter*-like organisms, gastritis, and peptic ulcer disease. *Gastroenterology* 93:371–383, 1987.

Curry CE Jr., Tatum-Butler D: Laxative products. In *Handbook of Prescription Drugs*, 10th ed. American Pharmaceutical Association, Washington, DC, 1993.

Demeester TR, Johnson LF, Joseph GJ, et al.: Patterns of gastroesophageal reflux in health and disease. *Ann Surg* 184:459– 470, 1976.

Dooley CP, Cohen H: The clinical significance of *Campylobacter pylori*. *Ann Intern Med* 108:70–79, 1988.

Ebell MH: Peptic ulcer disease. *Am Fam Phys* 46:217–227, 1992.

Feldman M, Burton ME: Histamine$_2$-receptor antagonists. Standard therapy for acid-peptic disease. Part II. *New Engl J Med* 325:1749–1755, 1990.

Goodman Gilman A, Rall TW, Nies AS, Taylor P (eds.): *Goodman and Gilman's The Pharmacological Basis of Therapeutics*. Pergamon Press, New York, 1990.

Graham DY, Lew GM, Klein PD, et al.: Effect of treatment of *Helicobacter pylori* infection on the long-term recurrence of gastric or duodenal ulcers. *Ann Intern Med* 116:705–708, 1992.

Hentschel E, Brandstatter G, Dragosics B, et al.: Effect of ranitidine an amoxicillin plus metronidazole on the eradication of *Helicobacter pylori* and the recurrence of duodenal ulcer. *New Engl J Med* 328:308–312, 1993.

Hixson LJ, Kelley CL, Harper WN, et al.: Current trends in the pharmacotherapy for peptic ulcer disease. *Arch Intern Med* 152:726–732, 1992.

Jensen DM: Economic and health aspects of peptic ulcer disease and H_2-receptor antagonists. *Am J Med* 81(Suppl 4B):42–48, 1986.

Koppelo KJ, Kaplan B: Management of gastroesophageal reflux disease. *J Amer Pharm Assoc* NS36:16–26, 1996

Longe RL: Antidiarrheal products. In *Handbook of Nonprescription Drugs*, 10th ed., American Pharmaceutical Association, Washington, DC, 1993.

Maton PN: Omeprazole. *New Engl J Med* 324:965–975, 1991.

NIH Consensus Development Panel on *Helicobacter pylori* in Peptic Ulcer Disease: *Helicobacter pylori* in peptic ulcer disease. *JAMA* 272:65–69, 1994.

Pinson JB, Weart CW: Antacid products. In *Handbook of Nonprescription Drugs*, 10th ed. American Pharmaceutical Association, Washington, DC, 1993, pp. 147–179.

Soll AH: Pathogenesis of peptic ulcer disease and implications for therapy. *N Engl J Med* 322:909–916, 1990.

Spechler SJ: Comparison of medical and surgical therapy for complicated gastroesophageal reflux disease in veterans. *N Engl J Med* 326:786–792, 1992.

Wilson DE: Antisecretory and mucosal protective actions of misoprostol. Potential role in the treatment of peptic ulcer disease. *Am J Med* 83(Suppl 1A):2–8, 1987.

CHAPTER 15

Treatment of Respiratory Disorders

Key Terms

Anticholinergic
Antitussive
Asthma
Beta-Adrenergic Agonists

Chronic Obstructive Pulmonary Disease
Corticosteroids
Expectorants
Methylxanthines

LEARNING OBJECTIVES

After completion of this chapter and its learning activities, the student should be able to:

1. Briefly define asthma and chronic obstructive pulmonary disease.
2. Briefly review the pathophysiology and prevalence of asthma.
3. Briefly review the classification of asthma.
4. Briefly review the pathophysiology, prevalence, and risk factors associated with chronic obstructive pulmonary disease.
5. Review the different classes of medications used to treat asthma including mechanism of action, adverse reactions, and drug interactions.
6. Review the different classes of medications used to treat chronic obstructive pulmonary disease including mechanism of action, adverse reactions, and drug interactions.
7. Discuss the oral adverse effects associated with oral metered-dose inhalers.
8. Counsel a patient on appropriate oral hygiene following the use of an oral metered-dose inhaler.
9. Define mucolytic, antitussive, expectorant, and decongestant.
10. List the different types of medications available to treat the different types of cough.

INTRODUCTION

Respiratory illnesses are common illnesses and the dental hygienist will encounter patients taking one or more medications to treat them. Several of these medications can effect oral hygiene and dental treatment. The dental hygienist should know about these medications and how they affect the patient and dental therapy.

ASTHMA AND CHRONIC OBSTRUCTIVE PULMONARY DISEASE

Asthma is a chronic illness associated with periods of remission and acute exacerbations. Approximately 12 million Americans are affected and 2–5 million cases are in children. The prevalence has increased 29% and deaths from asthma have increased 31% from 1980 to 1987 (Scheffer, 1991).

The signs and symptoms of asthma include coughing, wheezing, shortness of breath, chest tightness, and increased sputum production. Asthma is the result of exaggerated bronchoconstriction caused by a hyperresponsiveness of the airway resulting in a reversible airway obstruction. The hyperresponsiveness is due to inflammation of the air passages in which any one of the following stimuli can induce an attack: exercise, stress, cold weather, humidity, allergens, environmental irritants, pulmonary infections, chemicals, and other medications.

Aspirin and other nonsteroidal antiinflammatory drugs (NSAIDs) have been reported to precipitate asthma attacks. Patients should be carefully questioned about known precipitants of their asthma attacks and a history of use of aspirin and other NSAIDs. These medications should be avoided in patients with asthma.

More than 11 million people suffer from *chronic obstructive pulmonary disease* (COPD) (Lenfant, 1982). COPD is characterized by irreversible airway obstruction with either chronic bronchitis or emphysema. Eighty to ninety percent of all cases are due to cigarette smoking, pollution, and occupational irritants (Anon, 1986). Chronic bronchitis is a result of chronic inflammation of the airways with excessive sputum production. Emphysema is due to an irreversible destruction of the alveoli with air space enlargement and airway collapse. Cessation of cigarette smoking will halt the progression of emphysema.

Dental Concerns

Patients with severe COPD can develop pulmonary hypertension when in a stressful situation. This can place them at risk for developing cardiac arrhythmias. Avoid stressful situations by carefully questioning the patient about previous dental visits and experiences and schedule appointments early in the morning to help minimize stress. Also, keep the appointment as short as possible.

Pharmacotherapy of Asthma and COPD

Asthma therapy has evolved over the past several years from the use of oral medications to oral metered-dose inhalers (MDIs) as the mainstay of therapy. Almost all asthma medications are available as MDIs. Asthma can be treated with corticosteroids, β-adrenergic agonists, anticholinergic agents, nonsteroidal antiinflammatory drugs, or methylxanthines. The drug of choice is dependent on the patient and his symptoms.

Chronic bronchitis is treated with β-adrenergic agonists, anticholinergics, expectorants, and antitussives. Antibiotics are routinely used to treat acute exacerbations of chronic bronchitis and are reviewed in Chapter 6. Expectorants and antitussives provide symptomatic treatment for cough and other upper respiratory symptoms and are further reviewed later in this chapter. Emphysema is treated with methylxanthines, β-adrenergic agonists, and anticholinergic agents. The main goal of therapy is to allow the patient to breathe better with her remaining healthy lung capacity.

Corticosteroids. Among the more effective therapies available to treat asthma are corticosteroids They may be administered orally, intravenously, or much more safely, by oral inhalation. Steroids work by inhibiting airway inflammation at all levels of the respiratory passage and by increasing the number and responsiveness of β_2 receptors.

ACUTE THERAPY. Acute exacerbations of asthma can be treated with tapering "pulse" doses of systemic steroids.

MAINTENANCE THERAPY. At one time, steroids were limited to those patients who were nonresponsive to other therapies because of their adverse reactions, which are discussed in detail in Chapter 17. Today, patients are treated primarily by oral inhalation and may receive alternate-day or daily doses of steroids if they have severe asthma.

INHALED STEROIDS. Inhaled steroids are indicated for maintenance therapy of mild to severe asthma and are reviewed in Table 15-1. It is recommended that inhaled steroids be added early on in the treatment of patients failing to attain adequate control with an antiinflammatory drug or a β-adrenergic agonist. Patients using inhaled steroids have a significant improvement in pulmonary function with decreased wheezing, shortness of breath, chest tightness, and cough. Oral, inhaled steroids are not indicated for treating an acute attack. They must be administered for at least 7 days to be therapeutically effective.

ADVERSE REACTIONS. Systemic adverse reactions are not seen as frequently with oral inhalation as with oral tablets or intravenous dose forms. Systemic adverse reactions are often due to the route of administration, frequency of intake, total dose, and preexisting conditions. Prolonged use of oral steroids can lead to adrenal suppression, poor wound healing, and immunosuppression. Prolonged use of oral, inhaled steroids does not appear to suppress adrenal function. Local, oropharyngeal adverse reactions are more common with oral, inhaled steroids. They include *dysphonia* or hoarseness, dry mouth, and cough.

DENTAL CONCERNS. Since continuous dosing of oral steroids can lead to adrenal suppression, poor wound healing, and immunosuppression, it is very

Table 15-1   Oral, Inhaled Corticosteroid Therapy for Asthma

Generic Name	*Trade Name*	*Usual Daily Dose*
Beclomethasone	Beclovent	2 puffs every 6–8 hours
	Vanceril	2 puffs every 6–8 hours
Flunisolide	Aerobid	2 puffs every 12 hours
Triamcinolone	Azmacort	2 puffs every 6-8 hours

important that the dental hygienist carefully review the patient's medication at each office visit. It may be necessary to temporarily increase the oral steroid dose of the patient prior to a dental procedure because of adrenal suppression. Also, an antibiotic may be warranted postprocedure because of the risk of poor wound healing and immunosuppression.

Dental hygienists should also counsel patients about the proper use of MDIs. They should carefully examine patients using oral inhalers for oral candidiasis. Counsel patients about the need to rinse and gargle after each use of the MDI. Good oral hygiene will help to reduce the incidence of oral candidiasis, dysphonia, dry mouth, and cough.

Beta-Adrenergic Agonists. The mainstay of asthma therapy, *β-adrenergic agonists* are also used in the treatment of COPD. Table 15-2 reviews available oral, inhaled β-adrenergic agonists. The older, catecholamine compounds are nonspecific for α, β_1, and β_2 receptors and include **epinephrine, isoproterenol,** and **isoetharine.** The majority of the noncatecholamine compounds are selective for β_2 receptors. The selective β_2 agonists are available orally, parenterally, by inhalation, and by nebulizer.

The therapeutic effects of β-adrenergic agonists include (1) relaxation of airway smooth muscle, (2) increased ciliary movement, which can improve secretion clearance, and (3) effects on the mast cell to moderate mediator release, thereby causing bronchodilation in the lungs.

ACUTE THERAPY. Beta-adrenergic agonists are important medications for the control of breakthrough (acute) asthma symptoms. Oral, inhaled β-adrenergic agonists provide a rapid reversal of acute asthmatic symptoms within minutes. The nebulizer dose form provides an effective means of delivering medication to the lower air passages during an acute attack or a viral infection. Intravenous epinephrine can also be used to treat an acute attack.

MAINTENANCE THERAPY. Beta-adrenergic agonists are indicated for mild or intermittent asthma. With intermittent asthma, the patient only uses the MDI when she is experiencing symptoms. The inhaled preparation is the preferred

Table 15-2 Oral, Inhaled β-Adrenergic Agonists

Generic Name	Trade Name	Usual Daily Dose
Albuterol	Proventil	2 puffs every 6 hours
	Ventolin	2 puffs every 4–6 hours
Bitolterol	Tornalate	2–3 puffs every 8 hours, no more than 3 puffs every 6 hours or 2 puffs every 4 hours
Metaproterenol	Alupent	2–3 puffs every 4 hours, no more than 12 puffs/day
	Metaprel	2–3 puffs every 3–4 hours, no more than 12 puffs/day
Pirbuterol	Maxair	2 puffs every 4–6 hours, no more than 12 puffs/day
Salmeterol	Serevent	2 puffs every 12 hours
Terbutaline	Brethaire	2 puffs every 4–6 hours

dose form because it provides a greater degree of bronchodilation, less adverse reactions, and a faster onset than oral preparations. The oral, sustained-release tablets are helpful for patients with nighttime symptoms or for patients who cannot tolerate the MDI.

Chronic therapy with MDIs and oral tablets may lead to receptor subsensitivity. This can be managed with a short course of oral steroid therapy or the concurrent use of an oral, inhaled steroid preparation.

PROPHYLACTIC THERAPY. Prophylactic therapy is indicated for exercise-induced asthma. Oral, inhaled β-adrenergic agonists are used approximately 10–15 minutes prior to exercise and as needed. β-adrenergic agonists are the drugs of choice and can prevent an attack from developing for at least 10–12 hours.

ADVERSE REACTIONS. Adverse reactions include nervousness, tachycardia, and insomnia. There have been concerns about the increased incidence of cardiac adverse reactions and deaths associated with oral, inhaled β-adrenergic agonists. The majority of the problems were associated with incorrect use of the MDI. Patients were not associating the increased attacks with poor control of their symptoms and continued to use the inhaler instead of returning to their physician. The correct use of the MDI and a good knowledge base about asthma has helped to reduce the number of patients experiencing problems.

DENTAL CONCERNS. Because these agents can increase heart rate, it is a good idea to measure a patient's blood pressure and pulse prior to administering a local anesthetic with a vasoconstrictor or prior to a dental procedure. Patients may also experience dry mouth with the inhalers. The patient should be counseled to rinse his mouth out after each use and to use good, daily oral hygiene.

Antiinflammatory Agents. **Cromolyn sodium** and **nedocromil sodium** (Table 15-3) are anti-inflammatory agents that prevent mast cell mediator release. Mast cells release histamine, leukotrienes, and other substances when exposed to antigens. Cromolyn sodium and nedocromil sodium prevent the influx of calcium ions into the cell, thereby preventing mast cell rupture.

MAINTENANCE THERAPY. Both drugs are indicated for the treatment of mild to moderate asthma. Cromolyn sodium is recommended as first-line therapy for children because of its safety profile and extensive clinical experience. The MDI, spinhaler, and nebulizer are used in maintenance therapy. The nebulizer is use-

Table 15-3   Oral, Inhaled Antiinflammatory Agents

Generic Name	Trade Name	Symptomatic Therapy	Maintenance Therapy
Cromolyn sodium	Intal	2–4 puffs qid for approximately 1–3 weeks or until symptoms stabilize	2 puffs qid
Nedocromil sodium	Tilade	2 puffs qid	2 puffs bid to qid

ful for patients who cannot use an MDI, young children, patients with upper respiratory inflammation, or patients intolerant to the aerosol propellant or spinhaler powder.

PROPHYLACTIC THERAPY. Cromolyn sodium has been shown to be clinically effective in the prophylactic treatment of seasonal and perennial allergic asthma as well as animal, occupational, and irritant-induced asthma. Drug therapy should be started 7–10 days prior to seasonal or perennial or other allergen exposure to gain maximum therapeutic effects. Cromolyn sodium and nedocromil are second line for the treatment of exercise-induced asthma. They should be inhaled approximately 10–15 minutes prior to exercise or prior to cold weather exposure. Neither medication is indicated for the treatment of acute asthmatic symptoms.

ADVERSE REACTIONS. Adverse reactions include bronchospasm, wheezing, and cough. There have been reports of dizziness, headache, and nausea.

DENTAL CONCERNS. The patient should be counseled to rinse carefully after each use. The spinhaler and MDI can cause dry mouth and the powder from the spinhaler may leave a bitter aftertaste. Remind the patient about the importance of good oral hygiene.

Anticholinergic Agents. Anticholinergic agents, such as **ipratroprium bromide** (Atrovent), decrease intrinsic vagal tone to the airway, which results in bronchodilation. This medication also helps to block reflex bronchoconstriction.

MAINTENANCE THERAPY. Ipratroprium bromide can reduce the hyperactivity present in patients with asthma, emphysema, and chronic bronchitis. It appears to be effective in patients with cold air or humid air-induced asthma. It can be used alone or in combination with a β_2-adrenergic agonist and is administered as a metered-dose inhalation of 2 puffs every 6 hours.

ADVERSE REACTIONS. Ipratroprium bromide has a much lower adverse reaction profile than oral anticholinergic medications (Chapter 3). Adverse reactions include dry mouth and bad taste.

DENTAL CONCERNS. Dry mouth and bad taste can be minimized by counseling the patient to gargle and rinse well after each use. Remind the patient about the need for good oral hygiene. The patient should also be instructed to drink water or suck on sugarless candy or chew sugarless gum for lingering dry mouth or bad after taste.

Metered-Dose Inhalers. The current trend in asthma treatment involves the use of a number of pharmacologic agents administered orally via an MDI or a dry-powder inhaler (Figure 15-1). When used correctly, MDIs are equally as effective as nebulizers and spacers. MDIs deliver the medication directly to the bronchioles, thereby minimizing systemic effects and producing greater bronchodilation than a comparable oral dose. The onset of action of medication administered via an MDI is rapid and predictable as compared to oral medications. Lastly, MDIs are compact, portable, and sterile.

The main problem with MDIs is that many patients do not use them correctly. Most patients require repeated instructions and review of their technique at follow-up visits. Spacer devices are available to help improve delivery of MDI medication. Spacers reduce hand-lung coordination requirements, decrease oropharyngeal deposition, and enhance pulmonary deposition of medication. They are indicated for any-one having difficulty with proper MDI technique, especially preschool-age children and the elderly. They are also recommended for patients receiving inhaled steroids. Spacers help to decrease the risk of developing oropharyngeal candidiasis and en-hance efficacy even if the MDI technique is optimal.

Methylxanthines. **Theophylline,** along with caffeine and theobromine, belong to the class of medications called the *methylxanthines*. Theophylline administration pro-duces mild to moderate bronchodilation and decreases respiratory muscle fatigue. Theophylline is thought to produce its bronchodilatory effect by inhibiting the action of phosphodiesterase, which indirectly increases the available levels of cAMP (cyclic adenosine monophosphate).

ACUTE AND MAINTENANCE THERAPY. In the 1970s and 1980s theophylline was the primary choice for the treatment of acute and chronic asthma. Theo-phylline is available in tablet, capsules, and liquid dose forms and is available as the generic equivalent or by various trade names (Theodur, Theobid, Slobid, Slo-phyllin). Today, theophylline is considered to be second- or third-line therapy because of our better understanding of the pathophysiology of asthma and the availability of safer, more effective medications. It is used to control nocturnal asth-ma symptoms and for those asthmatic patients not easily controlled by oral, inhaled cromolyn sodium or oral, inhaled steroids. Theophylline is also used as maintenance therapy for patients with emphysema.

ADVERSE REACTIONS. Patients taking theophylline must have their blood drawn periodically to make sure that they are being dosed appropriately. The early signs of theophylline toxicity include nausea, vomiting, restlessness, and anxiety. Severe signs of toxicity include seizures and arrhythmias. The early signs of toxi-city do not always precede severe toxic effects.

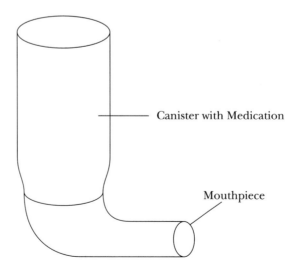

Figure 15-1   *Metered-dose inhaler*

DRUG INTERACTIONS. Theophylline is metabolized in the liver via the P450 hepatic system. Theophylline clearance decreases with increasing age, liver disease, congestive heart failure, and during febrile illnesses. Theophylline clearance increases with children, in cigarette smokers, and in people with cystic fibrosis. Medications such as **cimetidine,** quinolone antibiotics, **erythromycin,** oral contraceptives, **allopurinol,** and **propranolol** decrease theophylline clearance. **Rifampin, carbamazepine, phenobarbital,** and **phenytoin** increase theophylline clearance.

DENTAL CONCERNS. One should consider not using erythromycin or any one of the quinolone antibiotics in patients taking theophylline. These medications can decrease the clearance of theophylline, causing an increase in theophylline blood levels. This may place the patient at increased risk for developing theophylline toxicity. If any one of these antibiotics must be used, the patient should have his theophylline level checked and should be educated as to what to look for in terms of toxicity. The patient's physician should be notified about the addition of the antibiotic. The patient should contact his physician should he notice any signs of toxicity. The best way to avoid toxicity is not to use these medications.

RESPIRATORY COUGH AND COLD PRODUCTS

Americans spend billions of dollars each year in order to alleviate the symptoms of a cold, the flu, or chronic bronchitis. Many of your patients will be taking prescription and nonprescription medications. Question the patient carefully about the use of over-the-counter (OTC) medications. The patient does not always consider them to be medication because they can be purchased without a prescription. The following is a brief review of these respiratory products.

Pharmacotherapy

Nasal Decongestants. Nasal decongestants are α-adrenergic agonistss that act by constricting the blood vessels of the nasal passages. An example of a popular nasal decongestant is **pseudoephedrine.** These medications are available as oral tablets, capsules, or liquids, or as a nasal spray. Chronic use (greater than 3 days) of a nasal spray can cause a rebound nasal congestion. Agents such as beclamethasone (steroid), are used to treat nasal stuffiness due to allergies. They work by reducing inflammation in the nasal passages.

Expectorants. Expectorants are thought to work by decreasing sputum viscosity and by promoting the release of exudate from the respiratory passages. **Guaifenesin** is the most commonly used expectorant and is available in many OTC cough and cold products. Maintaining fluid intake and adequate humidity promote the release of exudate from the respiratory passages.

Antitussives. Antitussive medications are used to provide symptomatic relief from dry, nonproductive coughs. Opioid and nonopioid antitussives cause CNS depression of the cough center in the medulla.

CODEINE. **Codeine** is the most commonly used opioid antitussive and is safe and effective when used appropriately. Codeine-containing products should be avoided in patients with chronic pulmonary disease and in patients sensitive to histamine.

DEXTROMETHORPHAN. **Dextromethorphan** is the active ingredient in most OTC antitussive medications either alone or in combination with other agents. It is safe and effective with no apparent contraindications, unless the patient is hypersensitive to it.

Mucolytics. Mucolytics are enzymes that are able to digest mucus and decrease its viscosity. The most commonly used mucolytic is **acetylcysteine** which loosens secretions in pulmonary disease. It is also used to treat **acetaminophen** overdose.

Dental Concerns

Both opioid and nonopioid antitussives can cause sedation and dry mouth. Counsel the patient about the increased risk of sedation, confusion, and fatigue with an antianxiety agent, opioid pain reliever, or a general anesthetic. The patient should have someone drive him to and from the dental appointment and the patient should be instructed not to perform any activities that require thought or concentration after taking these medications.

Dry mouth can be treated with water, sucking on tart, sugarless candy, or chewing on sugarless gum. Counsel the patient about the importance of good oral hygiene.

Summary

The dental hygienist plays an important role in the oral health care of patients with respiratory illnesses. Chronic obstructive pulmonary disease is treated with β_2-agonists, theophylline, anticholinergic drugs, and antibiotics. The treatment of asthma includes β_2-agonists, steroids, anticholinergic drugs, antiinflammatory drugs, and theophylline. Many of these medications are available in metered-dose inhalers that deliver medication directly to the lungs. These medications stay in the oral cavity and can cause dry mouth, hoarseness, change in taste, and some can cause oral candidiasis. The dental practitioner should review with the patient the importance of good oral hygiene and the correct way of using the inhaler.

Theophylline clearance is decreased when given with erythromycin. Extreme caution should be used if this combination must be given. Oral β_2-agonists can increase blood pressure and make the patient nervous and anxious. These feelings can be exacerbated by the addition of a vasoconstrictor to a local anesthetic. Aspirin and other NSAIDs can precipitate an asthma attack and should be avoided in patients with asthma. Stress has been known to precipitate an asthma attack which makes it all the more important to provide the patient with a dental experience that is as stress-free as possible.

Many patients self-medicate with cough and cold preparations. Some cough and cold products are only available with a prescription. Both prescription and nonprescription products have adverse reactions and drug interactions that can affect oral health. These medications cause dry mouth and many are sedating. Patients should be made aware of side effects and the dental practitioner should help the patient learn how to avoid or minimize them.

Case Study: Jamil Jones

Jamil Jones is 5 years old and has been coming to your practice for 2 years. His medication/health history is significant for asthma. He is being treated with a cromolyn sodium spinhaler and a β_2-adrenergic agonist (albuterol inhaler). He is quite proud of the fact that he has "mastered" the use of his inhalers. He has done this with the assistance of a spacer. He is in today for a scheduled maintenance visit.

1. What is cromolyn sodium and what is its role in the treatment of asthma?
2. What are the adverse reactions associated with cromolyn sodium?
3. What are the dental concerns associated with cromolyn sodium? What would the dental practitioner tell Mrs. Jones about them?
4. What are the adverse reactions associated with albuterol?
5. What are the dental concerns associated with albuterol and what would the dental practitioner tell Mrs. Jones about them?
6. What is the rationale behind spacers?

Case Study: Lucky Savoy

Lucky Savoy is a 27-year-old who has been coming to your practice for close to 10 years. His medication/health history is significant for asthma. He is being treated with ipratroprium bromide and metaproterenol inhalers. He is at the office today to have a cavity filled. The dentist will be using a local anesthetic with a vasoconstrictor.

1. What is ipratroprium bromide and what is its role in the treatment of asthma?
2. What are the adverse reactions associated with ipratroprium bromide?
3. What are the dental concerns associated with ipratroprium bromide and what would the dental practitioner tell Mr. Savoy about them?
4. What are the potential drug interactions between metaproterenol and a vasoconstrictor?
5. What is the potential drug interaction between ipratroprium bromide and the vasoconstrictor?
6. What should be done about these potential drug interactions?

Review Questions

1. Define COPD. Compare and contrast between emphysema and bronchitis.
2. Do patients with COPD respond to steroids?

3. What is theophylline and what is its role in treating COPD?
4. What are some of the signs and symptoms of theophylline toxicity?
6. Are decongestants beneficial in the treatment of COPD? Why or why not?
7. What is an expectorant and how does it work? Why is it beneficial in the treatment of COPD?
8. What are the different types of antitussives and how do they work? Include adverse reactions and dental concerns.
9. Define mucolytic and give an example.

BIBLIOGRAPHY

Anon: Deaths due to chronic obstructive pulmonary disease and allied conditions. *MMWR* 35:507–510, 1986.

Barnes PJ: Inhaled glucocorticoids for asthma. *N Engl J Med* 332:868–875, 1995.

Blumenthal R, Selcow J, Spector S, et al.: A multicenter evaluation of the clinical benefits of cromolyn sodium aerosol by metered-dose inhaler in the treatment of asthma. *J Allergy Clin Immunol* 81:681–687, 1988.

Bryant BG, Lombardi TP: Cold, cough, and allergy products. In *Handbook of Nonprescription Drugs,* 10th ed. American Pharmaceutical Association, Washington, DC, 1993.

Hill MR, Kamada AK: Pathogenesis of asthma: Therapeutic implications. *Ann Pharmacother* 25:993–1001, 1991.

Kelly HW, O'Connell MB: Asthma products. In *Handbook of Nonprescription Drugs,* 10th ed. American Pharmaceutical Association, Washington, DC, 1993.

Lenfant C: Lung research: Government and community. *Am Rev Respir Dis* 26:753–757, 1982.

McFadden ER Jr., Gilbert IA: Exercise-induced asthma. *N Engl J Med* 330:1362–1367, 1994.

Nelson HS: Bronchodilator therapy for reversible obstructive airway disease. *J Respir Dis,* Suppl:S58–S65, 1989.

Nelson HS: β-adrenergic bronchodilators. *New Engl J Med* 333:499–506, 1995.

Persson CGA: Xanthines as airway inflammatory drugs. *J Allergy Clin Immunol* 81:615–617, 1988.

Scheffer AL: Guidelines for the diagnosis and management of asthma: National Heart, Lung, and Blood Institute National Asthma Educational Program Expert Panel Report. *J Allergy and Clin Immunol* 88 (Part 2):425–534, 1991.

Self TH, Rumbak MJ, Kelso TM: Correct use of metered-dose inhalers and spacer devices. *Postgrad Med* 92:95–96, 99–100, 102–106, 1992.

CHAPTER 16

Histamine and H$_1$-Receptor Antagonist Drugs

Key Terms

Allergy

Anaphylaxis

Antihistamine

Autacoids

Histamine

Sedation

LEARNING OBJECTIVES

After completion of this chapter and its learning activities, the student should be able to:

1. Define autacoid.
2. Describe the pharmacologic effects and clinical uses of histamine.
3. Describe the pharmacologic effects of both first- and second-generation H$_1$-receptor antagonists.
4. Discuss the clinical uses of both first and second generation H$_1$- receptor antagonists.
5. Describe the adverse reactions and drug interactions associated with first- and second-generation H$_1$-receptor antagonists.
6. Discuss the dental concerns associated with first- and second-generation H$_1$-receptor antagonists.

INTRODUCTION

Many patients self-treat with H$_1$-receptor antagonists and many others are prescribed the newer, second-generation H$_1$-receptor antagonists. They take these medications in an attempt to treat symptoms of the common cold, the flu, or seasonal rhinitis (allergies). It is important for the dental hygienist to have a sound knowledge base about these drugs because they have adverse reactions and drug interactions that can alter dental treatment.

AUTACOIDS

The term *autacoid* is defined as an organic substance that is produced in one part of the body and travels by blood to another part of the body where it produces its effect. It is derived from the Greek *autos* (self) and *akos* (remedy). Some examples of autacoids include histamine, serotonin, angiotensin, kinin, and prostaglandin.

HISTAMINE

Histamine is a biogenic amine that is found in almost every part of the body, with the most found in mast cells. It is localized and stored in granules in the mast cells and only released and activated when the cells are lysed. Histamine is released in response to allergic reactions, the common cold, trauma, infection, or drugs, and the amount released determines the severity of the reaction in the patient.

Histamine Receptors

There are two, and possibly three, types of histamine receptors: H_1, H_2, and H_3. Histamine stimulation of H_1-receptors produces vasodilation, bronchoconstriction, pain or itching at nerve endings, and increased capillary permeability. Stimulation of H_2-receptors can increase gastric acid secretions, and the actions of H_3-receptors are unknown.

Pharmacologic Effects

The pharmacologic effects of histamine primarily pertain to the cardiovascular system, exocrine glands, and smooth muscles. Pharmacologic effects include vasodilation, increased capillary permeability, bronchoconstriction, pain or itching in cutaneous nerve endings, and increased gastric acid secretions.

Clinical Effects

During allergic reactions or anaphylaxis an antigen-antibody reaction occurs and histamine is released. The most serious consequences are *anaphylaxis,* in which the patient experiences bronchoconstriction, hypotension followed by shock, and cardiovascular collapse. Other symptoms include apprehension, paresthesia, urticaria, edema, choking, coughing, and wheezing. Patients can proceed to fever, shock, loss of consciousness, coma, convulsions, and death.

Clinical Use

Histamine is used in the diagnosis of achlorhydria and pheochromocytoma.

FIRST-GENERATION ANTIHISTAMINES (H_1-RECEPTOR ANTAGONISTS)

The first-generation *antihistamine* drugs have been in use since the 1940s and are widely used drugs. They not only block histamine receptors but also block acetylcholine and serotonin receptors. Table 16-1 reviews some of these drugs.

Table 16-1   Selected First-Generation H₁-Receptor Antagonists

Generic (Trade Name)	Adult Dose (mg)	Dosing Interval (hours)
Diphenhydramine (Benadryl)	25–50	6–8
Clemastine (Tavist)	1	12
Dimenhydrinate (Dramamine)	50–100	4–6
Doxylamine (Unisom)	25–50	4–6
Chlorpheniramine (Chlor-Trimeton)	4	6–8
Brompheniramine (Dimetane)	4–8	6–8
Hydroxyzine hydrochloride (Atarax)	25–50	4–6

Pharmacologic Effects

The pharmacologic effects of antihistamines are due to their ability to block histamine and other receptor sites. These drugs are effective in treating motion sickness and nausea and vomiting. **Diphenhydramine** is used topically or locally (by injection) for anesthesia.

Clinical Use

Antihistamines are used to control the symptoms of allergic rhinitis and seasonal hay fever. These medications are also used to treat the symptoms of allergic reactions such as acute urticaria and are sometimes used as second-line treatment for anaphylaxis. Although they are often in many combination products for colds, they are not useful in the treatment of colds.

Other uses include the treatment of nausea and vomiting, motion sickness, preoperative sedation, sleep aid, and as local anesthesia.

Adverse Reactions

The adverse reactions of antihistamines are discussed next.

CNS Effects. The most common CNS adverse reactions are *sedation*, drowsiness, and confusion. Excitability and restlessness can occur in the elderly and small children. Other CNS adverse reactions include tinnitus, incoordination, and fatigue.

Anticholinergic Effects. These adverse reactions include dry mouth, blurred vision, constipation, urinary retention, and tachycardia.

Gastrointestinal (GI) Effects. GI adverse reactions include anorexia, nausea, and vomiting.

Toxicity. Toxicity is normally characterized by sedation in adults and excitability in small children. The most predominant signs and symptoms are anticholinergic. Cardiac arrest and death may occur.

Drug Interactions

Antihistamines enhance the sedative and depressant effects of other CNS depressant drugs. They also enhance the effects of anticholinergic drugs and enhance the effects of antiemetics.

Dental Concerns

Since many patients take over-the-counter cold and *allergy* medications that contain antihistamines, it is inevitable that the dental hygienist will treat these patients. The dental hygienist should counsel the patient on the importance of good oral hygiene and how to treat or minimize the xerostomia associated with these drugs. Patients should be instructed to drink plenty of water and stay away from juices and caffeinated beverages. Juices can lead to an increased risk of dental caries and caffeine can exacerbate xerostomia. Patients can also chew tart, sugarless gum or suck on tart, sugarless candy.

The dental practitioner should also instruct the patient to use caution if an antianxiety drug or an opioid analgesic is prescribed. These drugs are sedating and can cause increased sedation and confusion in patients taking antihistamines. Patients should not drive and should use caution when operating heavy machinery or equipment or doing anything else that requires thought or concentration.

SECOND-GENERATION H_1-RECEPTOR ANTAGONISTS

The newer, second-generation H_1-receptor antagonists are nonsedating antihistamines that do not cross the blood-brain barrier in therapeutic doses. These drugs work by blocking histamine action at H_1-receptor sites, in the periphery, and by inhibiting histamine release from mast cells and basophils. They are relatively free of antiserotonergic, anticholinergic, and α-adrenergic blocking effects. Table 16-2 reviews these drugs.

Clinical Use

Peripheral, nonsedating antihistamines are used in the treatment of seasonal and perennial rhinitis and certain forms of urticaria.

Table 16-2   Second-Generation H_1-Receptor Antagonists

Generic (Trade Name)	Adult Dose (mg)	Dosing Interval (hours)
Terfenadine (Seldane)	60	12
Astemizole (Hismanal)	10	24
Loratadine (Claritin)	10	24

Adverse Reactions

These drugs are relatively free of the adverse reactions associated with the first-generation antihistamines; however, some patients do complain of sedation. **Terfenadine** (Seldane) in high doses can have cardiotoxic effects and **astemizole** (Hismanal) can cause appetite stimulation and inappropriate weight gain.

Drug Interactions

Both terfenadine and astemizole can have cardiotoxic effects when given with erythromycin or ketoconazole. These drugs should not be given together as a result of this fatal drug interaction.

Dental Concerns

The dental hygienist should question the patient about his use of either terfenadine or astemizole in order to determine if erythromycin can be prescribed. This will help to avoid problems with cardiotoxicity.

Summary

Many patients are taking either first- or second-generation antihistamine drugs and a general understanding of their differences will help the dental practitioner to better treat the patient. The second-generation antihistamines do not penetrate the blood-brain barrier as well as the first-generation antihistamines and cause little sedation. The second-generation drugs do not cause the anticholinergic effects and tachycardia of which first-generation antihistamines are capable. Two second-generation antihistamines, terfenadine and astemizole, interact with erythromycin and can cause cardiac abnormalities. This combination of drugs should be avoided. Patients who are penicillin allergic should be given something other than erythromycin if an antibiotic is needed. The dental practitioner should be able to counsel patients on how to treat these adverse reactions and how to avoid the drug interactions associated with first- and second-generation antihistamines.

Case Study: Jan Smith

Jan Smith is a 25-year-old patient with a long history of allergic rhinitis. She is continually trying old and new over-the-counter (OTC) allergy medications to treat her symptoms. The OTC medications do work though she often has problems staying awake during the day and she is always very thirsty. Ms. Smith works as a schoolteacher and the sedating effects of the drug are bothersome. Her only other medications include oral contraceptives and a multivitamin.

1. What are first-generation antihistamines and how do they work?
2. What are the pharmacologic effects of first-generation antihistamines?

3. What are the adverse reactions associated with first-generation antihistamines and can they lead to toxicity?
4. What would the dental practitioner tell Ms. Smith about these adverse reactions with a special emphasis on those with dental implications?
5. What are the drug interactions associated with first-generation antihistamines that are of dental concern?
6. What should Ms. Smith be told about these adverse reactions and drug interactions?

Case Study: John Esposito

John Esposito is 55 years old and has a history of rheumatic heart disease. His only prescription medications include erythromycin prophylaxis for his dental appointments and over-the-counter analgesics and allergy medications. Mr. Esposito is allergic to penicillin antibiotics. He calls your office today to let you know that his physician has placed him on terfenadine for his allergies. It seems as if the over-the-counter products were making him so dizzy that he could not function at work. Mr. Esposito is concerned about this because he heard about a "terrible" interaction between terfenadine and erythromycin.

1. What is the interaction between terfenadine and erythromycin?
2. What other second-generation antihistamine interacts with erythromycin?
3. What should Mr. Esposito be told and what should he receive for prophylaxis?
4. What is the mechanism of action of second-generation antihistamines?
5. What are the adverse reactions of second-generation antihistamines?
6. What are the advantages of the second-generation antihistamines over the first-generation antihistamines?

Review Questions

1. What does *autacoid* mean and where does the word come from?
2. What are the pharmacologic effects of histamine?
3. What are the clinical uses of histamine?
4. Compare and contrast the first- and second-generation antihistamines.
5. What are the clinical uses of the first-generation antihistamines?
6. Name three nonsedating antihistamines and their clinical uses.

BIBLIOGRAPHY

McTavish D, Goa KL, Ferrill M: Terfenadine: An updated review of its pharmacological properties and therapeutic efficacy. *Drugs* 39:552–574, 1990.
Meltzer EO: Antihistamine- and decongestant-induced performance decrements. *J Occup Med* 32:327–334, 1990.

Richards DM, Brogden RN, Heel RC, et al.: Astemizole. A review of its pharmacodynamic properties and therapeutic efficacy. *Drugs* 28:38–61, 1984.

Simons FER: H₁-receptor antagonists. Clinical pharmacology and therapeutics. *J Allergy Clin Immunol* 84:845–861, 1989.

Simons FER: Loratadine, a non-sedating H₁-receptor antagonist (antihistamine). *Ann Allergy* 63:266–268, 1989.

Simons FER, Simons KJ: Histamine and H₁-receptor antagonists. In Smith CM, Reynard AM (eds.), *Textbook of Pharmacology,* 1st ed. W. B. Saunders Company, Philadelphia, 1992.

CHAPTER 17

Treatment of Endocrine Disorders

Key Terms

Androgenic
Diabetes
Estrogen
Hormone
Hypothalamus

Pancreas
Pituitary Gland
Progesterone
Thyroid

LEARNING OBJECTIVES

After completion of this chapter and its learning activities, the student should be able to:

1. Describe the relationship between the pituitary gland and hypothalamus in the regulatory mechanism of hormones in the body.
2. Describe the negative feedback mechanism of the hypothalamus, pituitary gland, and adrenal cortex system.
3. List the pharmacologic effects, clinical uses, adverse reactions, and dental concerns associated with glucocorticoids and mineralocorticoids.
4. Describe the overall function of the thyroid gland and compare and contrast hypothyroidism and hyperthyroidism.
5. Describe the symptoms of hypothyroidism, including dental concerns, and list the various drugs used to treat it.
6. Describe the symptoms of hyperthyroidism, including dental concerns, and list the various drugs used to treat it.
7. Describe the overall function of the pancreas and describe the pathogenesis of diabetes. Include dental concerns.
8. List the drugs used to treat both type I and type II diabetes including general mechanisms of action and adverse reactions.
9. Describe the overall function of estrogen and progesterone. Include clinical use, adverse reactions, and dental concerns.
10. Describe the overall function of male sex hormones including clinical use, adverse reactions, and dental concerns.

INTRODUCTION

The endocrine system regulates many functions of the body by releasing hormones directly into the bloodstream from various endocrine glands throughout the body. The amount of *hormone* released is regulated by a negative feedback system. Many patients take different drugs to correct hormonal imbalances or to mimic such conditions as pregnancy. Other uses of hormones include diagnostic procedures, cancer, and other systemic disorders. The dental hygienist will invariably treat patients taking hormonal replacement therapy or oral contraceptives. These medications or the hormonal imbalance may present dental implications of which the dental hygienist should be aware. The intent of this chapter is to provide a brief overview of a select group of hormones that are used therapeutically along with the diseases that they treat, their adverse reactions, drug interactions, and dental concerns.

HYPOTHALAMUS–PITUITARY GLAND SYSTEM

The pituitary gland is a small gland attached to the hypothalamus at the base of the brain and is often referred to as the "master" endocrine gland (Figure 17-1). The *hypothalamus* is the part of the central nervous system (CNS) that controls the functions of the autonomic nervous system, many somatic functions, and the pituitary gland.

The *pituitary gland* is made up of the anterior lobe (adenohypophysis) and the posterior lobe (neurohypophysis) and both contain different hormones that can be released into the bloodstream. The anterior lobe secretes growth hormone or somatotropin, adrenocorticotropic hormone (ACTH), follicle-stimulating hormone (FSH), prolactin (Prl), luteinizing hormone (LH), thyroid-stimulating hormone (TSH), and melanocyte-stimulating hormone (MSH). Many of the hormones located in the anterior lobe have effects on other endocrine glands located throughout the body.

The posterior lobe of the pituitary gland secretes antidiuretic hormone (ADH) and oxytocin. These hormones are actually synthesized in the hypothalamus and stored in the pituitary gland until they are released into the bloodstream.

Mechanism of Hormone Release

Hormones are released into the body when levels are low or there is a physiologic need to increase these levels. The control mechanism that allows for this is termed "negative feedback," meaning that once the hormone is released into the bloodstream and reaches a certain blood level, this appropriate blood level triggers mechanisms that inhibit further release of the hormone. An example would be when cortisol levels in the body were low or when a stressful situation stimulated the hypothalamus to release corticotropin-releasing factor (CRF), which then acts on the pituitary gland. The pituitary gland then secretes ACTH, which stimulates the adrenal cortex to release hydrocortisone. Sufficiently high hydrocortisone levels then act on the pituitary gland and hypothalamus to stop releasing further ACTH and CRF.

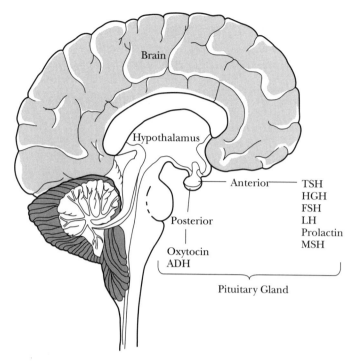

Figure 17-1   *Hypothalamus–pituitary gland system*

Corticosteroids

Corticosteroids or adrenocorticosteroids can be divided into two groups: the gluco-corticoids and mineralocorticoids (Table 17-1). The normal adult secretes about 20 mg of hydrocortisone each day with maximum secretion occurring between 4 A.M. and 8 A.M. in stress-free adults following a normal day–night schedule. There can be a 10-fold increase in the amount of hydrocortisone released when the patient is in a stressful situation.

MINERALOCORTICOIDS. The mineralocorticoids are responsible for maintaining water and electrolyte balance in the body. Aldosterone is the main substance that controls sodium reabsorption in the collecting tubule of the kidney in exchange for potassium. Increased sodium and water retention can lead to edema and hypertension.

GLUCOCORTICOIDS (STEROIDS). The glucocorticoids are available in many dose forms including oral tablets, oral and nasal inhalers, topical, intramuscular, and intravenous preparations. Systemic effects are usually seen when the drug is administered orally or parenterally. Systemic effects occur to a lesser extent with topical and inhaler dose forms.

Pharmacologic Effects. The pharmacologic effects of steroids can be either broad or catabolic. Broad effects include carbohydrate metabolism, antiinflammatory activity, antiallergenic activity, enzyme action, membrane function, and RNA (ribonucleic

Table 17-1   Selected Adrenocorticosteroids

Drug Name	Dose (mg)
Mineralcorticoids	Treatment of Addison's disease
Fludorcortisone (Florinef)	0.1
Glucocorticoids	Treatment of Antiinflammatory Processes
Betamethasone (Valisone)	0.60
Dexamethasone (Decadron)	0.75
Hydrocortisone	20
Prednisone (Deltasone)	5
Triamcinolone (Aristocort, Kenalog, Mycolog)	4

acid) synthesis. Catabolic effects include increased gluconeogenesis, decreased glucose use, increased protein catabolism, decreased growth, decreased bone density, and decreased resistance to infection.

Adverse Reactions. The adverse reactions to steroids are many and are related to dose form, dose, frequency, time of administration, and duration of treatment.

METABOLIC EFFECTS. Metabolic adverse reactions include a moon face and buffalo hump (fat deposits on the back of the neck); which is referred to as Cushing's syndrome, truncal obesity, weight gain, muscle wasting, and hyperglycemia may also be aggravated or initiated. Steroids decrease resistance to infections. They can also mask the signs and symptoms of infection.

CENTRAL NERVOUS SYSTEM EFFECTS. CNS effects include mood swings, changes in behavior and personality, agitation, psychosis, euphoria, and depression.

GASTROINTESTINAL (GI) EFFECTS. These drugs are irritating to the stomach and can increase the production of stomach acid and pepsin. Steroids can exacerbate existing peptic ulcers.

IMPAIRED WOUND HEALING. Steroids impair collagen synthesis, which can impair wound healing.

OSTEOPOROSIS. The catabolic effects of steroids break down bone and also impair collagen synthesis. This can lead to osteoporosis in adults and impaired growth in children.

OPHTHALMIC. EFFECTS. Steroids can increase intraocular pressure and can exacerbate existing glaucoma. They can also cause cataracts.

ELECTROLYTE AND FLUID IMBALANCE. Some steroids have mineralocorticoid effects and can cause sodium and water retention. Sodium and water retention may exacerbate hypertension or congestive heart failure.

ADRENAL CRISIS. Patients taking long-term steroids are often unable to secrete additional steroids in response to a stressful situation. Patients may experience weakness, syncope, cardiovascular collapse, or death.

ORAL EFFECTS. Oral steroid inhalers can cause oral candidiasis, which can be prevented by having the patient rinse after each inhaler use.

Clinical Uses. The therapeutic uses of steroids include replacement therapy for adrenal gland insufficiency, treatment of shock or adrenal crisis, and as an antiinflammatory drug. Steroids are used to treat such inflammatory conditions as rheumatoid arthritis, rheumatic fever, systemic lupus erythematosus, acute and chronic asthma, and severe and acute allergic reactions. Dental uses of steroids include the treatment of noninfectious inflammatory oral lesions, temporomandibular joint arthritis, and aphthous stomatitis.

Dental Concerns. The adverse reactions of steroids are of concern to the dental hygienist. A detailed medication/health history will reveal whether or not a patient is taking steroids, doses used, dose form, and duration of therapy. The dental practitioner should also take the patient's blood pressure prior to a procedure or the administration of a vasoconstrictor because steroids can increase blood pressure.

Nonsteroidal antiinflammatory drugs, aspirin, and opioid analgesics should be avoided because they can cause GI irritation which can exacerbate the GI irritation, seen with steroids.

Steroids can mask the symptoms of infection and can delay wound healing. The dental practitioner may want to consider prophylaxing a steroid-dependent patient with an antibiotic prior to a dental procedure because of the risk of bacterial endocarditis. The dental practitioner should also use caution when surgical procedures are performed in the oral cavity because of the risk of delayed wound healing. Steroid-dependent patients are at risk for developing osteoporosis, which may be demonstrated on dental radiographs.

Steroid-dependent patients may be at risk for adrenal crisis during a stressful dental procedure. Patients who are steroid dependent cannot naturally increase the amount of cortisol that the body needs during stressful situations. This is due to an inhibition of the negative feedback system of the hypothalamus–pituitary gland–adrenal cortex system. The dental practitioner may consider temporarily increasing the patient's steroid dose to meet the body's need for the dental procedure. This situation should first be reviewed with the patient's physician.

THYROID GLAND

Thyroid hormones are responsible for maintaining normal functioning of almost all organ systems, regulating metabolism, and controlling energy expenditure. The thyroid gland is located in the front of the trachea just below the larynx. The two thyroid hormones, triiodothyronine (T_3) and thyroxine (T_4), are synthesized and stored in the thyroid gland and their release into the bloodstream is controlled by the hypothalamus–pituitary–thyroid axis. Low levels of T_3 and T_4 trigger the release of thyroid-stimulating hormone (TSH) in the blood and the thyroid gland produces additional T_3 and T_4. Iodine is absolutely essential for the synthesis of these two hormones and it is added to table salt to help ensure adequate amounts in daily diets.

Hyperthyroidism

Hyperthyroidism is due to the excessive production of T_3 and T_4 and can be the result of tumors of the thyroid or pituitary glands, cancer of the hypothalamus, inflammatory disorders, or autoimmune disorders (Graves' disease). Signs and symptoms include fine hair, fine tremor and hyperreflexia, gynecomastia in men, onycholysis, retraction of the eyelids and lid lag, systolic ejection murmur, tachycardia, warm, smooth, moist skin, widened pulse pressure, easy fatigability, emotional lability, heat intolerance, and nervousness. Oral signs include accelerated tooth eruption, marked loss of the alveolar process, diffuse demineralization of the jawbone, and rapidly progressing periodontal destruction.

Treatment. The treatment of hyperthyroidism includes antithyroid drugs, iodide, radioactive iodide, or thyroidectomy.

ANTITHYROID DRUGS. They include **methimazole** (Tapazole) and **propylthiouracil** (PTU) and both drugs work by interfering with the synthesis of T_3 and T_4. The adverse reactions of these drugs include a mild transient leukopenia, skin reactions, and agranulocytosis. Other adverse reactions include arthralgias, hypoprothrombinemia, and GI disturbances.

IODIDES. **Iodide** inhibits thyroid hormone synthesis and prevents the release of thyroid hormones from the thyroid gland. It is usually given as a saturated solution of **potassium iodide** (SSKI) or Lugol's solution. Adverse reactions include skin rashes, conjunctivitis, metallic taste, burning in the mouth, sore throat, and head cold–like symptoms. Radioactive iodine is given as ^{131}I and is actively taken up by the thyroid gland and incorporated into thyroid hormone synthesis; it causes a localized destruction of thyroid tissue over time.

SURGERY. Surgery (thyroidectomy) is indicated in patients with autonomous adenomas, when drug therapy is ineffective or contraindicated, or if there is esophageal or respiratory compromise due to a large goiter. Surgery and radioactive iodide can make the patient hypothyroid and thyroid supplementation is often necessary.

Dental Concerns. The dental hygienist should carefully examine patients with suspected or known hyperthyroidism for any oral changes. These should be reported to the dentist and the patient's physician.

Epinephrine is contraindicated in hyperthyroid patients because of the ensuing increased sympathetic activity. The combination could result in angina, arrhythmias, or hypertension. Hyperthyroid patients have a low tolerance to pain and may require additional local anesthetics and higher doses of CNS depressant medications.

Hypothyroidism

Hypothyroidism is due to decreased thyroid hormone synthesis that is usually the result of primary thyroid gland failure. In adults, hypothyroidism is referred to as myxedema. Signs and symptoms include bradycardia, coarse skin and hair, cold skin, delayed reflexes, peripheral puffiness, cold intolerance, constipation, tiredness, weakness, and weight gain. In children and infants, hypothyroidism is referred to as cretinism and can lead to mental and physical retardation and dwarfism. Oral findings in children include delayed tooth eruption, malocclusion, increased tendency to develop periodontal disease, poorly shaped and carious teeth, and gingiva that are either inflamed or pale and enlarged.

Treatment. Hypothyroidism is treated by hormonal replacement that is given on a gradual and carefully monitored basis. Thyroid supplement products include crude hormones; **thyroid** strong, thyroid USP (various), and synthetic hormones; **levothyroxine** (Levothroid, Levoxine, Synthroid, Syroxine); **liothyronine** (Cytomel, Cyronine); and **liotrix** (Euthroid, Thyrolar). Adverse reactions are associated with overdose and can include symptoms similar to hyperthyroidism.

Dental Concerns. The dental hygienist should carefully examine children suspected of having hypothyroidism and children diagnosed with hypothyroidism. These patients and their families should be instructed on the importance of maintaining good oral care.

Hypothyroid patients are more sensitive to CNS depressant medications and caution should be used if opioid analgesics or an antianxiety drug is prescribed. The dose should be lowered in these patients and the patient should be counseled about the need to avoid driving or doing anything that requires thought or concentration while taking CNS depressants.

THE PANCREAS

The overall function of the *pancreas* is to produce insulin and glucagon that are secreted by islands of cells (located throughout the pancreas) called the islets of Langerhans. Insulin is released in response to high glucose levels and increases glucose absorption into tissues, stimulates the storage of glycogen, and stimulates the storage and synthesis of fat and proteins. Glucagon is released in response to low blood glucose levels and stimulates the breakdown of glycogen to glucose (glyconeolysis) and stimulates the breakdown of protein to glucose (gluconeogenesis).

Diabetes Mellitus

Diabetes mellitus is a common disease of the endocrine system that is caused by a failure of the β-cells to produce adequate insulin or poorly timed secretion of insulin from the pancreas. The production of insulin may be totally absent or partial. The symptoms of diabetes include hyperglycemia, glucosuria, ketosis, polyphagia, polydypsia, polyuria, and dry mouth. Patients are usually weak and have weight loss and wasting despite the increase in appetite.

Diabetes is classified as insulin dependent (Type I) or noninsulin dependent (Type II). Type I diabetes begins early in life, the pancreas secretes no insulin, and the patient requires insulin therapy. Type I diabetes is thought to be due to virus or toxins that produce an autoimmune response or may be due to β-cell abnormalities. Type II diabetes begins during adulthood (over age 40). The pancreas secretes insulin, but the insulin is ineffective due to a number of factors, and the patient can be treated with either diet, oral hypoglycemic drugs, insulin, or a combination of diet and drugs. Type II diabetes is often due to decreased tissue sensitivity to insulin and/or a decreased response of β-cells to insulin.

Dental Concerns. The dental hygienist should counsel diabetic patients about the importance of good oral hygiene and question all patients regarding their last meal and dose of antidiabetic medication. A quick glucose source (cake frosting) should always be kept in case the patient experiences hypoglycemia. Other dental concerns associated with diabetes are as follows.

DENTAL CARIES. Uncontrolled diabetics appear to be at a greater risk for dental caries. This may be due to dry mouth caused by the excessive loss of water from the body. Treated or controlled diabetics do not seem to have this problem.

PERIODONTAL DISEASE. Periodontal changes include mild gingivitis, painful periodontitis, and increased tooth mobility due to the destruction of supporting alveolar bone.

DENTAL APPOINTMENTS. Dental appointments for oral surgery should be scheduled in the morning, 1.5–2 hours after breakfast and regular antidiabetic medication. Patients should consume an adequate caloric intake to prevent hypoglycemia. All other dental appointments should be scheduled around mealtime and should involve as little stress as possible.

WOUND HEALING AND INFECTION. Diabetics are more at risk for delayed wound healing and developing infections. Antibiotics may be necessary in some patients and infections should be aggressively treated if they occur.

DRUG INTERACTIONS. Epinephrine, steroids, and opioid analgesics can decrease insulin release or increase insulin requirements. These drugs should be used with caution in diabetic patients.

Treatment of Diabetes Mellitus

The overall goal of antidiabetic therapy is to control metabolic balance and return fluid and electrolytes to the body. Therapy is generally aimed at regulating glucose levels through diet and/or antidiabetic drug administration.

Insulin. Insulin is administered subcutaneously, intravenously, and intramuscularly. The most common form of administration is subcutaneously. Table 17-2 reviews the available insulin preparations. The older preparations of insulin were prepared from

Table 17-2   Insulin Preparations

Duration of Action	Insulin Preparation
Short acting	Regular insulin (Humulin R, Novolin R)
	Prompt insulin zinc suspension (Semilente, Semilente Insulin, Semitard)
Intermediate acting	Insulin zinc suspension (Lente, Humulin L)
	Isophane insulin suspension (Humulin N, NPH, Novolin N, Insulatard NPH)
Long acting	Protamine zinc insulin suspension (PZI)
	Extended insulin zinc suspension (Ultralente, Humulin U Ultralente)
Mixed preparations	Isophane insulin suspension and regular insulin injection (Humulin 70/30, Mixtard)

beef or pork pancreas and differed in terms of peak effect and duration of action. The problem associated with animal sources of insulin is the high rate of allergic reaction, which has led to the development of "human insulins." Human insulin is produced by two different mechanisms. Human insulin can be made through gene splicing of *Escherichia coli* through recombinant deoxyribonucleic acid (DNA). The other involves transpeptidation of pork insulin.

Adverse Reactions. The most common adverse reaction of insulin is hypoglycemia, which can be caused by insulin overdose, failure to eat, or increased exercise or stress. Symptoms include sweating, weakness, nausea, tachycardia, headache, blurred vision, mental confusion, incoherence, and eventually coma, convulsions, and death. Hypoglycemia can be treated with fruit juice, candy, or cake frosting if the patient is awake. Intravenous glucose, dextrose, or glucagon is used for unconscious patients.

Other adverse reactions include lipodystrophy at the site of injection and allergic reactions to noninsulin contaminants. Both have decreased with the development of more pure insulin preparations.

Oral Antidiabetic Drugs. The oral antidiabetic drugs consist of the sulfonylureas and the two new antidiabetic drugs, **metformin** and **acarbose,** which are unrelated pharmacologically to sulfonylureas (Table 17-3).

SULFONYLUREAS. Sulfonylureas stimulate the secretion of insulin from β cells and are indicated for adult-onset diabetics who cannot be treated by diet alone. The major adverse reactions of these drugs are hypoglycemia, blood dyscrasias, GI disturbance, muscle weakness, fatigue, dizziness, cutaneous reactions, and liver damage.

Table 17-3 Oral Antidiabetic Drugs

Drug	Dose (mg/day)
First-Generation Sulfonylureas	
Acetohexamide (Dymelor)	250–1500
Chlorpropamide (Diabinese)	100–500
Tolbutamide (Orinase)	500–3000
Tolazamide (Tolinase)	100–1000
Second-Generation Sulfonylureas	
Glyburide (DiaβEta, Micronase)	2.5–20
Glipizide (Glucotrol)	2.5–40
Glimepiride (Amaryl)	8
α-glucosidase Inhibitor	
Acarbose (Precose)	300
Biguanides	
Metformin (Glucophage)	850–2550

Sources: Rodger W, Non-insulin-dependent (type II) diabetes melitus. *Can Med Assoc J* 145:1571–1581, 1991; Lebovitz HE, Oral antidiabetic agents: The emergence of α-glucosidase inhibitors. *Drugs* 44(Suppl 3):21–28, 1992; Ponte CD, Non-insulin-dependent diabetes mellitus—current practice and future trends. *J Amer Pharm Assoc* NS36:50–59, 1996.

METFORMIN (GLUCOPHAGE). It is unrelated pharmacologically to sulfonylureas and does not increase insulin secretion or cause clinically significant hypoglycemia. Metformin is indicated as monotherapy for use as an adjunct to diet to lower blood glucose levels. It is also indicated for concomitant use with sulfonylureas when diet and metformin or a sulfonylurea alone does not produce adequate glycemic control. Adverse reactions include diarrhea, nausea, vomiting, abdominal bloating, flatulence, and anorexia, and tend to resolve spontaneously during continued treatment.

ACARBOSE (PRECOSE). This drug is an oral α-glucosidase inhibitor that reduces the intestinal absorption of carbohydrates, thus lowering postprandial blood sugar levels. It is recommended for patients who do not respond to diet therapy alone. Adverse reactions include GI disturbances and hypoglycemia.

ESTROGEN AND PROGESTERONE

Estrogen and *progesterone* are secreted by the ovaries and to some extent by the testes and placenta and are largely responsible for female sex characteristics, reproductive development, and preparing for conception. Changes in female sex hormone levels can cause gingival inflammation and plaque. Estrogen and progesterone levels change daily and Figure 17-2 reviews these changes.

Estrogens

Estrogens are responsible for the growth and development of the vagina, uterus, fallopian tubes, breasts, and axillary and pubic hair. They increase the amount of fat deposited in adipose tissue and increase salt and water retention. Estrogens also increase osteoblastic activity and cause early fusion of the epiphyses.

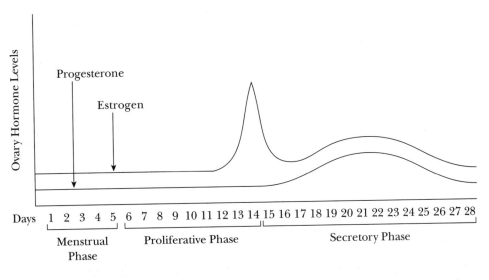

Figure 17-2   *The menstrual cycle*

Estrogens are available as oral tablets, creams, and transdermal patches. Examples include **ethinyl estradiol** (Estinyl), **esterified estrogens** (Estratab, Menest), **estradiol** (Estrace, Estraderm), **estradiol transdermal system** (Estra-derm), **conjugated estrogens** (Premarin), and **diethylstilbestrol** (DES). They are used as hormonal replacement therapy for the treatment of the symptoms of menopause or for young women with a failure to pubesce. They are also used to treat menstrual disturbances, osteoporosis, and atrophic vaginitis.

Adverse Reactions. Adverse reactions include nausea and vomiting, which usually disappear as the patient develops tolerance. Other adverse reactions include uterine bleeding, vaginal discharge, edema, thrombophlebitis, weight gain, headache, and hypertension. Estrogens can cause endometrial cancer in postmenopausal women, although this risk can be minimized by administering a progestin on the last 10 days of the cycle. There is still much debate about the risk of breast cancer and estrogen replacement therapy.

Progesterone

Progesterone is responsible for preparing the uterus for implantation of the fertilized egg. If this does not occur by the end of the menstrual cycle, progesterone levels decline and menarche begins. Other effects include suppression of uterine contractility, proliferation of the acini of the mammary gland, and the ability to prevent immunologic rejection of the fetus.

Progesterone is available in both oral and parenteral dose forms. They include **medroxyprogesterone** (Provera [oral], Depo-Provera [intramuscular]), progestin only, oral contraceptives containing either **norethindrone** (Micronor) or **norgestrel** (Ovrette), and **levonorgestrel** (Norplant) implants that are placed transdermally under the arm, for up to 5 years. Therapeutic uses of progesterone include the treatment of dysfunctional uterine bleeding, endometriosis, dysmenorrhea, and premenstrual tension. Adverse reactions include abnormal menstrual bleeding, breakthrough bleeding, spotting, change in the amount of flow, and amenorrhea.

Oral Contraceptives

Oral contraceptives inhibit the release of FSH and LH, which prevents ovulation and pregnancy. They also alter the endometrium and alter the secretions of the cervix, which helps to prevent the egg from implanting in the endometrium.

Oral contraceptives contain either progesterone alone (minipill) or a combination of estrogen and progesterone in varying doses. The most common estrogen found in oral contraceptives is **ethinyl estradiol** and the progesterones are **desogestrel, norgestrel, norethynodrel,** and **norethindrone.** Examples include Ortho-Novum, Norinyl, Lo-Ovral, Ovral, Nordette, TriLevlen, Levlen, Try-Cyclen, and Desogen. Therapeutic uses include the prevention of pregnancy and regulation of menstrual flow.

Adverse Reactions. The most common adverse reactions include nausea, dizziness, weight gain, headache, and breast tenderness, which are attributable to estrogen. Other more serious adverse reactions include hypertension, liver damage, and thrombophlebitis and thromboembolis. Oral adverse reactions include increased gin-

Chapter 17 ~ Treatment of Endocrine Disorders   247

gival fluid, gingivitis, gingival inflammation similar to that seen during pregnancy, and an increased risk for dry socket after extractions.

Dental Concerns. The dental hygienist should review the importance of good oral hygiene with all patients taking oral contraceptives because of the potential for gingivitis and gingival inflammation. Extractions should also be performed on days 23 through 28 of the oral contraceptive cycle in order to minimize the risk of developing dry socket. The patient's blood pressure should be taken prior to any procedure because of the oral contraceptive's ability to cause hypertension. "Breaks" should be scheduled during long procedures in order to minimize the incidence of thrombophlebitis. Allow the patient to get up, stretch her legs, and walk around to keep the circulation going in all parts of her body.

Drug Interactions. Antibiotics, particularly penicillin and the tetracyclines, decrease the effectiveness of oral contraceptives. The patient should be counseled about this and an additional method of contraception should be recommended until the end of that oral contraceptive cycle. This should be documented in the patient's dental record.

ANDROGENS AND ANABOLIC STEROIDS

Testosterone is the main male sex hormone and has both *androgenic* and anabolic capabilities. Testosterone is responsible for secondary male sexual characteristics and its anabolic capabilities include increased osteoblastic activity, epiphyseal closure, increased sebaceous gland activity, an increase in tissue protein, and nitrogen retention. Therapeutic uses include the treatment of breast cancer or hormonal replacement therapy.

Anabolic steroid use has increased notably in sports and its use is no longer limited to elite athletes or adult males (Yesalis et al., 1993). Women and children as young as grade school have been illicitly using these drugs, to enhance their athletic performances. Examples include **methyltestosterone** (Metandren), **stanozol** (Winstrol), and **nandrolone decanoate** (Deca-Durabolin). This list does not include anabolic steroids from veterinary sources or foreign countries. These drugs are controlled substance Schedule III because of their relatively high incidence of abuse. The only legal use for these drugs in the medical field is in the treatment of cancers or the wasting associated with immunocompromising illnesses. Adverse reactions are many and include the following.

Hepatic Effects. Hepatitis, cancer, cholestatic jaundice, elevated liver function tests.

Endocrine Effects. Testicular atrophy, acne, gynecomastia, altered glucose tolerance, hyperinsulinism, decreased spermatogenesis, masculinization of women including deepening voice, hirsutism, menstrual irregularities, enlarged clitoris, decreased breast size, and alopecia.

Cardiovascular Effects. Increased blood pressure, increased cholesterol, increased sodium and water retention.

CNS Effects. Aggressiveness, mood swings, depression, euphoria, irritability, headache, and dizziness.

Summary

Steroids are used to treat asthma, chronic obstructive pulmonary disease, degenerative joint diseases, sepsis, and allergic rhinitis. These drugs can adversely affect alveolar bone development, mask symptoms of infection, and delay wound healing. They can exacerbate the GI adverse reactions associated with nonsteroidal antiinflammatory drugs that are often prescribed for dental pain.

Both diabetes and thyroid gland disorders can affect alveolar bone growth and development. It is thought that patients with diabetes may be at an increased risk for dental caries. Patients with diabetes may sometimes experience hypoglycemia in the dental office, especially if they have taken their antidiabetic medications without eating. This can be treated by immediately administering a sugar source to the patient. The drugs used to treat these disorders, and the disorders themselves, may interact with drugs used in the dental office. Epinephrine can increase heart rate and should be used with caution in patients with controlled hyperthyroidism, thyroid supplements, and with diabetes.

Women take estrogen supplements for the treatment of symptoms of menopause or in combination with progesterone for birth control. These hormones can increase gingival swelling and inflammation similar to pregnancy. Antibiotics prescribed in a dental office can interact with oral contraceptives and make them less effective. Women taking oral contraceptives are at a higher incidence for developing dry socket. They are also at risk for developing thrombophlebitis if they lie in one position for too long. These women should be allowed to get up and stretch their legs during a long procedure.

Anabolic steroids have become drugs of abuse. Signs and symptoms of their use may include mood swings that could make the patient uncooperative during an oral examination.

The dental hygienist will treat many patients with these endocrine disorders or conditions. These disorders or conditions may have oral manifestations or the medications used to treat them may adversely impact on oral hygiene and dental therapy. The dental hygienist should learn about these disorders, their oral manifestations, adverse reactions, and drug interactions to more effectively treat patients.

Case Study: Carter Edwards

Carter Edwards is a 10-year-old who has been coming to your practice for close to 6 years. He tries his best to brush his teeth at least twice a day (just like you told him). However, he is an active child and brushing his teeth isn't always on his agenda. He does floss at least three times a week and he is quite proud of this. About 4 years ago, however, Carter was diagnosed with juvenile-onset (Type 1) diabetes. Carter is fortunate in that his physician is working with him and his parents to maintain good control of his blood glucose levels without restricting his diet too much. Carter receives a combination of regular and intermediate-acting insulin and was just switched to the combination product Humulin 70/30 (this means two insulin injections a day instead of four). Carter and his parents are pleased with this and he is here today for a general oral examination and cleaning. He did remember to eat before coming in for his appointment and brought some juice just in case.

1. What is diabetes and what are its signs and symptoms?
2. Compare and contrast Type I and Type II diabetes.
3. What are some of the dental concerns associated with diabetes and how would the dental practitioner counsel Carter and his parents about them?
4. When should Carter's dental appointments be scheduled and why?
5. What is the rationale for Carter bringing juice to his dental appointment?
6. Compare and contrast the different types of insulin.
7. What are the adverse reactions associated with insulin?
8. Should Carter be treated with an antibiotic after his dental procedure? Why or why not?

Case Study: Ted Hamilton

Ted Hamilton is a 45-year-old with a history of myasthenia gravis. He takes oral steroids to treat the myasthenia gravis. Mr. Hamilton is otherwise healthy and takes occasional over-the-counter analgesics and cough and cold preparations. He is at your practice today for a maintenance oral examination.

1. Should steroid-dependent patients be prophylaxed with antibiotics prior to a dental procedure? Why or why not?
2. Mr. Hamilton needs to have a root canal and new crown. Should he receive an antibiotic after this procedure? Why or why not?
3. What are the adverse reactions associated with steroids?
4. What are the dental concerns associated with steroids?
5. Are there any drug interactions of which Mr. Hamilton needs to be aware?
6. What should the dental practitioner tell Mr. Hamilton about the dental concerns associated with steroids?

Review Questions

1. What are the functions of the hypothalamus and the pituitary gland?
2. How are hormones released into the body and what mechanism inhibits their release into the body?
3. Compare and contrast glucocorticoids and mineralcorticoids in terms of pharmacologic effects.
4. Compare and contrast hyperthyroidism and hypothyroidism including treatment and dental concerns.
5. Compare and contrast the oral antidiabetic medications.
6. What are the adverse reactions of oral antidiabetic medications?
7. What are the legal and illegal uses of male sex hormones?

BIBLIOGRAPHY

Bond WS: Toxic reactions and side effects of glucorticoids in man. *Am J Hosp Pharm* 34:479–485, 1977.

Colditz GA, Hankinson SE, Hunter DJ, et al.: The use of estrogens and progestins and the risk of breast cancer in postmenopausal women. *New Engl J Med* 332:1589–1593, 1995.

Felson DT, Zhang Y, Hannan MT, Kiel DP, Wilson PWF, Anderson JJ: The effect of postmenopausal estrogen therapy on bone density in elderly women. *N Engl J Med* 329:1141–1146, 1993.

Franklyn JA: The management of hyperthyroidism. *New Engl J Med* 330:1731–1738, 1994.

Hatcher RA, Trussell F, Stewart F, et al.: *Contraceptive Technology,* 16th rev. ed., Irvington Publishers, New York, 1994.

Kibble MW, Ross MB: Adverse effects of anabolic steroids in athletes. *Clin Pharm* 6:686–692, 1987.

Lebovitz HE: Oral antidiabetic agents: The emergence of α-glucosidase inhibitors. *Drugs* 44(Suppl 3):21–28, 1992.

Lefebvre PJ, Scheen AJ: Management of non-insulin-dependent diabetes mellitus. *Drugs* 44(Suppl 3):29–38, 1992.

McGuinness ME, Talbert RL: Management of thyroid disorders. *Am Pharm* NS34:36–47, 1994.

Ponte CD: Non-insulin-dependent diabetes mellitus–current practice and future trends. *J Amer Pharm Assoc* NS36:50–59, 1996.

Rodger W: Non-insulin-dependent (type II) diabetes mellitus. *Can Med Assoc J* 145:1571–1581, 1991.

Smith CM, Reynard AM (eds.): *Textbook of Pharmacology,* 1st ed. W. B. Saunders Company, Philadelphia, 1992.

Stanford JL, Weiss NS, Voight LF, Daling JR, Habel LA, Rossing MA: Combined estrogen and progestin hormone replacement therapy in relation to risk of breast cancer in middle-aged women. *JAMA* 274:137–142, 1995.

Stumvoll M, Nurjhan N, Perriello G, Dailey G, Gerich JE: Metabolic effect of metformin in non-insulin-dependent diabetes mellitus. *New Engl J Med* 333:550–554, 1995.

Toft AD: Thyroxine therapy. *New Engl J Med* 331:174–180, 1994.

Yesalis CE, Kennedy NJ, Kopstein AN, Bahrke MS: Anabolic-androgenic steroid use in the United States. *JAMA* 270:1217–1221, 1993.

CHAPTER 18

Infectious Disease Pharmacology

Key Terms

AIDS
Antiretroviral
CD4 T-Cells
Hepatitis

HIV
Opportunistic Infections
Tuberculosis

LEARNING OBJECTIVES

After completion of this chapter and its learning activities, the student should be able to:

1. Understand the difference between HIV and AIDS.
2. Describe the antiretroviral drugs used in the treatment of HIV infection including mechanism of action, adverse reactions, and drug interactions.
3. Discuss the dental concerns associated with HIV and AIDS.
4. List the different opportunistic infections associated with HIV and AIDS and their treatment(s).
5. List the different drugs used to treat tuberculosis including mechanism of action and adverse reactions.
6. Discuss the dental concerns associated with tuberculosis and its treatments.
7. Discuss the differences between hepatitis A, hepatitis B, hepatitis delta, and non-A, non-B hepatitis.
8. Describe the preexposure prophylaxis for hepatitis A and hepatitis B.
9. Describe the postexposure prophylaxis for hepatitis A and hepatitis B.
10. Describe the dental concerns associated with hepatitis.

INTRODUCTION

The dental hygienist will treat many patients with either acquired immunodeficiency virus (AIDS) and its related opportunistic infections, tuberculosis, or hepatitis. Although the dental hygienist cannot directly ask patients if they have AIDS, it is still important to obtain a medication/health history. Most patients will tell what medications they are taking and may often tell you the reason for taking them. The intent of this chapter is to briefly review these illnesses, the medications used to treat them, and the dental concerns associated with them.

ACQUIRED IMMUNODEFICIENCY SYNDROME (AIDS)

AIDS is the end result of the human immunodeficiency virus (HIV) when the symptoms of *HIV* infection become very severe. Once HIV infection is diagnosed, the purpose of treatment is to prolong survival, prevent opportunistic infections, and manage the symptoms of the disease in order to improve the patient's quality of life.

Antiretroviral Drugs

There are currently two classes of *antiretroviral* drugs used to treat HIV and AIDS. The first is the class of drugs known as nucleoside analogues and they include **zidovudine, didanosine, zalcitabine,** and **lamivudine.** They work by inhibiting HIV reverse transcriptase, the enzyme responsible for viral replication. Once the antiretroviral drug enters the *CD4 T-cell,* the nucleoside analogue is converted into an active triphosphate moiety by cellular enzymes and viral replication is inhibited by (1) competition between the drug and the naturally occurring nucleoside triphosphate for binding to the active site of HIV reverse transcriptase and (2) termination of deoxyribonucleic acid (DNA) synthesis (Skowron, 1992). Table 18-1 reviews the indications and adverse reactions of the these drugs.

The second, and new, class of drugs is known as HIV protease inhibitors. **Saquinavir mesylate** (Table 18-1) is first of the this class and was approved for use by the Food and Drug Administration (FDA) in December 1995. HIV protease inhibitors work by blocking the enzyme protease. Saquinavir can only be used with other nucleoside analogues at this time. The combination of the HIV protease inhibitor and

Table 18-1. Antiretroviral Drugs

Drug	Indication	Adverse Reactions
AZT: Zidovudine (Retrovir)	HIV-infected adults with CD4 counts <500 cells/mm^3 HIV-infected children more than 3 years old, with or without symptoms HIV-infected pregnant women HIV-infected women during labor and delivery Neonates during the first 6 weeks of life	Bone marrow suppression Anemia Neutropenia Myositis Fever Abdominal pain Diarrhea and vomiting Mood disturbances
ddI: Didanosine (Videx)	HIV-infected adults and children more than 6 months old with advanced HIV infection who have not responded to or cannot tolerate AZT	Pancreatitis (nausea, vomiting, abdominal pain, elevated amylase levels) Peripheral neuropathy Dizziness, headache Oral—stomatitis, taste loss/perversion, dry mouth

Table 18-1. Antiretroviral Drugs (*cont.*)

Drug	Indication	Adverse Reactions
ddC: Zalcitabine (Hivid)	HIV-infected adults who are failing AZT monotherapy and have CD4 counts ≤300 cells/mm^3	Peripheral neuropathy Pancreatitis Oral—Oral ulcers, dry mouth, glossitis, stomatitis
Indinavir* sulfate (Crixivan)	For use either alone or in combination with nucleoside analogues to treat HIV infection	Nephrolithiasis Flank pain with or without hematuria Rash Taste perversion Nausea Vomiting Diarrhea
3TC: Lamivudine (Epivir)*	For use as first-line therapy in combination with zidovudine for the treatment of HIV infections	Headache Nausea Malaise and fatigue Nasal symptoms Diarrhea Neuropathy Low white blood cell counts and anemia Pancreatitis in the pediatric population
Ritonavir (Norvir)**	For use either alone or in combination with nucleoside analogues to treat HIV infection	Asthenia Nausea Diarrhea Vomiting Anorexia Abdominal pain Taste perversion Circumoral and peripheral paresthesias
Saquinavir mesylate (Invirase)*	The first of a new class of protease inhibitors that is to be used in combination with nucleoside analogues such as zidovudine. It is indicated for the treatment of advanced HIV infection in selected patients.	Diarrhea Abdominal discomfort Nausea

*Both drugs were reviewed under the FDA's accelerated approval program that permits the early release of drugs based on laboratory results. Additional safety and efficacy data must be provided once the drugs are marketed in order for the drugs to remain on the market.

**Clinical trails were performed in patients with advanced stages of HIV. Additional data on patients with early-stage HIV are requested.

Sources: AED 1994; Saag MS, Nucleoside analogues: Adverse effects. *Hosp Pract* 27(Suppl 2):26–36, 1992; APhA Editorial Board on Pharmaceutical Care for Patients with HIV Infection: Pharmacotherapy of HIV. *Am Pharm* NS34:60–69, 1994. Anon, Drug updates. *J Amer Pharm Assoc* NS36:7–8, 289, 1996; Anon, First of new class of drugs approved for AIDS treatment. *Pharmacy Today* 2:3, January 15, 1996.

nucleoside analogue blocks two of the enzymes needed for the HIV virus to replicate. Saquinavir should not be used in combination with **rifampin** and caution should be used if it is used in combination with **rifabutin** or any other drug that increases hepatic enzyme systems. **Indinavir sulfate** (Crixivan) and **ritonavir** (Norvir) are also protease inhibitors which were approved by the FDA in 1996 for the treatment of HIV infection either alone or in combination with a nucleoside analogue.

Drug Interactions

Several of the antiretroviral drugs can interact with some of the drugs prescribed in the dental office, and cause toxicity or decreased therapeutic effect. The dental hygienist should carefully question patients about any medications that they may be receiving and decisions to treat should be made upon patient response to those questions. Drug interactions are as follows.

Nonopioid Analgesics. **Acetaminophen** and **aspirin** may potentiate the toxicity of zidovudine and concurrent administration should probably be avoided or used with great caution. (APhA Editorial Board on Pharmaceutical Care for Patients with HIV Infection, 1994). All three antiretroviral drugs have GI adverse reactions that could be potentiated with the addition of aspirin, nonsteroidal antiinflammatory drugs, or opioid analgesics.

Antianxiety Drugs.

LORAZEPAM. An increase in the toxicity of zidovudine (AEB, 1994) has been reported in connection with **Lorazepam.** Caution should be exercised if an antianxiety drug is prescribed.

TETRACYCLINE. The aluminum and magnesium in didanosine tablets chelate with **tetracycline,** making it less active. The problem can can avoided by giving tetracycline and didanosine at different times.

Dental Concerns

HIV infection is a concern for both dental personnel and the patient. HIV infection cannot be spread through casual contact and dental personnel can take precautions to prevent its spread during dental procedures. This can be accomplished by using universal precautions—that is, gloves and masks.

Both didanosine and zalcitabine have oral manifestations that include oral ulcerations and dry mouth. The dental hygienist should stress the importance of good oral hygiene with patients taking these drugs and suggest ways to treat oral manifestations and to minimize dry mouth. This topic is discussed in other chapters.

Opportunistic Infections

As a patient's CD4 T-cell count drops, he becomes more at risk for the development of any number of *opportunistic infections*. Table 18-2 reviews some opportunistic infections and the drugs used to treat them.

Table 18-2   Treatment of Selected Opportunistic Infections

Infection	Treatment

Pneumocystis carinii pneumonia	SMZ-TMP or
	    Pentamidine or
	    Dapsone + Trimethoprim or
	    Atovaquone or
	    Primaquine + Clindamycin

Toxoplasmosis	Pyrimethamine + Sulfadiazine or
	    Pyrimethamine + Clindamycin or
	    Atovaquone

Cryptosporidosis	Paromomycin or Azithromycin
Coccidioidomycosis	Amphotericin B or Fluconazole or Ketoconazole or Itraconazole
Cryptococcosis	Amphotericin B ± Flucytosine or Fluconazole or Itraconazole
Histoplasmosis	Amphotericin B or Itraconazole
Cytomegalovirus	Ganciclovir or Foscarnet

Disseminated *Mycobacterium avium* complex (MAC)	Clarithromycin or Azithromycin + one or more of the following:
	    Ethambutol, Clofazimine, Ciprofloxacin, Amikacin
	    Rifabutin + one or more of the above drugs
	    Prophylaxis - Rifabutin

Source: Anon, Drugs for AIDS and associated infections. *Med Lett* 35:79–86, 1993.

TUBERCULOSIS

Tuberculosis is caused by the acid-fast bacterium *Mycobacterium tuberculosis* that is highly communicable (infectious). The intent of therapy is to cure the patient of infection, make her noncontagious as soon as possible, and avoid relapse or failure. The majority of patients require the concomitant administration of two drugs to treat tuberculosis because of the problems with drug resistance. AIDS patients often require the concomitant administration of four drugs because of the increase in multiple-drug-resistant tuberculosis. Table 18-3 reviews drugs used to treat tuberculosis.

Dental Concerns

Since the dental hygienist may not know that her patient has tuberculosis, she should take precautions with all patients. The dental hygienist should always wear a mask and gloves when working with a patient. This should help to prevent the transmission of tuberculosis from the patient to dental personnel and vice versa.

HEPATITIS

Acute viral *hepatitis* is among the most common causes of liver disease and jaundice. There are four distinct causative agents responsible for causing hepatitis: hepatitis A virus (HAV), hepatitis B virus (HBV), delta hepatitis caused by the HBV-associat-

Table 18-3   Drugs Used in the Treatment of Tuberculosis

Drug	Adverse Reactions
Isoniazid (INH)	Lightheadedness, peripheral neuropathies (give vitamin B_6) hepatoxicity, gastrointestinal effects, dry mouth
Rifampin (Rifadin)	Anorexia, nausea, vomiting, diarrhea, GI discomfort, red-orange color to all body fluids (including saliva)
Pyrazinamide (PZA)	Rash, hyperuricemia, GI effects, hepatotoxic
Ethambutol (Myambutol)	Optic neuritis, rash, joint pain, GI discomfort, malaise, headache, dizziness

Source: Anon, Drugs for AIDS and associated infections. *Med Lett* 35:79–86, 1993.

ed delta agent (HDV), and non-A, non-B hepatitis, whose cause is unknown. Table 18-4 reviews the mode of transmission, incubation period, onset, preexposure prophylaxis, and postexposure prophylaxis from an infected source for the different types of hepatitis.

Dental Concerns

Both hepatitis type A and type B can be transmitted orally. The dental hygienist should use caution with any patient who has hepatitis. Gloves should be worn when treating patients and the dental hygienist should always wash his hands after each patient. Caution should also be used if a patient with hepatitis B, hepatitis delta, or hepatitis non-A, non-B requires an injection. All three types can be transmitted via a "needle-stick."

Table 18-4   A Comparison of the Different Types of Hepatitis

	Hepatitis A	Hepatitis B	Delta Hepatitis	Non-A, Non-B Hepatitis
Mode of transmission	Fecal-oral Contaminated shellfish, food, water	Parenteral, oral-oral, venereal	Parenteral	Parenteral
Incubation period (mean)	28 days	75 days	35 days	50 days
Onset	Sudden	Insidious	—	Insidious
Preexposure prophylaxis	Hepatitis A vaccine	Hepatitis B vaccine	Hepatitis B vaccine	No specific recommendations
Postexposure prophylaxis	Immune globulin or hepatitis A vaccine	Hepatitis B vaccine or hepatitis B immune globulin	Hepatitis B vaccine or hepatitis B immune globulin	No specific recommendations

Source: Anon, Hepatitis A vaccine. *Am Pharm* NS35:5–6, 1995.

Summary

Patients with infectious diseases are of concern to the dental hygienist. The illnesses themselves and their medications can impact on dental treatment. Patients with HIV are living longer and can take many different medications to control their disease as well as a host of potential opportunistic infections. Zidovudine, an antiretroviral drug, interacts with both aspirin and acetaminophen. All antiretroviral drugs have GI adverse reactions that could be exacerbated by the addition of a nonsteroidal antiinflammatory drug. Extreme caution should be used if an analgesic is necessary. Saquinavir is the first in a new class of anti-AIDS drugs called HIV protease inhibitors. The extent of its adverse reaction and drug interaction profile is unknown. The dental practitioner should work with HIV and AIDS patients to make sure that they have optimal oral health care.

Tuberculosis and hepatitis are two other infectious diseases that dental patients may have. Both can occur in HIV and AIDS patients and tuberculosis occurs in others with immunocompromised health (e.g., alcoholics). Both are contagious, though the use of universal precautions will help to decrease their spread. The dental hygienist can better treat these patients by becoming knowledgeable about HIV, tuberculosis, and hepatitis including modes of transmission, ways to minimize or prevent transmission, and medications used to treat these diseases.

Case Study: Susan Brown

Susan Brown is 26 years old and has been coming to your practice for close to 10 years. She is an administrative assistant with a local finance company. Ms. Brown had noted a definite deterioration in her health over the past year and a half and went to numerous physicians to find out what was wrong. You have noted the definite decline in her health. Ms. Brown comes in today for her regular oral examination and cleaning. Prior to starting the examination you review Ms. Brown's medication/health history. Ms. Brown proceeds to tell you what has happened to her over the past 6 months. She was finally referred to an infectious disease specialist who diagnosed her with HIV (previous tests were negative) and a CD4 count of about 500 cells/mm^3. Ms. Brown was immediately placed on zidovudine therapy and has had several bouts of esophageal candidiasis and numerous vaginal yeast infections.

1. What is the difference between HIV and AIDS?
2. How do nucleoside analogue antiretroviral drugs work?
3. Compare and contrast the four nucleoside analogue antiretroviral drugs in terms of indications and adverse reactions.
4. What are the different drug interactions associated with nucleoside analogue antiretroviral drugs and how do they impact on dental therapy?
5. Which nucleoside analogue antiretroviral drugs have oral manifestations and what are the oral manifestations?
6. What are the dental concerns with HIV and AIDS?

7. What are some of the different opportunistic infections associated with HIV and AIDS?
8. What are some of the drugs used to treat esophageal candidiasis?

Case Study: Walter Phillips

Walter Phillips is a 32-year-old who is new to your practice. He is somewhat emaciated and appears to be in poor health. During the medication/health history you learn that he is on the following medications: zidovudine, saquinavir, SMZ-TMP, rifabutin, and itraconazole. Mr. Phillips tells you that he is HIV positive and has a series of other HIV-related infections as well.

1. What can you do to prevent the transmission of viruses/bacteria to Mr. Phillips? (You have a head cold.)
2. How can the dental hygienist minimize the transmission of HIV disease during a dental procedure?
3. What is saquinavir and how does it differ from zidovudine?
4. What are some of the adverse reactions associated with saquinavir?
5. What are two drug interactions associated with saquinavir?
6. What are opportunistic infections and which ones does Mr. Phillips have?

Review Questions

1. What is tuberculosis and what are the main goals of therapy?
2. Why do patients receive more than one drug to treat tuberculosis?
3. What are the dental concerns associated with tuberculosis?
4. Compare and contrast antituberculosis drugs in terms of mechanisms of action.
5. Compare and contrast antituberculosis drugs in terms of adverse reactions.
6. Compare and contrast the different types of hepatitis.
7. How is hepatitis transmitted?
8. What are the dental concerns associated with hepatitis?
9. How can one prophylaxis against hepatitis A and hepatitis B?

BIBLIOGRAPHY

Anon: Hepatitis A vaccine. *Am Pharm* NS35:5–6, 1995.
Anon: Drugs for AIDS and associated infections. *Med Lett* 35:79–86, 1993.
Anon: Drug updates. *J Amer Pharm Assoc* NS36:7–8, 289, 1996.
Anon: First of new class of drugs approved for AIDS treatment. *Pharmacy Today* 2:3, January 15, 1996.
APhA Editorial Board on Pharmaceutical Care for Patients with HIV Infection: Pharmacotherapy of HIV. *Am Pharm* NS34:60–69, 1994.
Beam TR Jr.: Drugs used in the treatment of tuberculosis: Antimycobacterial agents. In Smith

CM, Reynard AM (eds.), *Textbook of Pharmacology* 1st ed. W. B. Saunders Company, Philadelphia, 1992.

Lee BL, Safrin S: Interactions and toxicities of drugs used in patients with AIDS. *Clin Infect Dis* 14:773–779, 1992.

Saag MS: Nucleoside analogues: Adverse effects. *Hosp Pract* 27(Suppl 2):26–36, 1992.

Skowron G: Nucleoside analogues: Monotherapy. *Hosp Pract* 27 (Suppl 2):5–13, 1992.

CHAPTER 19

Antineoplastic Drugs

Key Terms

Alkylating Drugs
Antimetabolites
Benign
Chemotherapy

Malignant
Metastasis
Neoplasia

LEARNING OBJECTIVES

After completion of this chapter and its learning activities, the student should be able to:

1. Describe the reproductive cycle of a cell.
2. Describe the general characteristics of cancer cells and define neoplasia, malignant, benign, and metastasis.
3. Discuss the rationale for the use of chemotherapy and its effectiveness in treating cancer.
4. List the different types of chemotherapeutic agents and describe their general mechanisms of action and adverse reactions.
5. List examples of the different classes of chemotherapeutic agents along with mechanisms of action and clinical use.
6. Discuss the dental concerns associated with chemotherapeutic agents and effectively counsel patients about them.

INTRODUCTION

The antineoplastic drugs are used to treat many different types of cancers and have helped many people live longer lives. As a result, the dental hygienist will treat many cancer patients in his practice. These drugs have adverse reactions that can affect dental treatment. The intent of this chapter is to briefly review the available chemotherapeutic agents and their mechanisms of action with emphasis on adverse reactions and their management.

CANCER CELL PATHOPHYSIOLOGY

Normal cells have the ability to reproduce (mitotic activity) at a steady rate, reproducing daughter cells that are exactly like them. Cancer cells differ from normal cells in that mitotic activity is accelerated and they no longer reproduce daughter cells that are exactly like them. These new cells are abnormal and can either be localized to a particular area (tumor) or can diffuse throughout the body (e.g., lymph related).

The terms describing both cancerous and noncancerous cells are as follows:

Neoplasia: overgrowth of cells; increased mitotic activity with the production of abnormal cells.

Benign: overgrowth of new cells, but the overgrowth is slower and localized to a specific area.

Malignant: rapid new overgrowth of cells that spreads locally or throughout the body.

Metastasis: abnormal cells have spread to distant sites throughout the body.

TREATMENT OF CANCER

Cancer therapy is dependent on the type of tumor (benign vs. malignant), stage of diagnosis (early vs. late), and degree of metastasis. Therapy consists of surgery, radiation, or chemotherapy (drug use). Surgery is used if the neoplasm is localized and easily accessible, especially if it is diagnosed early. Radiation therapy is often used if the tumor site is inaccessible or the tumor is inoperable and was not diagnosed early. *Chemotherapy* is used to destroy and suppress the growth and spread of malignant cells. One or a combination of all three may be used to completely suppress the tumor for a chance of a total cure.

Chemotherapy

The current philosophy of chemotherapeutic drugs is to aggressively use them in the initial stages of cancer for a more promising potential to control and cure the disease. However, this also involves more severe adverse reactions including oral manifestations.

Mechanism of Action. Chemotherapeutic or antineoplastic drugs work by interfering with cell mitotic activity at any one of the four stages of cell reproduction. The four stages are as follows:

- G_1 ("gap"1)—postmitotic or pre-DNA synthesis
- S—period of DNA synthesis
- G_2 ("gap"2)—premitotic or post-DNA synthesis
- M—period of mitosis

Cells that are at rest or not reproducing are in the G_0 stage and cells enter the reproductive cycle from this stage. Problems occur when a large portion of tumor cells are in this stage and unable to be destroyed by chemotherapy.

Adverse Reactions. Unfortunately, chemotherapeutic agents attack both cancerous and normal cells, which leads to many different adverse reactions. These drugs tend to attack cells in the bone marrow, gastrointestinal (GI) tract, and skin because they have a very high growth rate. The main adverse reactions are as follows.

BONE MARROW SUPPRESSION. Bone marrow suppression leads to leukopenia, agranulocytosis, thrombocytopenia, and anemia. This puts the patient at a greater risk for developing infections because of such a drastic drop in white blood cells. Patients may bleed more easily and are always tired.

GASTROINTESTINAL EFFECTS. GI adverse reactions include nausea, vomiting, diarrhea, stomatitis, and oral ulcerations.

DERMATOLOGIC EFFECTS. Skin adverse reactions can range from mild erythema to maculopapular eruptions to exfoliative dermatitis and Stevens-Johnson syndrome. Alopecia, or hair loss, occurs frequently and hair usually regrows once therapy has been stopped.

HEPATOXICITY. Liver problems can occur with almost all cancer chemotherapeutic drugs but occur more frequently with antimetabolites.

Nephrotoxicity. Many of these agents cause *hyperuricemia*, which can lead to renal tubular impairment.

GERM CELLS. Cancer chemotherapeutic drugs attack rapidly growing cells and inhibit spermatogenesis and oogenesis. These drugs are contraindicated in pregnancy because of their ability to attack, mutate, and destroy a rapidly growing fetus.

ORAL EFFECTS. These medications can cause dry mouth, altered sense of taste, sensitivity of the teeth and gums, mucosal pain and ulceration, and gingival hemorrhage.

CARDIOTOXICITY. Potential cardiovascular reactions include congestive heart failure, dysrhythmia, ischemia, and hypotension.

Classification of Chemotherapeutic Drugs. Chemotherapeutic drugs are classified according to their mechanism and site of action. Table 19-1 lists these chemotherapeutic drugs.

ALKYLATING DRUGS. These drugs bind with DNA (deoxyribonucleic acid) and inhibit cell reproduction during the S phase of the cell reproductive cycle.

PLANT ALKALOIDS. These drugs are mitotic inhibitors and stop cell growth during the metaphase.

ANTIBIOTICS. These drugs are cell-cycle nonspecific and are effective against solid tumors.

HORMONES. Hormones work by interrupting cell cycle reproduction during the G_1 stage.

ANTIMETABOLITES. These drugs are similar to the metabolites found in the body that cells use for normal growth and function. *Antimetabolites* compete with metabolites needed by the cell and are incorporated into the normal synthesis pathway, which blocks the growth and normal reproduction.

Table 19-1   Selected Cancer Chemotherapeutic Drugs

Category	Examples
Alkylating Agent	**Nitrogen Mustards** Mechlorethamine (Mustargen) Cyclophosphamide (Cytoxan) Chlorambucil (Leukeran) **Nitrosureas** Carmustine (BiCNU) Semustine (MethylCcnu) **Miscellaneous** Busulfan (Myleran) Cisplatin (Platinol)
Antimetabolites	**Folic Acid Analog** Methotrexate (Amethopterin) **Pyrimidine Analog** Fluorouracil (5-FU) Cytarabine (Cytosar) **Purine Analog** Mercaptopurine (Purinethol, 6-MP)
Miscellaneous	**Plant Alkaloids** Vinblastine (Velban) Vincristine (Oncovin) **Antibiotics** Dactinomycin (Actinomycin-D) Doxorubicin (Adriamycin) **Hormones** Prednisone Antiestrogen (Tamoxifen [Nolvadex]) Estrogen **Immune Modulators** Interferon **Other** Hydroxyurea (Hydrea) Paclitaxel (Taxol)

Source: Calabresi P, Chabner BA, Antineoplastic drugs. In Goodman Gilman A, Rall TW, Nies AS, Taylor P (eds.), *Goodman and Gilman's The Pharmacological Basis of Therapeutics,* 8th ed. Pergamon Press, New York, 1990.

Dental Concerns Associated with Cancer Chemotherapeutic Drugs. Patients taking cancer chemotherapeutic drugs must to be treated carefully. The dental hygienist needs to work with her patient prior to, during, and after chemotherapy to ensure optimal oral hygiene. The best defense for these patients is to obtain maximum oral hygiene and dental health prior to chemotherapy. Dental procedures should be avoided during chemotherapy because the patient is at risk for infection because of low white blood

Table 19-2   Proper Oral Care for Patients Undergoing Cancer Chemotherapy

Stage of Chemotherapy	Oral Care
Prior to chemotherapy	1. Maximize oral health care. 2. Treat any existing infections. 3. Control periodontal disease. 4. Provide patients with information on good oral hygiene.
During chemotherapy	1. Treat only if necessary and after consulting with the patient's oncologist. 2. Document hematologic status. 3. Treatment should only be given if the neutrophil count is ≥1000/mm. 4. Prophylaxis for bacterial endocarditis if a venous catheter is present. 5. Institute good oral hygiene measures (brush properly; rinse with baking soda, saline, or chlorhexidrine). Use baking soda or saline rinses after vomiting. Do not brush teeth. No dentures at night. Do not use commercial mouthwashes. Use topical fluorides if there is prolonged xerostomia. 6. Culture any lesions.
After chemotherapy	1. Perform necessary dental treatment. 2. Continue to maintain oral health.

cell counts. Platelets may also be low and this puts the patient at increased risk for bleeding. Patients should come in for dental care just prior to any type of chemotherapeutic regimen because they are feeling their best and their white counts are normal. Table 19-2 reviews the oral care necessary for patients receiving cancer chemotherapeutic drugs.

Summary

There are a number of different drugs used to treat cancer and many patients are taking these drugs. Many patients experience dry mouth or an altered sense of taste as a result of the drugs. Vomiting is an adverse reaction of all cancer chemotherapeutic drugs and this can adversely affect oral hygiene. Patients should be instructed about the best way to perform oral hygiene once they have vomited. Cancer chemotherapeutic drugs can lower a patient's white blood cell count, which could make it difficult for the patient to fight off infections. It is very important for patients to be treated when their white blood counts are within normal ranges. It is also important for the dental hygienist to work with the patient to ensure that he maintains optimal oral hygiene during chemotherapy.

Case Study: Mary Jones

Mary Jones is a 55-year-old of mixed European descent who has been a patient of yours for close to 15 years. Her daughter came in for her scheduled appointment and told you that Mrs. Jones underwent surgery for breast cancer 2 months ago. Mrs. Jones has an appointment with you next month and plans on keeping that appointment. Her daughter would like to know if there is anything her mother can do to "get a running start" on preventing or minimizing the oral adverse reactions associated with the chemotherapy that she is starting next week.

1. What are the oral adverse reactions associated with cancer chemotherapeutic drugs?
2. What should Mrs. Jones do for oral care prior to chemotherapy and how can you help in this matter?
3. Counsel Mrs. Jones on the appropriate oral hygiene program during chemotherapy.
4. Why sould you be concerned about bone marrow suppression in someone receiving oral care?
5. Do GI adverse reactions affect oral hygiene? If so, how?

Review Questions

1. Compare and contrast the following terms: benign, malignant, neoplasia, and metastasis.
2. What are the general mechanisms of action of cancer chemotherapeutic drugs?
3. Compare and contrast the different approaches to treating cancer.
4. What are the major classifications of cancer chemotherapeutic drugs? Give one example of each.
5. What are the adverse reactions associated with cancer chemotherapeutic drugs (excluding bone marrow suppression, GI, and oral)?

BIBLIOGRAPHY

Calabresi P, Chabner BA: Antineoplastic drugs. In Goodman Gilman A, Rall TW, Nies AS, Taylor P (eds.), *Goodman and Gilman's The Pharmacological Basis of Therapeutics,* 8th ed. Pergamon Press, New York, 1990.

Calabresi P, Schein PS, Rosenberg SA: *Medical Oncology: Basic Principles and Clinical Management of Cancer.* Macmillan, New York, 1985.

CHAPTER 20

Treatment of Seizure Disorders

Key Terms

Barbiturates
Carbamazepine
Clonazepam
Ethosuximide
Felbamate

Focal Seizure
General Seizure
Hydantoin
Lamotrigine
Valproate

LEARNING OBJECTIVES

After completion of this chapter and its learning activities, the student should be able to:

1. Define epilepsy.
2. Describe the two categories of seizures and give a brief description of the different classifications of seizure disorders.
3. Describe the diagnosis and overall management of epilepsy.
4. Discuss the mechanism of action, clinical use, and adverse reactions associated with phenytoin.
5. Discuss the relationship of gingival hyperplasia with phenytoin including ways to minimize it.
6. Discuss the mechanisms of action, clinical use, and adverse reactions of phenobarbital and primidone.
7. Discuss the mechanisms of action, clinical use, and adverse reactions associated with ethosuximide, carbamazepine, and valproate.
8. Discuss the use of benzodiazepines in the treatment of seizure disorders.
9. Be familiar with the newer antiseizure medications; know their therapeutic effects and mechanism of action.
10. Review and counsel patients on the dental concerns associated with all antiseizure drugs.

INTRODUCTION

Epilepsy has been defined as a state of recurrent single or multiple seizures accompanied by motor activity or changes in sensory or emotional behavior. It is a common disorder that affects a large number of individuals with an estimated prevalence ranging from 0.5% to 3% of the population (Garnett, 1992a; 1992b; Pugh and Garnett, 1991). The dental hygienist will perform oral care on many patients with seizure disorders. Both seizure disorders and the medications used to treat them can impact on oral health care. The intent of this chapter is to review seizure disorders and the medications used to treat them including a brief review of mechanisms of action, clinical use, adverse reactions, and dental concerns.

ETIOLOGY

The etiology of epilepsy is varied. Seizures may be a result of trauma, infection, toxins, fever, congenital malformation, vascular disease, metabolic or nutritional imbalance, neoplasm, hereditary factors, drugs, and degenerative disorders. The majority of patients, however, have seizures for which there is no known cause (idiopathic).

CLASSIFICATION OF SEIZURE DISORDERS

Most seizures can be divided into two categories: *general* and partial *(focal)*. Generalized seizures are bilaterally symmetrical and do not have a local onset. The seizures are usually accompanied by a loss of consciousness and may or may not be accompanied by convulsive movements. For example, absence seizures are nonconvulsive, primarily affect children, and are characterized by brief periods of "staring off." Generalized tonic-clonic, clonic, and tonic seizures are characterized by convulsive movements.

Partial seizures begin in a local area in one hemisphere of the brain and are further classified as simple or complex. Patients remain conscious during simple partial seizures and have impaired consciousness during complex partial seizures. Both types can evolve into generalized tonic-clonic seizures and the process is referred to as "secondary generalization."

PHARMACOTHERAPY OF SEIZURE DISORDERS

The intent of drug therapy is to prevent the recurrence of seizures without compromising the patient's quality of life because of adverse reactions. If therapy is required, one should attempt to treat the patient with single drug therapy at a low dose with gradual dosage increases over 3–4 weeks. Multiple drug therapy should be reserved for individuals who cannot tolerate high doses of single therapy or who have not responded to at least two different drugs (Garnett, 1992b). Table 20-1 lists the different seizures and medications used to treat them, and Table 20-2 reviews the drugs and doses used to treat seizure disorders.

Barbiturates

Phenobarbital is the most common *barbiturate* used to treat generalized tonic-clonic and focal seizures, and status epilepticus. It can be used alone or in combination with

Table 20-1   Treatment of Seizure Disorders

Seizure Disorder	Drug of Choice	Alternatives
Tonic-clonic	Phenytoin Carbamazepine Valproic Acid	Phenobarbital Primidone
Absence	Ethosuximide Valproic Acid	Clonazepam Trimethadione
Simple partial	Carbamazepine Felbamate Phenytoin Phenobarbital	Gabapentin Phenobarbital Primidone
Complex partial	Carbamazepine Felbamate Phenytoin Valproic Acid	Gabapentin Phenobarbital Primidone
Status epilepticus	Diazepam	Phenytoin Phenobarbital

Source: Data from Garnett WR, Epilepsy. In DiPiro JT, Talbert RL, Hayes PE, et al., eds., *Pharmacotherapy: A Pathophysiologic Approach,* 2nd ed. Elsevier, New York, 1992; Meyer MC, Cloyd J, Garnett WR, Holmes GL, Schiffer JR, Practical considerations in anticonvulsant therapy—Parts 1 and 2. *Am Pharm* NS35:22–26, 31–34, 1995.

other seizure medications. Phenobarbital is discussed in detail as it is the prototype for its class.

Mechanism of Action. It is thought that barbiturates work by elevating the seizure threshold of both the epileptogenic and normal neurons by nonselectively depressing neuronal excitation and preventing seizure spread.

Adverse Reactions. The most common adverse reactions affect the central nervous system (CNS). Sedation is the most common CNS effect and most patients develop tolerance to it. Though sedation is common in adults, phenobarbital may cause hyperactivity in children and may cause confusion, excitation, or depression in the elderly.

Other adverse reactions include such skin reactions as exfoliative dermatitis, erythema multiforme, Stevens-Johnson syndrome, and pruritus.

Hydantoins

Phenytoin is the most commonly used *hydantoin* and is discussed as the prototype of this group. Phenytoin is the drug of choice for generalized tonic-clonic seizures, partial seizures, and tonic-clonic status epilepticus. It is not used to treat absence seizures and may actually aggravate them.

Mechanism of Action. Phenytoin is thought to work by preventing the spread of the seizure discharge.

Table 20-2 Antiepileptic Drug Therapy*

Generic Name	Trade Name	Dose
Barbiturates		
Phenobarbital	Luminal	60–200 mg/day
Hydantoins		
Phenytoin	Dilantin	300–400 mg/day
Succinimides		
Ethosuximide	Zarontin	250–3000 mg/day
Oxazolidinediones		
Trimethadione	Tridione	900–2400 mg/day
Benzodiazepines		
Clonazepam	Clonopin	1.5–20 mg/day
Diazepam*	Valium	5–10 mg IV, repeatable up to 30 mg
Other Agents		
Carbamazepine	Tegretol	600–1600 mg/day
Felbamate	Felbatol	1200–3600 mg/day
Gabapentin	Neurontin	900–1800 mg/day
Primidone	Mysoline	350mg–1400 mg/day
Valproic acid	Depakene/Depakote	1000–3000 mg/day

Source: Garnett WR, Epilepsy. In DiPiro JT, Talbert RL, Hayes PE et al., eds., *Pharmacotherapy: A Pathophysiologic Approach*, 2nd ed. Elsevier, New York, 1992; Meyer MC, Cloyd J, Garnett WR, Holmes GL, Schiffer JR, Practical considerations in anticonvulsant therapy—Parts 1 and 2. *Am Pharm* NS35:22–26, 31–34, 1995

*Treatment of status epilepticus

Adverse Reaction. Phenytoin's narrow therapeutic index allows for many adverse reactions that affect many body systems. The chance for an adverse effect is also increased because phenytoin demonstrates saturated pharmacokinetics, which means that a small increase in dose can cause large increases in blood levels.

GASTROINTESTINAL EFFECTS. The most common adverse reactions associated with phenytoin are nausea, vomiting, loss of taste, and anorexia.

CENTRAL NERVOUS SYSTEM EFFECTS. CNS adverse reactions include sedation, confusion, nystagmus, ataxia, slurred speech, blurred vision, diplopia, amblyopia, dizziness, and insomnia.

OTHER EFFECTS. Other adverse reactions include hirsutism, rash, rarely exfoliative dermatitis, systemic lupus erythematosus (SLE), and Stevens-Johnson syndrome. Phenytoin use may also lead to vitamin D and folate deficiency characterized by oral mucosal changes such as stomatitis or glossitis.

Oral Adverse Reactions. Gingival hyperplasia (gingival overgrowth) may occur from shortly after the patient has started therapy to after several years of therapy. Most patients usually develop gingival hyperplasia after 2–3 months of therapy with a maximal hyperplastic state within 9–12 months.

The management of gingival hyperplasia involves the patient, dental personnel, and the patient's physician. Patients should be instructed to continue to take their phenytoin and only discontinue it under the direct supervision of their physician. Improved oral hygiene may reduce the rate of formation of the hyperplasia and a reduction in phenytoin dose or changing to another seizure medication should help reduce the amount of hyperplasia. A gingivectomy may be used when gingival hyperplasia interferes with plaque control, esthetics, chewing, or when improved oral hygiene has failed. However, hyperplasia can return after a gingivectomy if the patient remains on phenytoin. A gingivectomy should not be performed until at least 18 months postphenytoin therapy because a number of individuals can continue to experience a decrease in hyperplasia past the first year.

Valproate

Valproic acid is used in the treatment of absence seizures, generalized tonic-clonic seizures, and complex partial seizures. It is structurally unrelated to other anticonvulsants.

Mechanism of Action. It is thought that valproic acid works by increasing the inhibitory neurotransmitter γ-aminobutyric acid (GABA).

Hematologic Effects. Adverse reactions include hepatoxicity and bleeding, and the patient may present with petcchia, bruising, hematoma, or thrombocytopenia. Bleeding time may be prolonged due to the inhibition of platelet aggregation.

Gastrointestinal Effects. The most common adverse reactions associated with valproic acid are nausea, vomiting, and indigestion. Other GI effects include hypersalivation, anorexia, increased appetite, cramping, diarrhea, and constipation.

Central Nervous System Effects. CNS reactions include sedation and drowsiness. Hyperactivity, aggression, and behavioral disturbances have been reported in children. This may make it more difficult to treat a child who cannot sit still or becomes aggressive during a dental procedure.

Carbamazepine

Carbamazepine is structurally related to tricyclic antidepressants and is used to treat generalized tonic-clonic seizures, temporal lobe epilepsy (TLE), and mixed seizures.

Mechanism of Action. Carbamazepine is thought to work by limiting seizure propagation by reducing postetanic potentiation of synaptic transmission.

Adverse Reactions. Adverse reactions include sinus tachycardia, atrioventricular conduction delay, urinary frequency and retention, oliguria, and impotence.

HEMATOLOGIC EFFECTS. Carbamazepine therapy can cause agranulocytosis, thrombocytopenia, leukopenia, and aplastic anemia. Frequent carbamazepine blood levels are necessary at the initiation of therapy or after a dose increase. Signs of a low white blood cell count include fever, chills, aches, and pains. The patient should be advised to contact her physician should she have any of these symptoms.

CENTRAL NERVOUS SYSTEM EFFECTS. CNS reactions include dizziness, vertigo, drowsiness, fatigue, ataxia, confusion, headache, nystagmus, and visual and speech disturbances.

DERMATOLOGIC EFFECTS. Dermatologic reactions include rashes, urticaria, erythema multiforme, exfoliative dermatitis, photosensitivity, altered skin pigmentation, reports of aggravation of SLE, and alopecia.

GASTROINTESTINAL EFFECTS. Nausea, vomiting, diarrhea, gastric distress, abdominal pain, constipation, and anorexia are indicative of gastrointestinal adverse reactions.

ORAL ADVERSE REACTIONS. Oral adverse reactions include dry mouth, glossitis, and stomatitis.

Dose Forms. The pediatric dose form (chewable tablet) of carbamazepine is 63% sugar. The dental practitioner should discuss this with both parent and child. Both parent and child should be counseled on the importance of good oral hygiene, especially after the child has chewed the tablet.

Ethosuximide

Ethosuximide is used to treat absence seizures. It has no positive clinical effects against tonic-clonic and partial complex seizures.

Adverse Reactions. Serious adverse reactions include positive direct Coombs test, SLE, Stevens-Johnson syndrome, parkinsonian symptoms, and psychotic episodes.

GASTROINTESTINAL EFFECTS. Adverse reactions include anorexia, gastric upset, nausea, vomiting, diarrhea, and abdominal pain.

CENTRAL NERVOUS SYSTEM EFFECTS. CNS effects include drowsiness, dizziness, lethargy, headache, hiccups, and hyperactivity.

Oral Adverse Reactions. Oral adverse reactions include gingival hypertrophy and swelling of the tongue.

Trimethadione

Because of its high rate of toxicity, **trimethadione** is mainly used to treat absence seizures unresponsive to other available therapies. It is sometimes used in combination with other antiepileptic medications to treat combination seizure disorders.

Adverse Reactions. Adverse reactions include drowsiness and visual disturbances. Ataxia, sedation, and incoordination occur at high doses. Other adverse reactions include rash, exfoliative dermatitis, erythema multiforme, neutropenia, pancytopenia, fetal malformations, nephrotic syndrome, hepatitis, SLE, and myasthenia gravis.

Benzodiazepines

Several benzodiazepines (Chapter 9) used to treat seizure disorders include intravenous **diazepam** and **lorazepam** for recurrent tonic-clonic seizures and **clorazapate** as adjunctive therapy for the treatment of partial seizures. *Clonazepam,* another benzodiazepine (Chapter 9), is used as adjunct treatment for seizures not responsive to ethosuximide. It is effective in the treatment of infantile spasms and myoclonic and atonic seizures, and it has shown some efficacy against simple and complex partial seizures and tonic-clonic seizures.

Oral Adverse Reactions. Oral adverse reactions associated with clonazepam therapy include coated tongue, dry mouth, encopresis, abnormal thirst, and tender gums.

Primidone

Primidone is structurally related to phenobarbital and is effective against tonic-clonic and partial seizures. It is also used as adjunctive therapy to phenytoin and carbamazepine. Most of the adverse reactions associated with primidone are the same as those with phenobarbital.

Gabapentin

Gabapentin was approved in 1993 by the Food and Drug Administration (FDA) for use in combination with other antiepileptic medications for the treatment of partial seizures with or without secondary generalizations in persons over the age of 12. Its exact mechanism of action is unknown and it is structurally related to the neurotransmitter GABA acid. Gabapentin is unique among seizure medications in that it does not interfere with the metabolism of other seizure medications and should not require as much laboratory monitoring; it should require fewer dose adjustments. It is not metabolized by the liver and is excreted unchanged in the kidneys, which leads to a favorable drug interaction profile. Adverse reactions include sleepiness, nystagmus, decreased muscular coordination, dizziness, and fatigue.

Felbamate

Felbamate, structurally similar to meprobamate, was recently approved by the FDA (1993) for single therapy or in combination with other antiepileptic medications for the treatment of partial seizures with or without secondary generalization in adults. It has also been approved for the treatment of seizures associated with Lennox-Gastaut syndrome in children.

Mechanism of Action. The exact mechanism of action of felbamate is unknown. It has been observed in neuronal cultures that felbamate blocks sustained, repetitive neuronal firing, possibly through an effect on sodium channels.

Adverse Reactions. Headache, insomnia, fatigue, nausea, vomiting, dyspepsia, weight loss, constipation, and diarrhea were the more frequently reported adverse reactions during clinical trials (Sorensen and Farrington, 1993). Other adverse reactions include somnolence, ataxia, rash, fever, and agitation. There have been reports of leukopenia, thrombocytopenia, agranulocytosis, and Stevens-Johnson syndrome when felbamate was given with other drugs.

Warning. Patients taking felbamate have an increased risk (up to 100 times greater) of developing aplastic anemia. The risk of death due to aplastic anemia is dependent on the severity and etiology of the anemia, with an estimated fatality rate of 20–30%. Felbamate has also been associated with a high risk of liver failure. Prescribers are aware of this risk and patients must now sign a patient information/consent form before they can receive this medication (*F-D-C Reports,* October 3, 1994; Pokalo Jones, 1995).

Lamotrigine

Lamotrigine is a new antiepileptic drug that is structurally unrelated to other antiseizure medications. It was recently approved as adjunct therapy in the treatment of partial seizures in adults with epilepsy.

Adverse Reactions. The adverse effects reported from available studies include diplopia, dizziness, somnolence, headache, ataxia, and asthenia (Matsu et al., 1993).

DENTAL CONCERNS ASSOCIATED WITH ANTIEPILEPTIC DRUGS

Seizure disorders and antiepileptic drugs can interfere with good oral hygiene and dental procedures. A detailed medication/health history will help to determine patients with seizure disorders and those taking antiepileptic drugs. The dental hygienist can help by educating the patient about oral adverse reactions and drug interactions with medications that may be prescribed in the dental office.

Seizure Episode

Seizure disorders may interfere with the dental hygienist's ability to treat a patient if the seizure should occur during the office visit. The dental hygienist should know what to do if a patient has a seizure while in the dental office (see Chapter 22).

Oral Adverse Reactions

Many of the antiepileptic drugs can cause gingival hypertrophy, glossitis, stomatitis, altered sense of taste, and xerostomia. Patients should be carefully evaluated for these adverse reactions and counseled on how to best minimize them. Gingival hypertrophy is discussed in a previous section. Patients experiencing glossitis and stomatitis should be referred to their treating physician for appropriate care.

Xerostomia. Xerostomia can be treated by having the patient drink plenty of water or by sucking on tart sugarless candy and chewing sugarless gum. Caffeine-containing beverages only intensify dry mouth and juices contain added sugar, which can increase the risk of dental carries.

Other Adverse Effects

Central Nervous System Stimulant Effects. Several of the antiepileptic drugs can stimulate young children and the elderly. This may make it difficult to treat a patient who cannot sit still. Appointments may need to be rescheduled if the patient is overly stimulated.

Gastrointestinal Effects. Some antiepileptic drugs cause nausea and vomiting, which may interfere with good oral hygiene since patients may not be able to brush and floss their teeth. Persistent nausea and vomiting need to be reported to the patient's physician because this is a sign of toxicity. Almost all antiepileptic drugs cause some degree of GI irritation. Caution should be used if an opioid analgesic, aspirin, or NSAID is prescribed to treat dental pain. Patients should be counseled about the increased risk of GI irritation and should take their medication with food or milk or after meals.

CNS Depressant Drug Interactions. Sedation, confusion, and other CNS depressant effects are common to almost all antiepileptic drugs. Caution should be used if an opioid analgesic or antianxiety drug is prescribed. Patients should have someone drive them to and from dental appointments and they should refrain from doing anything that requires thought or concentration. This includes driving, operating heavy machinery, and taking care of children.

Summary

The dental hygienist should be familiar with the available antiepileptic drugs and how they impact on oral health care. All antiepileptic drugs cause gastrointestinal adverse reactions and most are also sedating. Both types of adverse reactions can cause drug interactions with medications that are prescribed or used in a dental office. Be familiar with these adverse reactions and drug interactions and learn how to effectively discuss them with the patient.

Gingival hyperplasia occurs with phenytoin and can be a major cause of noncompliance. The dental hygienist should work with all patients taking phenytoin in order to ensure that the patient is doing all that she can to minimize this risk. This includes good oral hygiene and frequent visits with the dentist and dental hygienist to maintain optimal plaque control.

Other oral adverse reactions of almost all antiepileptic drugs include glossitis, stomatitis, and dry mouth. The dental hygienist should carefully examine the patient for oral adverse reactions and carefully question each patient about them.

Three new drugs have been recently approved for the treatment of different types of seizure disorders. Felbamate now carries a warning with it because of the high risk for developing aplastic anemia.

Case Study: Sammy Jones

Sammy Jones is 11 years old and has been coming to your practice for close to 6 years. His medication/health history is significant for generalized tonic-clonic seizures. He was receiving phenytoin, but could not tolerate it, so his physician changed him to the pediatric dose form of carbamazepine. He is in your ofnce for a scheduled maintenance oral examination.

1. What is carbamazepine and what is its role in treating seizure disorders?
2. What are the major classes of adverse reactions associated with carbamazepine therapy?
3. Can any of the central nervous system adverse reactions affect oral health care?
4. Why should Mrs. Jones be concerned about the pediatric dose form of carbamazepine?
5. What would you tell Mrs. Jones about the pediatric dose form of carbamazepine?
6. What are the dental concerns associated with carbamazepine and what should Mrs. Jones be told about them?

Case Study: Lydia Mitchell

Lydia Mitchell is 36 years old and has been coming to your practice for many years. Her medication/health history is significant for seizures for which she was being treated with a combination of phenytoin and phenobarbital. She comes in today and tells you that her physician switched her to a new drug called felbamate. Mrs. Mitchell was beginning to have seizures while on phenytoin and phenobarbital and other seizure medications made her very ill.

1. Where would you find information about felbamate?
2. What is its role in the treatment of seizure disorders?
3. What are the adverse reactions associated with felbamate?
4. Why do patients need to sign a consent form before starting felbamate therapy?
5. Does this drug have any adverse reactions or drug interactions that could interfere with oral health?

Review Questions

1. What are the two categories of seizures?
2. Compare and contrast the different types of seizure disorders.
3. What is the objective of drug therapy in the treatment of seizure disorders?
4. How do barbiturates work in treating seizure disorders?
5. What are the more common adverse reactions of phenobarbital?
6. What drug interactions should you be concerned about in a patient receiving valproic acid? Why?
7. What are the oral adverse reactions associated with ethosuximide?
8. What is the role of benzodiazepines in the treatment of seizure disorders?
9. Compare and contrast gabapentin and lamotrigine.

BIBLIOGRAPHY

Anon: Felbamate. *Med Let* 35:107–109, 1993.

Btaiche IM, Woster PS: Gabapentin and lamotrigine: Novel antiepileptic drugs. *Am J Health-Syst Pharm* 52:61–69, 1995.

Carter-Wallace: Felbatol should stay on market as second-line therapy: FDA committee recommends boxed warning for aplastic anemia, liver failure. *F-D-C Reports: The Pink Sheet* 4:3–4, October 3, 1994.

Chan AWK: Drugs used in the treatment of epilepsy. In Smith CM, Reynard AM (eds.), *Textbook of Pharmacology* 1st ed. W. B. Saunders Co, Philadelphia, 1992.

Garnett WR: Epilepsy. In DiPiro JT, Talbert RL, Hayes PE, et al. (eds.), *Pharmacotherapy: A Pathophysiologic Approach,* 2nd ed. Elsevier, New York, 1992a.

Garnett WR: Epilepsy: Controlling seizure activity is the first goal of drug therapy, but not all patients respond to treatment. *US Pharmacist* 42:43–46, 1992b.

Hammond-Tooke GD: The management of epilepsy in adults. *NZ Med J* 106:455–457, 1993.

Hussar DA: New drugs of 1993. *Am Pharm* NS34:37–38, 1994.

Hussar DA: New drugs of 1994. *Am Pharm* NS35:16–42, 1995.

Matsu F, Bergen D, Faught E, et al.: Placebo-controlled study of the efficacy and safety of lamotrigine in patients with partial seizures. *Neurology* 43:2284–2291, 1993.

Meyer MC, Cloyd J, Garnett WR, Holmes GL, Schiffer JR: Practical considerations in anticonvulsant therapy—Part 1. *Am Pharm* NS35:22–26, 1995.

Meyer MC, Cloyd J, Garnett WR, Holmes GL, Schiffer JR: Practical considerations in anticonvulsant therapy—Part 2. *Am Pharm* NS35:31–34, 1995.

Pokalo Jones C: Signed informed consent form required before dispensing felbamate. *Pharmacy Today* 7:12, 1995.

Pugh CB, Garnett WR: Current issues in the treatment of epilepsy. *Clin Pharm* 10:335–358, 1991.

So E: Update on epilepsy. *Med Clin North Am* 77:203–214, 1993.

Sorensen SJ, Farrington E: Felbamate (Felbatol). *Pediatr Nursing* 19:630–632, 1993.

CHAPTER 21

Treatment of Psychiatric Disorders

Key Terms

Antipsychotics
Depression
Lithium
Mania
Monoamine Oxidase Inhibitor

Schizophrenia
Selective Serotonin Reuptake Inhibitor
Serotonin/Norepinephrine Reuptake Inhibitor
Tricyclic Antidepressant

LEARNING OBJECTIVES

After completion of this chapter and its learning activities, the student should be able to:

1. Describe psychopharmacology and briefly describe the therapeutic approach to psychiatric disorders.
2. List the different classes of psychopharmacologic agents and their prototypes.
3. List the therapeutic uses and adverse effects of the class of medications known as antipsychotics.
4. List the categories of antidepressant medications used to treat depressive disorders.
5. Describe the mechanism of action of tricyclic antidepressants, monoamine oxidase inhibitors, older second-generation antidepressants, and newer second-generation antidepressants; also, indicate therapeutic uses and adverse effects of each group.
6. Describe the mechanism of action of the third-generation antidepressants: the selective serotonin reuptake inhibitors and the serotonin/norepinephrine reuptake inhibitors.
7. Give examples of selective serotonin reuptake inhibitors and serotonin/norepinephrine reuptake inhibitor antidepressants and be able to discuss their therapeutic uses and adverse effects.
8. Describe such mood-stabilizing drugs as lithium, carbamazepine, and valproic acid. Know their mechanisms of action, therapeutic uses, and adverse effects.
9. Describe the dental concerns associated with drugs used to treat psychiatric disorders and effectively counsel patients about them.

INTRODUCTION

There are many drugs available to treat psychiatric disorders and the dental hygienist will more than likely treat patients taking one or several of these medications. Many of these medications have oral adverse effects or other adverse effects that may interfere with the patient's or dental hygienist's ability to perform oral care.

The medications used to treat schizophrenia, major depression, and mania are discussed in this chapter. Medications used to treat anxiety and insomnia are reviewed in Chapter 9. This chapter briefly reviews the pharmacologic effects of each class of medication, adverse effects, dental effects, and information for the patient.

SCHIZOPHRENIA

Schizophrenia is a devastating disease characterized by such positive symptoms as delusions, hallucinations, and changes in thought content. Some patients will present with negative symptoms such as low levels of emotional arousal, mental activity, and social drive. Although it affects only 1% of the American population, schizophrenia has serious economic consequences. Schizophrenics consume about 2.5% of healthcare expenditures each year and comprise 10% of the totally and permanently disabled, a group that is highly dependent on public assistance (Rupp and Keith, 1993).

Dental Concerns Associated with Schizophrenia

It is highly likely that the dental hygienist will treat a patient with schizophrenia. The dental hygienist should keep in mind that the schizophrenic or psychotic patient may perceive the hygienist or other dental personnel as threatening. Dental personnel should discuss ways to handle such a situation. This may include canceling the appointment, calling 911, contacting the patient's caregiver or mental health provider, or simply reassuring the patient. Patients who are mentally ill are also less likely to take their medication as prescribed. It is important to review medication with the patients caregiver or mental health provider.

ANTIPSYCHOTIC THERAPY

Prior to the introduction of *antipsychotic* medications there was little available to treat schizophrenia. Available treatment included hydrotherapy, insulin therapy, electroconvulsive therapy, and institutionalization. Therapy was revolutionized in the late 1950s with the introduction of the phenothiazine antipsychotics. No single antipsychotic is superior to another. Therapy is based on a patient's previous experience with a particular medication, what the patient thinks of the medication, and the adverse effect profile of the medication. In many instances several medications are tried before one is chosen. Table 21-1 reviews available antipsychotic drugs and their adverse reaction profiles.

Mechanism of Action

Antipsychotic medications are thought to work by blocking dopamine$_1$ and dopamine$_2$ receptors, the reuptake of norepinephrine, and the reuptake of serotonin in the brain in varying degrees.

Table 21-1 Selected Antipsychotic Therapy

Generic Name	Maintenance Dose (mg/day)	Adverse Reactions
Phenothiazines		
Aliphatic		
Chlorpromazine (Thorazine)	100–400	ACH-3, Sedation-4, EPS-3, CV-4
Piperidine		
Thioridazine (Mellaril)	200–800	ACH-4, Sedation-4, EPS-2, CV-4
Piperazine		
Perphenazine (Trilafon)	16–48	ACH-2, Sedation-2,-3, EPS-3, CV-2
Trifluoperazine (Stelazine)	4–40	ACH-2, Sedation 2–3, EPS-3, CV-2
Fluphenazine (Prolixin)	5–4	ACH-1, Sedation-2, EPS-4, CV-1
NonPhenothiazines		
Thioxanthene		
Thiothixene (Navane)	5–40	ACH-2, Sedation-2, EPS-4, CV-2
Butyrophenone		
Haloperidol(Haldol)	5–20	ACH-1, Sedation-1, EPS-4, CV-1
Dibenzoxazepine		
Loxapine (Loxitane)	5–40	ACH-2, Sedation-3, EPS-4, CV-3
Dibenzazepine		
Clozapine (Clozaril)	50–400	ACH-4, Sedation-4, EPS-1, CV-4
Benzisoxazole		
Resperidone (Risperdal)	4–16	ACH-2, Sedation-2, EPS-1-2, CV-3

Sources: Gerlach J, New antipsycotics: Classification, efficacy, and adverse effects. *Schizophrenia Bull* 17:289–309, 1991; Baldessarini RJ, Drugs and the treatment of psychiatric disorders. In Goodman Gillman A, Rall TW, Nies AS, Taylor P (eds.), *Goodman and Gilman's The Pharmacologic Basis of Therapeutics*, 8th ed. Pergamon Press, New York, 1990.

ACH = anticholinergic, EPS = extrapyramidal, CV = cardiovascular, 1 = very low, 2 = low, 3 = moderate, 4 = high.

Adverse Reactions

The many adverse effects of antipsychotics are a result of their ability to block other receptors. These medications can block *a*-adrenergic, acetylcholine, and histamine receptors, thus causing a wide range of adverse reactions.

Cardiovascular Effects. Hypotension and tachycardia are a result of *a*-adrenergic receptor blockade.

Central Nervous System Effects. Sedation is one of the most common adverse effects and the patient usually develops tolerance to this effect. Other CNS effects include fatigue, confusion, and dizziness.

Anticholingeric Effects. These adverse reactions are the result of cholinergic receptor blockade. Anticholinergic adverse effects include dry mouth, blurred vision, constipation, and urinary retention.

Extrapyramidal Effects. The most common adverse effects associated with antipsychotics are extrapyramidal effects. They are thought to be a result of dopamine blockade in the extrapyramidal system in the brain. They usually occur at the onset of therapy or after a dose increase. Acute dystonia, which consists of muscle spasms of the face, back, neck, or tongue, usually occurs within 72 hours of starting therapy or a dose increase. Parkinsonian symptoms occur as therapy progresses and include resting tremor, rigidity, akathesia (inability to sit still), and akinesia (loss of muscle movement).

Tardive Dyskinesia. Tardive dyskinesia consists of involuntary abnormal movements of the tongue, lips, face, jaw, arms, legs, and trunk. It is usually seen in patients who have been on antipsychotics for a minimum of 6 months to 2 years. Its onset is gradual and the movements are coordinated and rhythmic. Discontinuing the drug initially exacerbates the symptoms while dose increases mask symptoms. Some patients demonstrate a reduction in tardive dyskinesia after a period of time.

Other Effects. Other adverse effects include photosensitivity, blood dyscrasias, skin eruptions, cholestatic jaundice, and neuroleptic malignant syndrome that is characterized by extrapyramidal symptoms and fever. The photosensitivity reactions are exaggerated by sunlight and light from a dental unit and the patient should always be encouraged to wear a sunblock with a skin protection factor greater than 15.

Dental Concerns Associated with Antipsychotic Drugs

Some of the adverse reactions associated with antipsychotic drugs can interfere with the dental hygienist's ability to treat the patient and with the patient's ability to perform his own oral care. Antipsychotics may also interact with drugs often prescribed in the dental office.

Anticholingeric Adverse Reactions. Antipsychotic drugs can cause dry mouth, which may cause many patients to be noncompliant. Dental hygienists should review ways to minimize dry mouth with their patients. Methods include drinking plenty of water and sucking on tart, sugarless candy or chewing tart, sugarless gum. Many patients tend to drink caffeinated beverages and juices. Caffeine-containing beverages only exacerbate dry mouth and sodas and juices are high in sugar and can increase the risk of dental caries.

Extrapyramidal Adverse Reaction. Many patients complain of tremors, akathesia, or other extrapyramidal symptoms that may make it impossible for a patient to sit for an oral examination and cleaning. It may make it very difficult for patients to brush and floss their teeth at home. Medication adjustments by the appropriate health-care provider may help to reduce some of these symptoms.

Tardive Dyskinesia. Tardive dyskinesia can make it almost impossible for the patient to perform self-care or sit for a dental appointment. The dental hygienist should be aware of this and work with the patient as best as possible.

Cardiovascular Effects. These drugs can cause hypotension and tachycardia. The dental chair should be raised slowly after the patient has been lying in it for her dental appointment. The patient should sit in the chair for several minutes before slowly rising.

CNS Depressant Drugs

Opioid analgesics and antianxiety drugs are sedating and can intensify the sedating effects of antipsychotic drugs. If any one of these drugs is prescribed, the patient, family member, or caregiver should be warned about the increased risk for sedation and confusion. Patients should have someone drive them to and from their dental appointment and they should not drive or operate heavy equipment or machinery. They should also refrain from anything that requires thought or concentration while taking a CNS depressant drug.

Epinephrine can cause CNS excitation and this may exacerbate some of the positive symptoms of schizophrenia. This drug should be used with caution or avoided if possible.

DEPRESSION

Depression is one of the most common psychiatric disorders, affecting approximately 13 million Americans (Grothe and Cohen, 1992). When it occurs, depression is very debilitating. Patients with depressive disorders are more likely to seek care for concomitant problems and have physical functioning levels worse than those with such chronic conditions as arthritis, diabetes, and hypertension (Kupfer, 1991) . Because it is such a common disorder, the dental hygienist should be familiar with the many medications used to treat it.

Antidepressant Pharmacotherapy

There are many different medications available to treat depression. Antidepressants are thought to work by blocking the reuptake of norepinephrine, serotonin, or both. The side-effect profile is what differentiates one antidepressant from another. The choice of antidepressants is based on the patient's past experience with a particular medication, side-effect profile, and physician familiarity with a particular antidepressant. The average onset of antidepressant action is approximately 4 weeks. Table 21-2 reviews selected antidepressant medications and their adverse reaction profiles.

Tricyclic Antidepressants. The **tricyclic antidepressants** (TCAs) are the oldest drugs used in the treatment of depression. They are very effective and their use is limited by their adverse reaction profile. They are inexpensive and still considered to be first-line therapy in the treatment of depression.

Monoamine Oxidase Inhibitors (MAOIs). Effective in treating depression, the use of MAOIs is limited because of their adverse effect profile. MAOIs interact with tyramine found in many foods, and sympathomimetic drugs causing a hypertensive crisis which is characterized by flushing, intense headache, and elevated blood pressure. MAOIs should not be given with TCAs or selective serotonin reuptake inhibitors.

Second Generation Antidepressants. The older and newer second-generation antidepressants differ from TCAs in terms of their adverse effect profile. Some may have a more favorable adverse effect profile than the TCAs.

Selective Serotonin Reuptake Inhibitors (SSRIs). With a much lower incidence of anticholingeric sedating, and cardiovascular adverse effects than TCAs, SSRIs also have

Table 21-2   Selected Antidepressant Therapy

Generic Name	Dose (mg/day)	Adverse Reactions
Tricyclic Antidepressants		
Amitriptyline (Elavil)	75–300	ACH = 3, S = 3, OH = 3, CV = 3, I = 0
Desipramine (Norpramin)	75–300	ACH = 1, S = 1, OH = 1, CV = 3, I = 0
Imipramine (Tofranil)	75–300	ACH = 2, S = 2, OH = 3, CV = 3, I = 0
Nortriptyline (Pamelor)	75–150	ACH = 1, S = 2, OH = 1, CV = 3, I = 0
Monoamine Oxidase Inhibitors		
Phenelzine (Nardil)	15–90	ACH = 0, S = 2, OH = 3, CV = 1, I = 1
Tranylcypromine (Parnate)	30–60	ACH = 0, S = 2, OH = 3, CV = 1, I = 2
Selected Older Second-Generation Antidepressants		
Trazodone (Desyrel)	50–60	ACH = 0, S = 4, OH = 2, CV = 1, I = 0
Selected Newer Second-Generation Antidepressants		
Buproprion (Wellbutrin)	300–450	ACH = 0, S = 1, OH = 0, CV = 0, I = 2
Selective Serotonin Reuptake Inhibitors		
Fluoxetine (Prozac)	20–80	ACH = 1, S = 1, OH = 1, CV = 1, I = 2
Sertraline (Zoloft)	50–200	ACH = 1, S = 1, OH = 1, CV = 0, I = 1
Paroxetine (Paxil)	20–50	ACH = 1, S = 1, OH = 0, CV = 0, I = 1
Serotonin/Norepinephrine Reuptake Inhibitors		
Venlafaxine (Effexor)	75–375	ACH = 1 +, S = 1 +, OH = 0, CV = 1 +, I = 1 +
Nefazodone (Serzone)	300–600	ACH = 1 +, S = 1 +, OH = 0, CV = 1 +, I = 0

Sources: American Psychiatric Association, Practice guideline for major depressive disorder in adults. *Am J Psychiatry* 150(Suppl 4):1–26, 1993; Wells BG, Jann MW, Marken P, Stimmel GL, Therapeutic options in the treatment of depression. *J Amer Pharm Assoc* 1–18, 1994

ACH = anticholinergic, S = sedation, OH = orthostatic hypotension, CV = cardiovascular, I = insomnia, 0 = nonexistent, 1 = very low, 2 = low, 3 = moderate, 4 = high.

a much more favorable adverse effect profile than TCAs, MAOIs, and second-generation antidepressants.

Serotonin-Norepinephrine Reuptake Inhibitor. The **serotonin-norepinephrine reuptake inhibitors** (SNRIs), have a lower incidence of anticholinergic and cardiovascular adverse reactions than TCAs but a somewhat higher incidence than SSRIs. They also have a lower incidence of sedation and venlafaxine may actually cause insomnia.

Adverse Reactions

As with antipsychotics, some of the adverse reactions of antidepressants are a result of blockade of other receptors.

Central Nervous System Effects. The most common CNS adverse reaction is sedation, which may be of benefit in a depressed patient with insomnia. Most patients develop tolerance to sedation over time. Other CNS adverse reactions include dizziness, fatigue, and confusion.

Anticholinergic Effects. All antidepressants block cholinergic receptors to varying degrees. Many patients complain of dry mouth, blurred vision, constipation, and urinary retention.

Cardiovascular Effects. The tricyclic antidepressants (TCAs) have been known to cause a quinidine-like slowing of cardiac conduction. Patients with heart block or bradycardia should not receive TCAs. TCAs also potentiate the pressor effects of sympathomimetics. Vasoconstrictors with a local anesthetic should be used with caution in patients taking TCAs because the combination may increase blood pressure.

Gastrointestinal Effects. Gastrointestinal adverse reactions include nausea, vomiting, and abdominal pain and occur more frequently with SSRIs and SNRIs.

Other Effects. Other adverse effects include orthostatic hypotension, weight gain, and insomnia. Insomnia can be avoided by giving the medication during the day.

Dental Concerns Associated with Antidepressants

As with antipsychotics, antidepressants have adverse reactions that can compromise oral care and interact with drugs prescribed in the dental office. Antidepressants have anticholinergic and cardiovascular adverse reactions and are also sedating, which can be intensified if CNS depressant drugs are prescribed. This is discussed in the section entitled "Dental Concerns Associated with Antipsychotics." The next section reviews those drug interactions relatively uncommon with antipsychotics.

Nonopioid Analgesics. The SSRIs and the SNRIs have GI adverse reactions that can be intensified with the addition of **aspirin** or nonsteroidal antiinflammatory drugs. Patients should be appropriately advised of this and should take these drugs with food or milk to avoid GI discomfort.

MAOIs and Epinephrine. This combination may cause a hypertensive crisis that can be fatal. This combination of drugs should be avoided.

MANIA

Mania is characterized by changes in mood that can range from euphoria to depression, or a combination of both. It affects approximately 1% of the population (Reiger et al., 1990). The early stages of mania often go unnoticed. The patient may sleep less, have more energy, and be very creative. As time goes on, the patient may sleep even less, go on spending sprees, and have an increased libido. Eventually, the patient becomes paranoid, aggressive, and may display schizophrenic symptoms.

Antimanic Pharmacotherapy

Lithium has been the cornerstone of therapy for mania with or without depression since the 1960s. It may take 2–4 weeks to be effective. Therefore, many manic patients require temporary treatment with an antipsychotic drug.

Adverse Reactions

The adverse effects of lithium are many and often lead to patient noncompliance. Nausea and fatigue occur during the first weeks of lithium therapy. Vomiting and diarrhea may indicate lithium toxicity. Other side effects, which can be minimized by adjusting lithium doses, include polyuria (frequent urination), fine hand tremor, increased thirst, edema, and weight gain. Other more severe adverse effects include ataxia, slurred speech, confusion, EKG (electrocardiogram) changes, and coarse hand tremor.

Dental Concerns

Polydipsia or increased thirst is a dental concern because patients attempt to quench their thirst with sodas and fruit juices. Patients should be instructed to drink water or sugar-free soft drinks in order to help minimize the risk of dental caries and weight gain.

Other Agents

There are patients who cannot tolerate lithium or who do not respond to it. Reports indicate that **carbamazepine** and **valproic acid** are viable alternatives to lithium and both drugs are discussed in Chapter 20 (Bowden et al., 1994; Small et al., 1991). Some patients respond to antipsychotic medications.

Summary

There are many drugs available to treat the different psychiatric disorders and many of these medications have oral adverse reactions or other adverse reactions that may interfere with the patient's or dental hygienist's ability to perform oral hygiene. Antipsychotic drugs differ in terms of their adverse reaction profile. Drugs such as haloperidol and fluphenazine have a higher incidence of extrapyramidal effects whereas drugs such as thioridazine and chlorpromazine have a higher incidence of dry mouth and sedation. Resperidone is the newest antipsychotic drug and it has very little extrapyramidal effects, sedation, dry mouth, and other adverse reactions associated with antipsychotics. Antipsychotic drugs cause extrapyramidal effects, dry mouth, and tardive dyskinesia, which can interfere with oral health care. The dental hygienist needs to know about side effects and how to counsel the patient. The symptoms of schizophrenia may also interfere with the dental hygienist's ability to treat patients.

Antidepressant drugs differ in terms of their adverse reaction profile. Antidepressant drugs are broken down into TCAs, MAOIs, second-generation antidepressants, SSRIs, and SNRIs. SSRIs and SNRIs do not have the dry mouth and sedation that is associated with the TCAs, MAOIs, and second-generation antidepressants. They also do not have the cardiac rhythm problems associated with the older drugs. The more common adverse reactions associated with the SSRIs and SNRIs are insomnia and gastrointestinal complaints.

Lithium has long been the mainstay of bipolar therapy. Patients experience polyphagia, polydipsia, and polyuria as a result of this drug. Patients must have their blood levels for lithium checked. Lithium can cause cardiac rhythm problems. Carbamazepine and valproic acid are now being used to treat patients with bipolar disorder who have not responded to lithium or cannot tolerate it.

Antipsychotics, antidepressants, and antimanic medications interact with opioid analgesics, antianxiety agents, and epinephrine. Extreme caution should be used if any one of these drugs is prescribed or used in conjunction with any of the psychotropic drugs. The dental hygienist should know about psychiatric disorders and the drugs used to treat them, including adverse reactions and drug interactions.

Case Study: Suzanne Fernandez

Suzanne Fernandez is 44 years old and has been coming to your practice for close to 2 years. She has no medical problems and only takes over-the-counter analgesics and cough and cold products. Mrs. Fernandez has noticed that lately she has not been herself. She feels "blue" and nothing seems to make her happy. Mrs. Fernandez tells you that she went to her physician last week and she placed Mrs. Fernandez on fluoxetine. Mrs. Fernandez will be having a cavity filled today and the dentist plans to use a local anesthetic with a vasoconstrictor.

1. What was Mrs. Fernandez's diagnosis?
2. What are some of the signs and symptoms of depression and who does it affect?
3. How does fluoxetine work?
4. Are there any drug interactions of which you need to be aware?
5. Does fluoxetine have any dental adverse reactions or concerns?
6. What should Mrs. Fernandez be told about potential drug interactions or dental adverse reactions?

Case Study: Frank Almeida

Frank Almeida is 25 years old and is new to your practice. During the medication/health history you notice a very fine hand tremor. He complains of frequent thirst and, subsequently, a frequent need to urinate. Mr. Almeida's medications include lithium and occasional analgesics and cough and cold products. He is in your office for a badly needed oral examination.

1. What is lithium and what is it used to treat?
2. What are some of the symptoms of mania?
3. What are five adverse reactions to lithium?
4. Are there any dental adverse reactions/concerns associated with lithium therapy?
5. What are some things that Mr. Almeida should *not* do to alleviate his frequent thirst?

6. What should Mr. Almeida be told about dental concerns associated with lithium therapy?

Review Questions

1. What were some of the options available to treat schizophrenia prior to the introduction of antipsychotics?
2. What are the more common adverse reactions of chlorpromazine?
3. How does risperidone differ from haloperidol?
4. What differentiates one antidepressant from another?
5. Compare and contrast the TCAs with the second-generation antidepressants.
6. What are MAOIs and what are their adverse reactions?
7. Compare and contrast the TCAs with the SSRIs.
8. What are some alternatives to lithium therapy?

BIBLIOGRAPHY

American Psychiatric Association: Practice guideline for major depressive disorder in adults. *Am J Psychiatry* 150 (Suppl 4):1–26, 1993.

Baldessarini RJ: Drugs and the treatment of psychiatric disorders. In Goodman Gilman A, Rall TW, Nies AS, Taylor P (eds.), *Goodman and Gilman's The Pharmacologic Basis of Therapeutics,* 8th ed. Pergamon Press, New York, 1990.

Bowden CL, Brugger AM, Swann AC, et al.: Efficacy of divalproex vs lithium and placebo in the treatment of mania. *JAMA* 271:918–924, 1994.

Carpenter WT Jr., Buchanan RW: Schizophrenia. *New Engl J Med* 326:681–690, 1994.

Gerlach J: New antipsychotics: Classification, efficacy, and adverse effects. *Schizophrenia Bull* 17:289–309, 1991.

Grothe DR, Cohen LJ: Major depression: Its recognition and treatment. Part 1: First generation antidepressants. *Am Pharm* NS32:33–40, 1992.

Kupfer DJ: Long-term treatment of depression. *J Clin Psychiatry* 52:28–34, 1991.

Perry P: Clinical use of the newer antipsychotic drugs. *Am J Health- Syst Pharm* 52(Suppl 1):S9–S14, 1995.

Potter WZ, Rudorfer MV, Manji H: The pharmacologic treatment of depression. *New Engl J Med* 325:633–642, 1991.

Price LH, Heninger GR: Lithium in the treatment of mood disorders. *New Engl J Med* 331:591–598, 1994.

Reiger DA, Farmer ME, Rae DS, Locke BZ, Keith SJ, Judd LL: Comorbidity of mental disorders with alcohol and other drug abuse: Results from the Epidemiologic Catchment Area (ECA) Study. *JAMA* 264:2511–2518, 1990.

Rupp A, Keith SJ: The costs of schizophrenia. Assessing the burden. *Psychiatr Clin North Am* 16:413–423, 1993.

Small JG, Klapper MH, Milstein V, et al.: Carbamazepine compared with lithium in the treatment of mania. *Arch Gen Psychiatry* 48:915–921, 1991.

Wells BG, Jann MW, Marken P, Stimmel GL: Therapeutic options in the treatment of depression. *J Amer Pharm Assoc* 1–18, 1994.

PART IV

TOPICS OF GENERAL INTEREST

CHAPTER 22

Medical Emergencies in the Dental Office

Key Terms

Age
Dental Office
Emergencies
Emergency Medical Kit

Patients
Prevention
Treatment

LEARNING OBJECTIVES

After completion of this chapter and its learning activities, the student should be able to:

1. Describe the factors that can increase the incidence of medical emergencies.
2. Discuss the different methods of preventing medical emergencies in a dental office.
3. Describe the different ways dental personnel can prepare for medical emergencies.
4. Describe the medications and equipment necessary for an emergency medical kit.
5. Describe the general treatment of all emergencies that can occur in the dental office.
6. Describe the treatment of cardiovascular emergencies in the dental office.
7. Describe the treatment of central nervous system emergencies in the dental office.
8. Describe the treatment of respiratory emergencies in the dental office.
9. Describe the treatment of endocrine emergencies in the dental office.
10. Describe the treatment of drug-induced medical emergencies in the dental office.

INTRODUCTION

More and more *patients* are living longer as a result of advances made in medicine and these patients continue to seek oral-dental care. Advanced age, an increased use of medication, and longer dental appointments place the patient at risk for a medical emergency in the dental office. The dental hygienist can help to minimize or prevent this risk by becoming familiar with patients, their medical illnesses, and the emergency treatment of those illnesses. The intent of this chapter is to briefly review some of the more common medical emergencies and their treatments.

PREVENTION OF MEDICAL EMERGENCIES

The best way to minimize medical *emergencies* in the dental office is to prevent them. This can be accomplished by asking detailed questions during the medication/health history. Detailed medication/health histories can help to prevent drug interactions, adverse reactions, or allergic reactions. The dental hygienist can also take blood pressure and pulse measurements of all patients with known cardiovascular disease or any other disease that can increase pulse or blood pressure. The patient should be observed for his stature, build, gait, color, age, and respiration rate. Dental personnel can also consult with the patient's physician if necessary.

Stress reduction plays an important role in preventing or minimizing medical emergencies in the dental office. First and foremost the patient should be evaluated for her level of stress and should be appropriately treated for it. This includes premedicating with an antianxiety drug, scheduling appointments early in the day, and minimizing waiting times in the waiting room and in the dental chair. Other means of reducing stress include psychosedation during dental treatment, shorter dental appointments, and postoperative pain and anxiety control.

PREPARATION OF DENTAL PERSONNEL

Dental personnel can help to avoid or minimize medical emergencies in the dental office by preparing and training for them. All dental personnel should be currently certified in cardiopulmonary resuscitation (CPR). Dental personnel should have assigned duties during an emergency and emergency practice drills should be held at least yearly. The telephone number of the nearest hospital emergency room, physician, and ambulance service (911) should be posted by all telephones. Lastly, the emergency medical kit should be checked quarterly and after each use, for outdated drugs or for replacement of drugs used during an emergency.

EMERGENCY MEDICAL KIT

Emergency medical kits can either be purchased as completed commercial kits or made up of individual medications that are purchased separately. Table 22-1 reviews medications that should be included in all emergency medical kits. It also briefly reviews adult doses and therapeutic uses. The dental hygienist should refer to previous chapters for complete information on the medications listed.

MEDICAL EQUIPMENT

Medical equipment such as an oxygen mask, manual resuscitation bag, and oxygen tank with a flow gauge are necessary for the treatment of medical emergencies. Other equipment includes blood pressure cuff and stethoscope, disposable syringes

Table 22-1   Emergency Medical Kit

Drug	Adult Dose	Use
Epinephrine	0.2–0.5 mg	Allergic reaction, asthma, cardiac arrest
Diazepam	5–10 mg	Seizures, thyroid storm
Diphenhydramine	50 mg	Allergic reactions, extrapyramidal reactions
Naloxone	0.4 mg	Opioid overdose
Morphine	10 mg	Severe pain due to myocardial infarction
Hydrocortisone	50–250 mg	Adrenal insufficiency
Glucose	50 ml	Hypoglycemia
Oxygen	100%	Respiratory distress
Spirits of ammonia	0.3 ml	Syncope
Metaproterenol	2 puffs	Asthma
Phenylephrine	0.2–0.5mg	Hypotension, acute adrenal insufficiency
Nitroglycerin	0.4 mg	Angina pectoris

and needles, and a tourniquet. Equipment that requires advanced training includes laryngeal suction cannula, endotracheal tubes, laryngoscopes, syringes and equipment necessary for intravenous administration, and a cricothyrotomy kit.

GENERAL TREATMENT OF MEDICAL EMERGENCIES

Before emergency treatment can be administered, dental personnel must recognize that the medical emergency is occurring. This includes noting the patient's signs and symptoms and making an accurate diagnosis of the situation. Once this has been done, the patient should be positioned properly and dental personnel should then follow the "ABCs" of treating a medical emergency. They include A—maintaining an airway; B—administering oxygen (breathing); and C—monitoring vital signs (circulation). Another staff member should be calling emergency services (911). Lastly, symptomatic (drug and nondrug) treatment should be initiated while awaiting emergency services.

CARDIOVASCULAR EMERGENCIES

Cardiovascular emergencies include angina pectoris, myocardial infarction, cardiac arrest, arrhythmias, cerebrovascular accident, hypertensive crisis, and hypotension. The primary goal of treatment is to maintain adequate circulation, call emergency services, perform CPR, and administer oxygen, if necessary.

Angina Pectoris

Angina pectoris is characterized by substernal chest pain that radiates across the chest to the left arm or jaw. The patient also experiences a feeling of chest heaviness, rapid pulse, and tachypnea. Causes include stress due to the fear of the dental procedure, pain, or underlying cardiovascular disease. Angina pectoris can be treated with sublingual **nitroglycerin.** Patients with angina pectoris should be instructed to carry their nitroglycerin with them. Premedication with nitroglycerin can sometimes prevent an angina attack. Other treatments include opioid analgesics or **diazepam,** which are administered by emergency personnel or in the hospital.

Acute Myocardial Infarction

Acute myocardial infarction (MI) is also characterized by pain, pressure, or heaviness in the chest that radiates to other parts of the body. The pain is persistent and unrelieved by nitroglycerin. Patients can also experience sweating, nausea, and vomiting. Other signs and symptoms include irregular, short rapid pulse, shortness of breath, diaphoresis, and indigestion. Treatment includes oxygen, opioid analgesics, and transfer to the hospital.

Cardiac Arrest

The signs and symptoms of cardiac arrest include a sudden circulatory and respiratory collapse. The patient's pulse is absent and blood pressure is unmeasurable. CPR should be started and the patient should be transferred to the hospital.

Other Cardiovascular Emergencies

Other cardiovascular emergencies include arrhythmias, which are confirmed by electrocardiogram; hypertensive crisis, which is treated with intravenous antihypertensive drugs; and hypotension, which is usually treated by placing the patient in a modified Trendelenburg position and administering either oxygen, **hydrocortisone,** or a vasopressor drug. Cerebrovascular accident (stroke) is characterized by weakness on one side of the body and changes in speech and is treated with oxygen and transfer to a hospital.

CENTRAL NERVOUS SYSTEM EMERGENCIES

Central nervous system (CNS) emergencies include syncope and seizures. Treatment depends on the patient and the symptoms.

Syncope

Syncope is a result of a loss of normal motor tone and a pooling of blood in the periphery that results in a sudden fall in blood pressure. The patient becomes diaphoretic and the skin is ashen gray in color. It is usually a result of anxiety, fear, or apprehension of the dental treatment. Treatment includes placing the patient in the Trendelenburg position (head down), spirits of ammonia, and confidence on the part of the dental staff. A calm and confident dental hygienist can help the patient to feel less anxious about being at a dental office.

Seizures

Seizures can be a result of a seizure disorder (generalized tonic-clonic), trauma, or they can be drug-induced. Signs and symptoms include generalized tonic-clonic movements and the patient may lose consciousness. Seizures are generally self-limiting and treatment should focus on protecting the patient from self-harm. This includes moving sharp objects away from the patient, helping the patient to the floor if standing, and turning the patient's head to the side to prevent aspiration. Diazepam may be necessary if the seizure is continuous.

RESPIRATORY EMERGENCIES

Respiratory emergencies include hyperventilation, asthma, anaphylactic shock, acute airway obstruction, and aspiration.

Hyperventilation

Hyperventilation is characterized by tachypnea, tachycardia, and paresthesia. Patients present with nausea, faintness, perspiration, acute anxiety, lightheadedness, and shortness of breath. Most patients can be treated with calm reassurance by dental personnel. Others may need to "rebreathe" into a paper bag or unconnected face mask.

Asthma

Most patients who have asthma attacks have a history of asthma and usually carry their medication (inhaler dose form) with them. Signs and symptoms include wheezing with prolonged expiration. Treatment consists of having the patient treat with his own medication, which is usually a β_2-agonist. If the patient does not respond or does not have any medication, he should be transferred to a hospital. Hospital treatment can include **epinephrine,** intravenous **aminophylline,** or **albuterol** via a nebulizer.

Anaphylactic Shock

Anaphylactic shock is usually due to an allergic reaction to a medication. Signs and symptoms include weak and rapid pulse, profound decrease in blood pressure, dyspnea, bronchoconstriction, and coughing. Treatment includes the immediate administration of epinephrine. **Diphenhydramine** can also be used.

Acute Airway Obstruction

Acute airway obstruction can occur when a foreign body falls into the pharynx or larynx. It is characterized by acute signs of anxiety and cyanosis. The patient will gasp for breath, cough, and gag in an attempt to dislodge the foreign body. Treatment includes placing the patient in the Trendelenburg position on his right side and encouraging coughing. The patient should not be allowed to sit upright. One should clear the pharynx and pull the patient's tongue forward. The Heimlich maneuver should then be attempted. It can be repeated as necessary. The patient should be transferred to the hospital if the foreign body cannot be dislodged.

Suction, intubation, or even ventilatory assistance may be necessary if the patient aspirates (swallows the foreign body into the lungs) the object. This requires transfer to a hospital. Aspiration can be prevented by the use of rubber dams and throat packing when appropriate.

ENDOCRINE EMERGENCIES

This section discusses hypoglycemia, diabetic coma, adrenal insufficiency, and thyroid storm, which are some of the more common endocrine emergencies.

Hypoglycemia

Hypoglycemia is a result of a drop in blood glucose levels. It often happens when the patient takes her antidiabetic medication but fails to eat prior to the dental appointment. Signs and symptoms include a rapid pulse, decreased respiration, hunger, dizziness, weakness, and tremor. The patient may also present with diaphoresis, mental confusion, and nausea. The patient may appear to be intoxicated. Treatment includes the immediate administration of a glucose source. This includes orange juice, cake frosting, a piece of candy, or oral glucose.

Diabetic Coma

Diabetic coma is caused by elevated blood sugar and is characterized by frequent urination, loss of appetite, nausea, vomiting, and excessive thirst. The patient may also have acetone (fruity smelling) breath, hypercapnia, warm, dry skin, rapid pulse, and decrease in blood pressure. The patient should be transferred to the hospital where she will be treated with insulin.

Adrenal Insufficiency

Adrenal insufficiency usually occurs when steroid-dependent patients experience stress without an increase in their steroid dose. Signs and symptoms include nausea, vomiting, abdominal pain, and confusion. It can lead to cardiovascular collapse, shock, and death if untreated. Treatment includes parenteral hydrocortisone, oxygen, fluid replacement, and vasopressors if necessary.

Thyroid Storm

During thyroid storm, the patient's hyperthyroid condition is out of control. It is characterized by hyperpyrexia, increased sweating, hyperactivity, mental status changes, shaking, nervousness, and tachycardia. Congestive heart failure and cardiovascular collapse can occur if left untreated. Treatment is symptomatic and includes analgesics and tepid bath for fever, and β blockers for cardiovascular symptoms. Sodium iodide and propylthiouracil are given to treat the hyperactive thyroid.

DRUG-INDUCED EMERGENCIES

Drugs used in the dental office can sometimes cause medical emergencies. This section discusses the emergencies caused by opioid analgesics, local anesthetics, and epinephrine. It also briefly reviews the adverse drug events caused by antipsychotics that can adversely impact dental treatment.

Opioid Analgesics

Large doses of opioid analgesics can cause respiratory depression or arrest. The patient presents with shallow and slow respiration and pinpoint pupils. These effects can be reversed with the administration of **naloxone.**

Local Anesthetics

Local anesthetics can cause either central nervous system (CNS) stimulation or depression. Signs and symptoms of CNS stimulation include excitement or even seizures. CNS depression is characterized by drowsiness, dizziness, and unconsciousness. Both CNS stimulation and depression are treated based on the patient's symptoms.

Epinephrine

Epinephrine is an α- and β-adrenergic agonist with cardiovascular and CNS effects. Signs and symptoms of epinephrine toxicity include nervousness, tremors, and tachycardia. This can be best treated by calm reassurance of the patient.

Antipsychotic Drugs

Some patients may experience acute extrapyramidal reactions with dose increases or initial doses of antipsychotic drugs. The patient may experience acute dystonic movements, uncoordinated tongue movements, and grimacing. This is usually treated with intravenous or intramuscular **diphenhydramine** or intramuscular **benztropine mesylate.**

Summary

Medical emergencies in the dental office are best treated by preventing them from occurring. Well-trained and well-prepared office personnel can effectively treat emergencies that do occur. The dental hygienist should learn how to assess the patient for a medical emergency and the general measures used to treat them. Though most dental practices call 911 for medical emergencies, each dental office should have a medical emergency kit. In some instances, dental practitioners may need to begin therapy before the emergency people have arrived. Medical kits should include nitroglycerin, glucose, epinephrine, diphenhydramine, β_2-agonists, hydrocortisone, naloxone, morphine, and oxygen, to list a few items.

Dental practitioners need to learn the signs and symptoms of cardiac, respiratory, central nervous system, endocrine, and drug-induced emergencies. This will help the dental practitioner to better assess the situation and initiate appropriate treatment.

Case Study: Kirsty Bellows

Kirsty Bellows is a 16-year-old who is new to your practice. During the medication/health history you learn that she has type I diabetes mellitus that was diagnosed when she was 6 years old. Miss Bellows is treated with a combination of regular and NPH insulin and maintains fairly adequate control of her blood sugar levels. During the oral examination Miss Bellows starts to feel weak, dizzy, and appears to be somewhat confused.

1. What is happening to Miss Bellows and what is the cause?
2. How can this condition be treated?
3. What are different ways to prevent this situation from happening again?
4. What would happen if Miss Bellows's glucose levels became too high?
5. What are the signs and symptoms of elevated blood glucose levels?
6. How can elevated blood glucose levels be treated?
7. How could this situation be prevented?

Case Study: George Blumberg

George Blumberg is 52 years old and has been coming to your practice for close to 15 years. He is a nice man with no medical problems. His only medications include over-the-counter analgesics and Tagamet HB for heartburn. He is in the office to have a crown replaced. The procedure is going well until Mr. Blumberg moves his head, coughs, and dislodges the crown. He immediately starts to cough and gag.

1. What is acute airway obstruction and what are its signs and symptoms?
2. What it the treatment of acute airway obstruction?
3. What should happen if Mr. Blumberg aspirates the crown?
4. How could this situation have been avoided?
5. How can dental personnel train for this type of emergency?

Review Questions

1. What factors can lead to medical emergencies in the dental office?
2. What are the different ways of preventing medical emergencies in the dental office?
3. State the general measures dental personnel can take to respond to medical emergencies.
4. List the equipment necessary for the treatment of medical emergencies.
5. What drugs are found in a medical emergency kit and what are their uses?
6. For each of the following, state the signs, symptoms, and treatment: (a) syncope, (b) hyperventilation, and (c) seizures.

BIBLIOGRAPHY

Caroline NL: *Emergency Care in the Streets,* 4th ed. Little, Brown and Company, Boston, 1991.

Ho MT, Saunders CE, eds.: *Current Emergency Diagnosis and Treatment,* 3rd ed. Appleton and Lange, Norwalk, CT, 1990.

Kravis TC, Warner CG, Jacobs LM Jr., eds.: *Emergency Medicine: A Comprehensive Review,* 3rd ed. Raven Press, New York, 1993.

Malamed SF: *Handbook of Medical Emergencies in the Dental Office,* 3rd ed. Mosby, St. Louis, 1987.

CHAPTER 23

Substance Abuse

Key Terms

Addiction
Depressants
Drug/Substance Abuse
Drug Dependence
Hallucinogen
Narcotic

Physical Dependence
Psychologic Dependence
Stimulants
Tolerance
Substance Abuse
Withdrawal

LEARNING OBJECTIVES

After completion of this chapter and its learning activities, the student should be able to:

1. Define psychologic dependence, physical dependence, tolerance, addiction, and drug abuse.
2. Describe the effects of CNS stimulant abuse.
3. Discuss the pharmacologic effects, adverse reactions, and toxicity associated with cocaine and amphetamines.
4. Describe the abuse associated with caffeine and nicotine.
5. Describe the effects of CNS depressant substance abuse.
6. Discuss the patterns of abuse, management of overdose and withdrawal, and dental concerns associated with alcohol, opioid analgesics, and sedative-hypnotics.
7. Describe the abuse associated with the hallucinogens phencyclidine, marijuana, and lysergic acid diethylamide.

INTRODUCTION

The dental hygienist will come across patients, health professionals, family members, and friends who are abusing any number of drugs. Substance abusers may be long-time patients or strangers to the practice in search of drugs. The dental hygienist needs to have a general knowledge of the different types of drugs being abused including patterns of abuse, management of overdose and withdrawal, and how abuse can affect oral health care.

DEFINITIONS

Addiction: often equated with physical dependence and can be defined as the compulsive use of a substance despite adverse consequences and a loss of control (Seymour and Smith, 1987).

Drug/Substance Abuse: the continued use of a drug that is inconsistent with medical practice.

Drug Dependence: the need or compulsion to take a drug to prevent withdrawal symptoms or the downside of not taking the drug.

Physical Dependence: continued use of the drug in order to maintain certain body functions. Withdrawal can lead to physical signs and symptoms.

Narcotic: a drug such as morphine used to produce sleep, insensibility, or stupor. These drugs are addicting.

Psychological Dependence: continued use of the drug for pleasure or to prevent discomfort.

Tolerance: increasing doses of a drug to produce the same effect.

Withdrawal: occurrence of objective signs of physical distress when a person abruptly discontinues the drug.

CENTRAL NERVOUS SYSTEM STIMULANTS

Central nervous system (CNS) *stimulants* include such drugs as **cocaine,** amphetamines, **caffeine,** and **nicotine.** Small to moderate doses overstimulate the CNS which, in turn, energizes muscles, increases heart rate and blood pressure, and decreases appetite. They can also cause heart, blood vessel, and seizure problems. Moderate doses make a person feel more confident, outgoing, eager to perform, and excited. Euphoric feelings are dependent on the dose and the person taking the drug. Larger doses or prolonged use can lead to anxiety, paranoia, and mental confusion.

Cocaine

Cocaine is a stimulant and is used as a topical, local anesthetic drug. It is used to numb nasal passages during nose surgery and as a local anesthetic during eye surgery. Cocaine is abused for its stimulating effects though it interferes with other neurotransmitters in the body. It greatly increases the release of norepinephrine, which raises blood pressure and increases heart rate, breathing, and jitteriness. It can also increase dopamine levels, which can cause paranoia, and can decrease acetylcholine, which causes muscle tremors, memory lapses, mental confusion, and hallucinations. It can deplete serotonin levels making it difficult for a person to sleep.

Routes of administration for cocaine abusers include intravenous, intranasal (snorting or sniffing), and smoking (free-base form that goes by the street name of "crack" or "rock"). Cocaine stimulates the reward/pleasure center of the brain and causes a sense of euphoria that causes abusers to use the drug again and again. The drug produces psychological dependence but has not been shown to have physical dependence, tolerance, or withdrawal. People continue to abuse the drug in order to achieve the feelings of their first "high" and to prevent a downside or crash that is very intense. Adverse reactions to cocaine include elevated blood pressure, myocardial infarction, stroke, seizures, arrhythmias, gastrointestinal complaints, and obstetrical and neonatal complications for pregnant women.

Amphetamines

Amphetamines include **amphetamine, methamphetamine** (Desoxyn), **dextroamphetamine** (Dexedrine), and **dextromethamphetamine** and go by the street names of "speed," "meth," "crank," "crystal," "ice," and "glass." These drugs are put in a gelatin capsule or on a piece of paper when taken orally because of their bitter taste. Intravenous injections are irritating and cause pain in the blood vessels and snorting causes mucosal irritation.

Small to moderate doses increase heart rate, respiration, blood pressure, cause CNS stimulation, increase body temperature, and decrease appetite. They are abused because of their ability to produce a sense of euphoria, feeling of well-being, increased energy and alertness, and a feeling of omnipotence and self-confidence similar to cocaine. Prolonged use can lead to tolerance, xerostomia, anxiety, aggressiveness, hallucinations, paranoia, extreme depression, and lethargy.

Amphetamine overdose is characterized by dilated pupils, increased blood pressure, rapid pulse, cardiac arrhythmias, seizures, xerostomia, diaphoresis, hyperthermia, and anxiety. Anxiety can be treated with calm reassurance or with sedative-hypnotic drugs. Cardiovascular symptoms and seizures are treated with the appropriate medication.

Caffeine

Caffeine is the active ingredient in many over-the-counter medications, coffee, tea, sodas, and chocolate and it is the most popular stimulant in the world. In fact, many people are surprised to learn that it is a drug. Low doses of caffeine make us feel more alert, dissipate drowsiness or fatigue, and help us to think. Cardiovascular effects include increased heart rate and blood pressure. It can also irritate the stomach. Excessive use (equivalent to 8–12 cups of coffee per day) can lead to nervousness, mental confusion, irritability, muscle twitching, and insomnia. Physical dependence can occur with as little as 2–3 cups per day.

Millions of Americans are mildly addicted to coffee (Seymour and Smith, 1987). This fact is usually overlooked until the patient tries to cut back or stop drinking coffee. Withdrawal symptoms can occur even with only a two-cup-a-day habit and usually start 24 hours after the last cup of coffee. Signs and symptoms include lethargy, irritability, disorientation, working difficulty, constipation, and a general intense headache. They decrease rapidly and are usually resolve within 3 days.

Nicotine

Nicotine is a stimulant drug that is either smoked, chewed, or placed between the gum and lip and absorbed into the body. People use tobacco (most common form of nicotine) because they claim that it increases alertness, relaxes them, increases memory and concentration, and decreases appetite and irritability. Other effects include increased blood pressure and heart rate. Initial use can cause nausea and vomiting. Oral manifestations of chewing tobacco or snuff include chronic gingivitis, leukoplakia, and precancerous lesions. The dental hygienist should carefully question all patients about tobacco use and thoroughly examine all patients that use tobacco products.

Chronic use of tobacco can lead to heart disease, chronic obstructive pulmonary disease, oral and lung cancer, noncancerous mouth disease, gum and jawbone deterioration, GI disease, anorexia, eating disorders, and allergies. Secondary smoke can have adverse effects on nonsmokers.

Most people who start smoking become addicted and go through withdrawal if they try to stop. Withdrawal symptoms include nervousness, restlessness, sleep disturbances, sweating, reduced heart rate and blood pressure, inability to concentrate, compulsive eating, headaches, and intense irritability. Symptoms are rapid in onset and nicotine cravings may continue for life. Nicotine withdrawal can be made less intense with the aid of nicotine as a chewing gum (Nicorette) or in patches (Nicoderm, Nicotrol, Prostep, Habitrol)—which are now available without a prescription.

CENTRAL NERVOUS SYSTEM DEPRESSANTS

CNS *depressants* slow heart rate and respiration, decrease muscle coordination and energy, and dull the senses. Opioid analgesics can cause constipation, nausea, and sexual dysfunction. Initially, CNS depressants act as stimulants because they lower inhibitions, but as more is taken, they act as depressants. Examples of classes of CNS depressants include opiates and opioids, sedative-hypnotics, and alcohol.

Alcohol

Fifteen million people in the United States have problems with alcohol and 90% of all assaults are due to excessive alcohol intoxication. Also, 50–60% of all murders, over half the rapes and sexual assaults on children, and one-third to one-half of all arrests involve alcohol. It is the number one health problem in the United States and is associated with many medical problems (Seymour and Smith, 1987).

Pharmacokinetics. Alcohol is rapidly and completely absorbed by the gastrointestinal tract. It is metabolized at a continuous rate that is dependent on the person's body weight, amount of alcohol consumed, time passed since the last drink, and to a lesser extent, tolerance to alcohol after years of continuous drinking. Food delays absorption and peak levels occur within 40 minutes when ingested on an empty stomach.

Intoxication. Mild intoxication is characterized by impaired judgment and emotional liability, and nystagmus can occur. Dilated pupils, slurred speech, ataxia, and a staggering gait are signs of moderate intoxication. Severe intoxication or overdose can result in seizures, coma, and death.

Withdrawal. Withdrawal from incidental intoxication can cause headaches, nausea, loss of appetite, shakiness, and muddled thinking. Withdrawal after long-term drinking can result in generalized tonic-clonic seizures, psychosis with hallucinations, tremors, agitation, and death.

Acute Treatment. In most instances time is the best treatment for incidental acute intoxication and withdrawal. Caffeine-containing beverages should not be used because they only make the drunk individual wide awake. Liquids (water), moderate exercise (walking in fresh air), and sleep can help the person who is "hung over." Benzodiazepines may be required for individuals undergoing withdrawal after long-term consumption of alcohol.

Long-Term Treatment. Alcohol detoxification is undertaken in inpatient facilities and often incorporates benzodiazepines for the treatment of acute withdrawal. Chronic intoxication and compulsive drinking are best treated with programs like Alcoholics Anonymous.

Chronic Effects. The chronic effects of long-term consumption include poor diet, which leads to protein deficiency and mineral and water-soluble vitamin deficiencies. Physical effects include cirrhosis of the liver, gastritis, esophageal varices, arrhythmias, and hypertension. Chronic use can increase the risk of mouth, pharynx, larynx, esophagus, and liver cancer. Alcohol consumption by pregnant women can result in a variety of birth defects known as fetal alcohol syndrome (FAS).

Opiates and Opioid Analgesics

Opiates and opioid analgesics include such drugs as **heroin, codeine, morphine, hydromorphone** (Dilaudid), **meperidine** (Demerol), **oxycodone** (Percodan), and **pentazocine** (Talwin). These drugs are sold illegally on the streets and many users try to con physicians and dentists into prescribing them (see Chapter 8).

Physical and Mental Effects. Opiates and opioid analgesics activate the reward/pleasure center of the brain (limbic system), which elevates mood, causes euphoria, and can either relieve or produce feelings of fear and apprehension. These drugs can also cause cardiovascular and respiratory depression, delay menstruation, decrease testosterone levels in men, and decrease sexual desire. Other effects include constipation, urinary retention, and peripheral vasodilation.

Tolerance, Dependence, and Withdrawal. Opiate and opioid analgesic abusers develop tolerance to initial doses and much more is necessary to achieve that "high" feeling. The body adapts to opiate and opioid analgesic ingestion so much that tissues and organs become dependent on the drugs in a relatively short period of time. Withdrawal symptoms are noted within 2–3 weeks of continuous abuse.

Heroin. Heroin is used as the example from this group of medications. The opioid analgesics are discussed in great detail in Chapter 8. Heroin can be smoked, snorted, or injected subcutaneously, intramuscularly, or intravenously. Initial reactions to the drug are usually negative and include nausea, sweating, and a general feeling of discomfort. After a few doses the user experiences a rush of good feelings that lasts several minutes and is then followed by drowsiness. Acute overdose is characterized by fixed, pinpoint pupils, depressed respiration, hypotension, shock, slow or absent reflexes, drowsiness, or coma. Acute overdose can be treated with naloxone (Narcan), which should be administered immediately.

Heroin withdrawal occurs when the patient fails to take the drug after a sufficient period of time. Signs and symptoms include lacrimation, rhinorrhea, diaphoresis, and restless sleep. As time progresses, the user begins to experience anorexia, tremors, irritability, weakness, excessive GI activity, increased heart rate and blood pressure, and chills alternating with excessive sweating. These symptoms tend to clear up about 8 days after the last dose of heroin. Long-term treatment includes methadone maintenance programs, counseling, and self-help groups like Narcotics Anonymous.

Dental Concerns of Opiates and Opioid Analgesics. As discussed in Chapter 8, opioid abusers will come to a dentist's office in search of medications to supply their habit. These people will talk about pain that can only be treated with specific opioid analgesics and usually come in at closing or call on the weekends. Refer to Chapter 8 for more information on this topic. Many heroin abusers inject their medications, which makes them at a higher risk for contracting hepatitis B, human immunodeficiency virus (HIV) and acquired immune deficiency syndrome (AIDS), treatment-resistant tuberculosis, and sexually transmitted diseases. The dental hygienist should use special care when treating these patients to not only protect herself but to protect the patient from developing other infections.

Sedative-Hypnotics

The sedative-hypnotics include the barbiturates, benzodiazepines, and the nonbarbiturate sedative-hypnotics. Examples of this last class include **glutethimide** (Doriden), **methaqualone** (Quaalude), **ethchlorvynol** (Placidyl), and **methaprylon** (Noludar). Initial physical and mental effects of sedative-hypnotics include loss of inhibition, euphoria, emotional instability, arguing, difficulty in thinking, poor memory and judgment, slurred speech, and ataxia. Continued use and increasing doses can cause drowsiness and sleep, respiratory depression, decreased cardiac output, and decreased gastrointestinal (GI) and genitourinary (GU) activity. Some patients may experience elation and excessive stimulation.

Tolerance. Tolerance develops rapidly to the physical and mental effects of sedative-hypnotics. Tolerance to physical effects develops more slowly than to mental effects. As a result, high doses can have lethal effects on cardiovascular and respiratory function.

Withdrawal. Withdrawal symptoms can occur within 6–8 hours after the last dose of the sedative-hypnotic and include such symptoms as anxiety, agitation, loss of appetite, nausea, vomiting, increased heart rate, excessive sweating, abdominal cramps, and tremulousness. Withdrawal effects peak on or about days 2–3 after stopping the drug(s). Withdrawal may not occur for at least several days and peak 2–3 weeks after stopping diazepam or chlordiazepoxide. Severe withdrawal symptoms include seizures, delirium, uncontrolled heartbeat, and death.

Overdose. The signs and symptoms of overdose include respiratory and cardiovascular depression, hypotension, coma, unchanged or small pupils, and possibly nystagmus. Other signs and symptoms include cold, clammy skin, weak and rapid pulse, and slow to rapid but shallow breathing. Treatment includes establishing and maintaining an airway, gastric lavage, and dialysis to assist in the removal of the sedative-hypnotic from the body. Benzodiazepine overdose can be treated with **flumazenil** (Romazicon), which is a benzodiazepine-receptor antagonist.

HALLUCINOGENS

Hallucinogens can act as either stimulants or depressants and distort perception of reality. Sensory input is perceived with heightened awareness; colors are more brilliant, sounds are brighter and clearer, and taste, smell, and touch are more acute. **Marijuana** increases appetite and makes the eyes bloodshot, **lysergic acid diethylamide** (LSD) increases blood pressure and causes sweating, and **phencyclidine** (PCP) acts as an anesthetic. The effects of hallucinogens are dependent on the dose, mood at the time of use, basic emotional make up of the user, and the surroundings when taking the drug.

Lysergic Acid Diethylamide

LSD is an extremely potent hallucinogen that requires very little (micrograms) to produce its effects. LSD can increase heart rate and blood pressure and can increase body temperature and cause sweating. Users are open to extremes of euphoria and anxiety because of its effects on the emotional center of the brain. Signs and symptoms of LSD overdose include widely dilated pupils, flushed face, elevated blood pressure, visual and temporal distortions, hallucinations, derealization, panic, and paranoia and are often referred to as a "bad trip." Treatment includes "talking the patient down" by providing calm reassurance, gentle suggestions, subdued lighting and sounds, and restful environments. Chronic effects include prolonged psychotic reactions, severe, life-threatening depression, flashbacks, and exacerbation of preexisting psychiatric illnesses.

Phencyclidine

PCP is a dissociative anesthetic and was used by veterinarians as a tranquilizer to anesthetize large primates. PCP can be smoked, snorted, swallowed, or injected and is often referred to as "angel dust," "ice," or "peep." This drug blocks the reuptake of serotonin, dopamine, and norepinephrine. It has strong CNS effects and can produce mild depression and stimulation at low doses (2–5 mg), a desirable sensory-deprived state at moderate doses (10–15 mg), and elevated blood pressure and combative behavior. Other adverse reactions include inability to talk, confusion, agitation, and paranoid thinking. High doses (>20 mg) can cause catatonia, convulsions, coma, respiratory depression, and cardiovascular instability. It is not widely used by the street population because of the high incidence of "bad trips" and is often sold to unsuspecting novices as other drugs.

Marijuana

Marijuana is derived from the hemp plant and its chemical name is delta-9, tetrahydrocannabinol. It has been used for medicinal (treatment of resistant glaucoma and as an antiemetic for nausea associated with cancer chemotherapy) and recreational purposes for the past 2,000 years and is smoked, eaten, infused into tea, or swallowed in pills or capsules. Its effects include increased pulse rate, red eyes, and behavioral changes. Euphoria and enhanced sensory perceptions occur, which are followed by sedation and an altered sense of consciousness.

Adverse reactions or negative effects associated with marijuana include lowered testosterone levels, decreased ability to do complicated tasks, temporary disruption of short-term memory, impaired eye coordination, and a loss of the sense of time. Large quantities of marijuana can cause anxiety reactions, paranoia, and hallucinations. Chronic use can lead to apathy and a neglect of life's problems. Chronic marijuana users can suffer a withdrawal syndrome characterized by headache, anxiety, depression, restlessness, and sleep disturbances.

Summary

Substance abuse is a very large problem that affects all segments of society. Though legal, caffeine, alcohol, and tobacco are addictive substances with both toxicity and withdrawal. Opioid analgesics, sedative-hypnotics, cocaine, marijuana, PCP, and LSD continue to be abused at alarming rates. All can adversely effect oral health care either through abuser neglect, actual drug effects, or users seeking drugs at a dental office. The information furnished in this chapter should provide the dental hygienist with the ability to be familiar with those drugs that are commonly abused and their patterns of abuse.

Case Study: Sam Raphael

Sam Raphael is a 32-year-old who has been coming to your practice for close to 7 years. Lately he has been very nervous and anxious. His caffeine consumption has increased to the point that he is consuming 15–20 cups of coffee per day in addition to a six-pack of diet cola. Work has been rather stressful and he is in the middle of relationship problems. Unfortunately, he finds himself having several beers each evening to relax after all that coffee and soda. He tells you all of this as you review his medication/health history.

1. What physical effects occur at low and high doses of caffeine consumption?
2. Can one build tolerance or become "addicted" to caffeine?
3. What are the symptoms associated with caffeine withdrawal?
4. Is Mr. Raphael having caffeine toxicity? Is so, what is this and what are its signs and symptoms?
5. What factors influence the metabolism of alcohol?
6. What are the physiologic effects of alcohol?
7. What are the chronic, long-term effects of alcohol consumption?
8. Is caffeine effective in treating acute alcohol intoxication? What should be done?

Case Study: Peter Weston

Peter Weston is 42 years old and has been coming to your practice for close to 2 years. His medication/health history is significant for opiate drug addiction. He has been "clean" for close to 3 years. Unfortunately, you notice some changes in him during this office visit. He looks somewhat disheveled and has lost weight. He is nervous and can't sit still and claims to be in pain. He pushes his shirt sleeves back and you notice needle marks on his arms. It would appear that Mr. Weston is abusing heroin again.

1. What are the physical and mental effects of heroin addiction?
2. Can opiate abusers develop tolerance, dependence, and withdrawal to their drugs of abuse?
3. How is heroin administered into the body?
4. What are the signs and symptoms of an acute heroin overdose?
5. How can heroin addiction be treated?

Review Questions

1. Define psychologic dependence, physical dependence, tolerance, withdrawal, and substance abuse.
2. How can a person who has overdosed on an opioid analgesic be treated?
3. What drug is used to treat benzodiazepine overdose?
4. What are the major adverse reactions associated with cocaine use?
5. What are the different routes of administration used by cocaine abusers?
6. What are the dangers of phencyclidine abuse?
7. What are the adverse reactions associated with marijuana?
8. How can LSD overdose be treated?

BIBLIOGRAPHY

Baciewicz GJ: The process of addiction. *Clin Obstet Gynecol* 36:223–233, 1993.
Das G: Cocaine abuse in North America: A milestone in history. *J Clin Pharmacol* 33:296–310, 1993.
Gawin FH, Ellinwood EH Jr.: Cocaine and other stimulants. Actions, abuse, and treatment. *New Engl J Med* 318:1173–1182, 1988.
Inaba DS, Cohen WE: *Uppers, Downers, All Arounders*. Cinemed Inc. and WEC Films, San Francisco, 1989.
Seymour R, Smith DE: *Guide to Psychoactive Drugs*, 1st ed. Harrington Park Press, New York, 1987.

CHAPTER 24

Drug Use During Pregnancy and Lactation

Key Terms

Breast-Feeding
FDA Categories of Pregnancy
Fetus
Infant

Lactation
Pregnancy
Teratogenesis
Trimester

LEARNING OBJECTIVES

After completion of this chapter and its learning objectives, the student should be able to:

1. Define teratogenesis.
2. Discuss the implications of drug use during pregnancy and lactation.
3. List the Food and Drug Administration (FDA) pregnancy categories and give examples of each.
4. Discuss the three trimesters of pregnancy and their relationship to dental treatment.
5. Briefly review which dental drugs can be used by a pregnant woman.
6. Briefly review which dental drugs can be used by a lactating and breast-feeding mother.
7. Effectively counsel lactating mothers about drug use and lactation.

INTRODUCTION

The dental hygienist will treat many pregnant and lactating women during her practice years. Pregnant women often require additional dental treatment because of changes in estrogen levels that can cause gingival inflammation and other oral changes. Drug administration to pregnant and lactating mothers presents a unique problem because the mother is not the sole recipient of the drug and its effects. Both the fetus and nursing infant absorb the drugs and this may result in harmful effects to them. The dental hygienist can help to prevent any unnecessary drug administration or use by carefully questioning women of childbearing potential of their pregnancy and lactating status.

The intent of this chapter is to briefly review the drugs most commonly prescribed or used for dental treatments and their effects on the developing fetus and breast-feeding infant.

TERATOGENESIS

Teratogenesis is defined as the production of a deformity in the developing embryo or fetus. Teratogen is derived from the Greek word *terato,* which means monster. It was not until the middle of the 20th century that physicians realized the adverse effects of drugs on the developing embryo and fetus. Prior to this time it was thought that the uterus provided a barrier to external environmental factors including drugs. This concept, however, changed with the **thalidomide** tragedy of the 1950s. Unfortunately, it took several years and thousands of malformed infants before the relationship of thalidomide therapy to pregnancy and birth defects was recognized.

PREGNANCY TRIMESTERS

In order to avoid teratogenic effects a woman must know that she is pregnant. However, fetal development begins before the woman knows that she is pregnant. This first trimester is the critical stage of organogenesis when cells are actively dividing to form organs. Drug administration during this time period can adversely affect such organ development as the heart and central nervous system. Drug therapy should be avoided and only given if absolutely necessary. X-rays are contraindicated throughout pregnancy. Any type of elective dental procedures should be avoided, especially since many women may feel nauseated throughout the day and evening.

The second trimester is usually an excellent time for the patient to receive oral health care and other dental treatments if necessary. This is because the majority of pregnant women no longer feel sick and have more energy. Fetal development continues throughout the second and third trimesters of pregnancy and fetal brain development continues throughout pregnancy and the neonatal period.

During the third trimester the patient may feel uncomfortable and may not be able to lie prone for any length of time. Drugs that may affect labor and delivery and the newborn should not be given during this time.

Many of the drugs used in the dental office and prescribed by a dentist have teratogenic effects. The Food and Drug Administration (FDA) has proposed categories of fetal risk to help health professionals determine whether or not they should use a drug in a pregnant or lactating woman. Table 24-1 reviews the *FDA Categories of Pregnancy* that should be considered when selecting a drug for a pregnant or breast-feeding woman.

Table 24-1   FDA Pregnancy Categories

Category	Description
A	Controlled studies in pregnant women fail to demonstrate a risk to the fetus in the first trimester (no evidence of risk in the second and third trimester) and the possibility of fetal harm seems remote.
B	Animal studies have not demonstrated a fetal risk and there are no controlled studies in pregnant women or animal studies have shown an adverse effect but it has not been confirmed in women during the first trimester. (No evidence of risk during the second and third trimester.)
C	Animal studies have demonstrated a fetal risk and there are no controlled studies in pregnant women or studies in women and animals are not available. Drugs should only be used if the potential benefit outweighs the risk to the fetus.
D	Positive evidence that human fetal risk exists but the benefits may outweigh the risk to the fetus.
X	Animal and human studies have demonstrated fetal abnormalities and there is evidence of fetal risk based on human experience, or both, and the risk of using the drug in a pregnant woman clearly outweighs any possible benefits. These drugs are contraindicated in any woman who is or may become pregnant

Source: Briggs GG, Freeman RK, Yaffe SJ, *Drugs in Pregnancy and Lactation*, 4th ed. Williams and Wilkins, Baltimore, 1994.

BREAST FEEDING

More and more women are breast-feeding their newborns when they leave the hospital and a small number continue to breast feed their children for at least 6 months to 1 year of age. Almost all drugs given to lactating mothers pass into breast milk, which can be passed to the infant when he is nursing. The plasma concentration of the drug, its lipid solubility, degree of ionization, and protein binding determine how much drug is absorbed into breast milk. As with pregnancy, drugs should be given to a lactating and breast-feeding mother only if necessary. If a drug must be given, the mother should nurse the child prior to the dose or immediately after taking the drug. She should avoid nursing during peak drug levels. In some instances the mother must not breast-feed and should express and discard all milk until the drug is completely gone from her body.

DENTAL DRUGS DURING PREGNANCY AND LACTATION

In general, drugs should be used only if they are truly necessary and the benefits of using the drug outweigh the risks of not using it.

Analgesics

Analgesics should be used only for short durations and at the lowest possible doses to control pain or reduce fever.

Acetaminophen. **Acetaminophen** has an FDA pregnancy category risk factor of B and is routinely used during all stages of pregnancy. It crosses the placenta and is found in low concentrations in breast milk. It is safe for short-term use in both pregnant and lactating women. It has been associated with renal and liver changes in the newborn when given in toxic doses.

Aspirin. **Aspirin** has a risk factor rating of C and has been associated with birth defects involving the eyes, central nervous system (CNS), gastrointestinal (GI) tract, and skeleton in animals. Aspirin is sometimes used during pregnancy and can cause anemia, antepartum and/or postpartum hemorrhage, prolonged gestation, and prolonged labor in the mother. It may also cause fetal or newborn hemorrhage and premature closure of the patent ductus arteriosus which occur with chronic high-dose aspirin use. Aspirin and other salicylates are excreted into breast milk in low concentrations. The American Academy of Pediatrics recommends that aspirin should be used with caution in a lactating mother because of the risk of decreased platelet function to the nursing infant (Committee on Drugs, American Academy of Pediatrics, 1994).

Nonsteroidal Anti-inflammatory Drugs (NSAIDs). **NSAIDs** produce effects similar to aspirin and the outcome on the fetus is similar. They can delay and make delivery more difficult and can cause maternal and neonatal hemorrhage. They can also constrict the patent ductus arteriosus. NSAIDs should not be used during the third trimester because of their ability to interfere with labor and delivery and the increased risk of hemorrhage. The American Academy of Pediatrics considers **ibuprofen** to be compatible with breast-feeding (Committee on Drugs, American Academy of Pediatrics, 1994).

Opioid Analgesics. Retrospective studies of **opioid analgesics** have been associated with increased risks of inguinal hernias, cardiac and circulatory system defects, cleft palate and lip, dislocated hips, and other musculoskeletal defects (Bracken and Holford, 1981; Saxen, 1975). These drugs have a risk factor of C. The use of opioid analgesics during labor produces neonatal respiratory depression and withdrawal symptoms. Opioid analgesics appear in breast milk in small amounts. The American Academy of Pediatrics considers codeine to be compatible with breast-feeding (Committee on Drugs, American Academy of Pediatrics, 1994).

Anti-Anxiety Drugs

Anti-anxiety drugs are often used as preanesthetic agents and to provide the patient with relief from the fears associated with a dental appointment or procedure. Their use, however, is often contraindicated during pregnancy and lactation.

Barbiturates. **Phenobarbital** has been associated with minor congenital defects, hemorrhage at birth, and addiction in the newborn, and has a risk factor of D. Phenobarbital and other barbiturates can be given to nursing mothers. The nursing mother and other caregivers should observe the infant for signs of sedation.

Benzodiazepines. First-trimester use of **benzodiazepines** has been associated with cleft palate and lip and neural tube defects. **Temazepam** and **triazolam** have an FDA pregnancy category risk factor of X and the other benzodiazepines have an FDA pregnancy category risk factor of D. Chronic ingestion or high doses can cause floppy infant syndrome that is characterized by hypotonia, lethargy, sucking difficulties, and a withdrawal syndrome characterized by intrauterine growth retardation, tremors, irritability, hypertonicity, diarrhea, vomiting, and vigorous sucking. Benzodiazepines may accumulate in breast-fed infants and their use is not recommended in lactating women.

Nitrous Oxide. Operating room personnel chronically exposed to **nitrous oxide** have had high incidences of spontaneous abortions and birth defects in children. This drug should not be used in pregnant women and pregnant dental hygienists should use caution if nitrous oxide is used in their practice.

Antimicrobials

Antimicrobial drugs should be used only when absolutely necessary.

Cephalosporins. **Cephalosporin** antibiotics have an FDA Pregnancy Category risk factor of B and have not been associated with congenital birth defects. These drugs can be used by a lactating mother. The infant should be watched for signs of allergic reaction and GI adverse reactions.

Clindamycin. **Clindamycin** has an FDA pregnancy category risk factor of B and there have been no reports of congenital defects. It is excreted in breast milk and the infant should be watched for signs of allergic reaction and GI adverse reactions.

Clotrimazole. **Clotrimazole** has an FDA pregnancy category risk factor of B and there have been no reports of congenital defects. There are no data available on clotrimazole and breast-feeding.

Erythromycin. **Erythromycin** has an FDA pregnancy category risk factor of B and there have been no reports of congenital defects. However, the estolate salt has been reported to induce hepatoxicity in pregnant women (McCormack, et al., 1977). Though erythromycin is excreted in breast milk, the American Academy of Pediatrics considers it to be compatible with breast-feeding.

Nystatin. **Nystatin** has an FDA pregnancy category risk factor of B and can be used during both pregnancy and lactation.

Penicillin. **Penicillin** *V* has an FDA pregnancy category risk factor of B and there have been no reports linking it with congenital birth defects. Penicillin is excreted in breast milk and the infant should be watched for signs of allergic reaction, candidiasis, and GI adverse reactions.

Tetracycline. **Tetracycline** antibiotics have an FDA pregnancy category risk factor of D. Their use during pregnancy can stain deciduous teeth and inhibit fetal bone growth. They can also cause maternal hepatotoxicity. Tetracycline is excreted in breast milk and dental staining and bone growth inhibition are possibilities.

Local Anesthetics and Vasoconstrictors

Local anesthetic drugs with vasoconstrictors are used with great frequency in dental practices and their use may be warranted during pregnancy.

Lidocaine with Epinephrine. **Lidocaine** has an FDA pregnancy category risk factor of B/C and should be used only when absolutely necessary. **Epinephrine** has an FDA pregnancy category risk factor of C and its use should be avoided.

Summary

Pregnancy and lactation are special times in a woman's life that require particular attention if medications must be prescribed. The dental hygienist can help to determine a woman's health status by asking appropriate questions during the medication/health history. References are available that provide the dental hygienist with the FDA pregnancy categories, which will help when deciding whether or not to use a drug. The dental hygienist can help the lactating mother by suggesting that she nurse prior to drug administration or immediately afterward to avoid maximum drug concentration. The risk to benefit ratio of any drug should be carefully reviewed during pregnancy and lactation.

Case Study: Lynn Watson

Lynn Watson is a 32-year-old who has been coming to your practice for about 3 years. She is 8 months pregnant and feeling rather "large." She is in today for her scheduled oral examination and cleaning. During the examination both you and the dentist note several cavities. All three of you agree that the cavities can wait until the baby is about 6 weeks old. Mrs. Watson has been reading up on breast-feeding and formula feeding and has decided to breast-feed. She wants you to know this because she is concerned about the use of a local anesthetic if she is nursing the baby.

1. When would be the more appropriate time to perform an elective procedure on Mrs. Watson?

2. What are the concerns associated with medications and breast-feeding?
3. What factors determine the amount of drug that is absorbed in breast milk?
4. Can local anesthetics with vasoconstrictors be given to lactating women? Why or why not?
5. What would you tell Mrs. Watson about the use of a local anesthetic with a vasoconstrictor?

Case Study: Yolanda Dallas

Yolanda Dallas is 32 years old and is new to your practice. She comes in today for an oral examination and cleaning. She is looking rather ill and you learn that she is 10 weeks pregnant (first trimester). Ms. Dallas tells you that she has had "morning sickness" almost 24 hours a day. Ms. Dallas is also complaining of tooth and gingival pain. During the examination both you and the dentist note an infection that must be treated.

1. Which antibiotic would be acceptable for Ms. Dallas?
2. What would you tell Ms. Dallas about the antibiotic that was chosen for her?
3. Which antibiotics are contraindicated in pregnant women and why?
4. Ms. Dallas also requests something for the pain. What can she take and why?
5. What would you tell Ms. Dallas about the analgesic that was chosen for her?
6. What analgesics are contraindicated in pregnant women and why?

Review Questions

1. What does teratogenesis mean?
2. What happens to fetal development during each of the three trimesters of pregnancy?
3. When do most teratogenic effects occur during pregnancy?
4. How can teratogenic effects be avoided?
5. What are the different FDA pregnancy categories and what are their significance?
6. When should drugs be given during pregnancy?

BIBLIOGRAPHY

Bracken MB, Holford TR: Exposure to prescribed drugs in pregnancy and association with congenital malformations. *Obstet Gynecol* 58:336–344, 1981.

Briggs GG, Freeman RK, Yaffe SJ: *Drugs in Pregnancy and Lactation,* 4th ed. Williams and Wilkins, Baltimore, 1994.

Committee on Drugs, American Academy of Pediatrics: The transfer of drugs and other chemicals into human milk. *Pediatrics* 93:137–150, 1994.

Lourwood DL: Treatment of chronic diseases during pregnancy. *Am Pharm* NS35:17–24, 1995.

McCormack WM, George H, Donner A, et al.: Hepatotoxicity of erythromycin estolate during pregnancy. *Antimicrob Agents Chemother* 12:630–635, 1977.

Saxen I: Association between cleft palate: An attempt to rule out chance correlation. *Int J Epidemiol* 4:37–44, 1975.

APPENDIX A

List of Drugs by Generic Name

acarbose (Precose)

acebutolol (Sectral)

acetaminophen (Tylenol, Panadol, others)

acetohexamide (Dymelor)

acetylcholine

acetylcysteine (Mucomyst)

activated charcoal

albuterol (Proventil, Ventolin)

alcohol

alfentanil (Alfenta)

alprazolam (Xanax)

amikacin

amiloride (Midamor)

amiodarone (Cordarone)

amitriptyline (Elavil)

amlodipine (Norvasc)

amobarbital (Amytal)

amoxicillin (Amoxil, others)

amphetamine

amphotericin B (Fungizone)

ampicillin (Polycillin, Omnipen)

amyl nitrite

aspirin (Bayer, various)

astemizole (Hismanal)

atenolol (Tenormin, others)

atovaquone

atropine (Atripison)

azithromycin (Zithromax)

aztreonam (Azactam)

bacitracin

beclomethasone (Beclovent, Vanceril)

benazepril (Lotensin)

benztropine mesylate (Cogentin)

betamethasone (Valisone)

betaxolol (Kerlone)

bethanechol (Urecholine)

biperiden (Akineton)

bisacodyl (Dulcolax)

bismuth subsalicylate (Pepto-Bismol)

bisoprolol (Zebeta)

bitolterol (Tornalate)

bretylium (Bretylol)

brompheniramine (Dimetane)

bumetanide (Bumex)

bupivacaine (Marcaine)

buprenorphine

buproprion (Wellbutrin)

buspirone (Buspar)

busulfan (Myleran)

butibarbital (Butisol)

butorphanol (Stadol)

caffeine

calcium carbonate (Tums)

captopril (Capoten)

carbachol (Miostat)

carbamazepine (Tegretol)

carbapenem/imipenem (Primaxin)

carbenicillin (Geocillin, Geopen)

carmustine (BiCNU)

carteolol (Cartrol)

cefaclor (Ceclor)

cefadroxil (Duricef)

cefixime (Suprax)

cefpodoxomine (Van Tin)

cefprozil (Cefzil)

cefuroxime (Ceftin, Kefurox, Zinacef)

cephadrine (Velosef)

cephalexin (Keflex)

chloral hydrate (Noctec)

chlorambucil (Leukeran)

chlordiazepoxide (Librium)

chlorpheniramine (Chlor-Trimeton)

chlorpromazine (Thorazine)

chlorpropamide (Diabinese)

chlorthalidone (Hygroton)

cholestyramine (Questran)

choline salicylate (Arthrospan)

cimetidine (Tagamet, Tagamet HB)

ciprofloxacin (Cipro)

cisapride (Propulsid)

cisplatin (Platinol)

clarithromycin (Biaxin)

clemastine (Tavist)

clindamycin (Cleocin)

clofazimine

clonazepam (Clonopin)

clonidine (Catapress)

clorazepate (Tranxene)

clotrimazole (Mycelex)

cloxacillin (Tegopen, Cloxapen)

clozapine (Clozaril)

cocaine

codeine with acetaminophen (Tylenol #3, Empirin #3)

colestipol (Colestid)

cromolyn sodium (Intal)

cyclizine (Marezine)

cyclophosphamide (Cytoxan)

cytarabine (Cytosar)

dactinomycin (Actinomycin-D)

dapsone

desipramine (Norpramin)

dexamethasone (Decadron)

dextroamphetamine (Dexedrine)

dextromethamphetamine

dextromethorphan

diazepam (Valium)

diclofenac sodium (Voltaren)

dicloxacillin (Dynapen, Dycil)

dicyclomine (Bentyl)

didanosine (Videx)

diethylpropion (Tenuate)

digoxin (Lanoxin)

diltiazem (Cardizem, Dilacor, Cardizem SR, Cardizem CD, Dilacor XR)

dimenhydrinate (Dramamine)

dioctyl sodium sulfosuccinate (Colace)

diphenhydramine (Benadryl)

diphenoxylate (Lomotil)

dipivefrin (Propine)

dipyridamole (Persantine)

dirithromycin (Dynabac)

disopyramide (Norpace)

doxazosin (Cardura)

doxorubicin (Adriamycin)

doxycycline (Vibramycin)

doxylamine (Unisom)

dronabinol (Marinol)

droperidol plus fentanyl (Innovar)

edrophonium (Tensilon)

enalapril (Vasotec)

encainide (Enkaid)

enflurane (Ethrane)

ephedrine

epinephrine (Bronkaid Mist, Medihaler-Epi, Primatene Mist)

erythromycin (E-Mycin, ERYC, Ery-Tab, PCE Dispertab)

erythromycin estolate (Ilosone)

erythromycin ethylsuccinate (E.E.S., EryPed)

erythromycin lactobionate

erythromycin stearate (Erythrocin)

estazolam (ProSom)

estrogen

ethambutol (Myambutol)

ethchlorvynol (Placidyl)

ethosuximide (Zarontin)

etidocaine (Duranest)

etodolac (Lodine)

famotidine (Pepcid, Pepcid AC)

felbamate (Felbatol)

felodipine (Plendil, Plendil ER)

fenfluramine (Pondimin)

fenoprofen (Nalfon)

fentanyl (Sublimaze)

flecainide (Tambocor)

fluconazole (Diflucan)

flucytosine

fludorcortisone (Florinef)

flumazenil (Romazicon)

flunisolide (Aerobid)

fluorouracil (5-FU)

fluoxetine (Prozac)

fluphenazine (Prolixin)

flurazepam (Dalmane)

flurbiprofen (Ansaid)

fluvastatin (Lescol)

foscarnet

fosinopril (Monopril)

furosemide (Lasix)

gabapentin (Neurontin)

ganciclover

gemfibrozil (Lopid)

gentamicin

glimepiride (Amaryl)

glipizide (Glucotrol)

glutethimide (Doriden)

glyburide (Diaβeta, Micronase)

glycerin

guanethidine (Ismelin)

halazepam (Paxipam)

haloperidol (Haldol)

halothane (Fluothane)

heparin

heroin

hydrochlorothiazide (Esidrix, HydroDiuril, others)

hydrocodone (Vicodin, Lortab)

hydrocortisone

hydromorphone (Dilaudid)

hydroxyurea (Hydrea)

hydroxyzine hydrochloride (Atarax)

ibuprofen (Motrin, others)

imipramine (Tofranil)

indapamide (Lozol)

indomethacin (Indocin)

insulin

interferon

ipratroprium bromide (Atrovent)

isoetharine

isoflurane (Forane)

isoniazid (INH)

isoproterenol (Isuprel)

isosorbide dinitrate (Isordil)

isosorbide mononitrate (Ismo)

isradipine (DynaCirc)

itraconazole (Sporanox)

kanamycin

kaolin + pectin (Kaopectate)

ketamine (Ketalar)

ketoconazole (Nizoral)

ketoprofen (Orudis, Oruvail, Orudis KT, Actron)

ketorolac (Toradol)

labetalol (Normodyne, Trandate)

lamivudine (Epivir)

lansoprazole (Prevacid)

levonordefrin (Neo-Cobefrin)

levothyroxine (Levothroid, Levoxine, Synthroid, Syroxine)

lidocaine (Xylocaine)

liothyronine (Cytomel, Cyronine)

liotrix (Euthroid, Thyrolar)

lisonopril (Prinivil, Zestril)

loperamide (Imodium)

loracarbef (Lorabid)

lorazepam (Ativan)

losartan (Cozaar)

lovastatin (Mevacor)

loxapine (Loxitane)

lysergic acid diethylamide

magnesium and aluminum (Maalox)

magnesium citrate

magnesium salicylate (Doan's)

marijuana

mechlorethamine (Mustargen)

meclizine (Bonine)

meclofenamate (Meclomen)

mefenamic acid (Ponstel)

meperidine (Demerol)

mepivacaine (Carbocaine)

meprobamate (Equanil, Miltown)

mercaptopurine (Purinethol, 6-MP)

metaproterenol (Alupent)

metformin (Glucophage)

methacholine (Provocholine)

methadone (Dolophine)

methamphetamine (Desoxyn)

methandrostenolone (Dianobol)

methantheline (Banthine)

methaprylon (Noludar)

methaqualone (Quaalude)

methicillin (Staphcillin)

methimazole (Tapazole)

methohexital sodium (Brevital)

methotrexate (Amethopterin)

methyl salicylate (Ben Gay)

methyldopa (Aldomet)

methylphenidate (Ritalin)

methyltestosterone (Metandren)

metoclopramide (Reglan)

metoprolol (Lopressor)

metoprolol LA (Toprol XL)

metronidazole (Flagyl)

mexiletine (Mexitil)

mezlocillin (Mezlin)

midazolam (Versed)

mineral oil

minocycline (Minocin)

morphine

mupirocin (Bactoban)

nabilone (Cesamet)

nabumetone (Relafen)

nadolol (Corgard)

nafcillin (Unipen, Nafcil)

nalbuphine

nalorphine

naloxone (Narcan)

naltrexone

nandrolone decanoate (Deca-
   Durabolin)

naproxen (Anaprox, Naprosyn, Aleve)

nedocromil sodium (Tilade)

nefazodone (Serzone)

neomycin

neostigmine (Prostigmin)

netilimicin

niacin

nicardipine (Cardene, Cardene SR)

nicotine (Nicorette, Nicoderm,
   Nicotrol, Prostep, Habitrol)

nifedipine (Procardia, Adalat,
   Procardia XL, Adalat CC)

nitroglycerin (Nitrostat, Nitro-Bid,
   Nitrol, Nitro-Dur, Transderm Nitro)

nitrous oxide

nizatidine (Axid, Axid AR)

nortriptyline (Pamelor)

nystatin (Mycostatin, Nilstat)

omeprazole (Prilosec)

oxacillin (Prostaphlin, Bactocil)

oxaprozin (Daypro)

oxazepam (Serax)

oxycodone with acetaminophen
   (Percocet, Tylox)

oxycodone with aspirin (Percodan)

paclitaxel (Taxol)

paregoric

paromomycin

paroxetine (Paxil)

penbutolol (Levatol)

penicillin G (Pentids)

penicillin G benzathine (Bicillin L-A)

penicillin G procaine (Crysticillin)

penicillin V (Pen Vee K, V-Cillin K

pentaerythritol (Peritrate)

pentamidine

pentazocine (Talwin)

pentobarbital (Nembutal)

perphenazine (Trilafon)

phencyclidine

phendimetrazine (Plegine)

phenelzine (Nardil)

phenobarbital (Luminal)

phenoxybenzamine (Dibenzyline)

phentermine (Fastin)

phentolamine (Regitine)

phenylephrine

phenylpropanolamine

phenytoin (Dilantin)

physostigmine (Eserine)

pilocarpine (Adsorbocarpine)

pimoline (Cylert)

pindolol (Visken, others)

piperacillin (Piperacil)

pirbuterol (Maxair)

piroxicam (Feldene)

polymyxin

pravastatin (Pravachol)

prazepam (Centrax)

prazosin (Minipress)

prednisone (Deltasone)

prilocaine (Citanest)

primaquine

primidone (Mysoline)

probucol (Lorelco)

procainamide (Pronestyl)

procaine (Novocain)

prochlorperazine (Compazine)

procyclidine (Kemadrin)

progesterone

propafenone (Rythmol)

propantheline (Pro-Banthine)

propoxycaine 0.4% with procaine 2% (Ravocaine)

propoxyphene (Darvon, Darvocet)

propranolol (Inderal, Inderal LA)

propylthiouracil (PTU)

psyllium seed (Metamucil)

pyrazinamide (PZA)

pyridostigmine (Mestinon)

quazepam (Doral)

quinapril (Accupril)

quinidine (Quinaglute)

ramipril (Altace)

ranitidine (Zantac, Zantac 75)

reserpine (Serapasil)

resperidone (Risperdal)

rifabutin

rifampin (Rifadin)

saquinavir mesylate (Invirase)

salicylic acid (Compound W)

salmeterol (Serevent)

salsalate (Disalcid)

scopolamine (Transderm-Scop)

secobarbital (Seconal)

semustine (MethylCcnu)

senna (Senekot)

sertraline (Zoloft)

simvastatin (Zocor)

sodium bicarbonate

sodium salicylate (Trilisate)

spironolactone (Aldactone)

stanozol (Winstrol)

streptomycin

sucralfate (Carafate)

sufentanil (Sufenta)

sulfamethoxazole

sulindac (Clinoril)

tamoxifen (Nolvadex)

temazepam (Restoril)

terazosin (Hydrin)

terbutaline (Brethaire)

terfenadine (Seldane)

testosterone

tetracycline (Achromycin V, Actisite)

theophylline (Theodur, others)

thiamylal sodium (Surital)

thiopental sodium (Pentothal)

thioridazine (Mellaril)

thiothixene (Navane)

thyroglobulin (Proloid)

thyroid (USP)

ticarcillin (Ticar)

ticlopidine (Ticlid)

timolol (Blocarden, others)

tobramycin

tocainide (Tonocard)

tolazamide (Tolinase)

tolazoline (Priscoline)

tolbutamide (Orinase)

tolmetin (Tolectin)

tranylcypromine (Parnate)

trazodone (Desyrel)

triamcinolone (Azmacort, Aristocort, Kenalog, Mycolog)

triamterene (Dyrenium)

triazolam (Halcion)

trifluoperazine (Stelazine)

trihexyphenidyl hydrochloride (Artane)

trimethadione (Tridione)

trimethobenzamide (Tigan)

trimethoprim

trolamine

valproic acid (Depakene/Depakote)

venlafaxine (Effexor)

verapamil (Calan, Isoptin, Calan SR, Isoptin SR, Verelan)

vinblastine (Velban)

vincristine (Oncovin)

warfarin (Coumadin)

zalcitabine (Hivid)

zidovudine (Retrovir)

zolpidem (Ambien)

APPENDIX B

Answers to Case Studies

(*Note:* If a chapter contains two case studies, only one answer has been provided to serve as an example for you.)

CHAPTER 1

Case Study: Susan Jones

1. Do you take any medication for a specific illness?

   What are the names of your medicines and how many times a day do you take them?

   How many times a day did your doctor tell you to take your medicine?

   Do you take any medicine that you can buy without a prescription?

   Do you have any allergies to medicines?, If yes, what medicines?

   What happened to you when you took the medicine?

2. Medication/health histories are the first line in safely treating any patient. Medication/health histories help to prevent possible drug interactions, allergies, and adverse reactions.

3. The dental hygienist can find information about medroxyprogesterone can be found in the *Physicians' Desk Reference, AHFS Drug Information, USP DI,* or *Facts and Comparison.*

4. *APhA Handbook of Nonprescription Drugs, Facts and Comparison,* or the OTC companion to the *Physicians' Desk Reference.*

5. Mrs. Jones should be told to take one penicillin tablet 4 times a day for 10 days. She needs to complete the full course of therapy and should report any unusual occurrences to her dentist (rash, difficulty breathing). She should also take the prescription with a full glass of water.

CHAPTER 2

Case Study: Fannie Smith

1. Mrs. Smith's percentage of body fat to muscle mass has changed so that she has more fat than muscle because of her age. She also has lower protein stores in her body, again because of her age. Both could lead to an increased incidence of adverse and toxic reactions.

2. One need only know Mrs. Smith's age to know that her liver and kidneys have

slowed down and are not working at the same level as that of a 40-year-old person.

3. Local anesthetics are given intradermally.

4. The intravenous (IV) route of administration provides the patient with the most rapid drug response. It is used during emergency situations or for drugs that are destroyed or inactivated in the gastrointestinal (GI) tract, or too poorly absorbed by the GI tract to produce an adequate drug response. It is also used for patients who are unconscious, uncooperative, or otherwise can not take oral medication. Absorption by the IV route produces more predictable blood levels than oral dose forms. The main disadvantage to IV administration is that the drug is injected directly into the patient's bloodstream. This makes the reversal of toxic or overdose situations difficult.

5. The oral route is the most common route of administration and is considered the most convenient, acceptable, and safest means of drug administration. In cases of overdose or toxic reactions, an antidote or gastric lavage can be given to counteract the negative drug effects. Disadvantages include slow onset of drug action; irregular drug absorption as a result of food, pathologic disease states, or other drugs; gastrointestinal upset due to the irritating effects of the drug; and patient age. Younger children, elderly patients, and even some adults have a hard time swallowing tablets and capsules.

6. One should remember that elderly patients have more body fat, and drugs that are lipid soluble can cause adverse and toxic reactions. The dental hygienist should also remember that decreased liver function can put the patient at risk for drug interactions and increased toxicity.

7. Mrs. Smith should take her medication in the morning. One of the side effects of this drug is frequent urination. If Mrs. Smith took this at bedtime, she may be up all night going to the bathroom. This could affect drug absorption because Mrs. Smith may decide to stop taking the drug because it interrupts her sleep.

8. This can be done by taking detailed information during a medication/health history regarding Mrs. Smith's over-the-counter and prescription drug use. The medication/health history can also be used to visually evaluate Mrs. Smith for any possible problems.

CHAPTER 3

Case Study: Rolanda Elliot

1. Uncontrolled heart disease and uncontrolled hyperthyroidism are two examples of contraindications to epinephrine therapy.

2. The drug interactions can be minimized or avoided by giving the lowest possible dose of epinephrine.

3. Propranolol is a β-adrenergic antagonist. It is a nonselective β-blocking agent used to treat hypertension, angina, cardiac arrhythmias, myocardial infarction, open-angle glaucoma, essential tremors, and for the prophylactic treatment of migraine headaches. It is also used to treat anxiety due to public speaking and stage fright.

4. It also lowers cardiac output and heart rate and should be avoided in people

with congestive heart failure, hypotension, and bradycardia. Other adverse reactions include hypoglycemia and sedation.

5. Medications such as propranolol can cross the blood-brain barrier and cause sedation and other CNS effects. Caution should be used if an opioid analgesic or antianxiety agent is prescribed. Someone should drive the patient to and from the appointment and the patient should avoid working with or operating heavy machinery, or anything that requires thought or concentration.

6. Albuterol is a β-adrenergic agonist that causes bronchodilation. It is used to treat asthma.

7. Albuterol can cause tachycardia and insomnia.

8. Albuterol inhalers can cause dry mouth and leave the patient with an aftertaste. Mrs. Elliot should be instructed to rinse and spit after each inhaler use. She should also brush and floss regularly and maintain good oral hygiene. Mrs. Elliot should drink plenty of water and suck on tart, sugarless candy and chew sugarless gum to help treat dry mouth.

CHAPTER 4

Case Study: Louisa Mendoza

1. The dental hygienist would ask about Mrs. Mendoza's health since having the baby and if she is taking any medications. The dental hygienist should also ask about potential drug allergies. She should ask Mrs. Mendoza if there is a possibility that she may be pregnant again.

2. Lidocaine would probably be the drug of choice because Mrs. Mendoza is nursing her baby. This drug has an FDA pregnancy rating category of B/C and can be used by nursing mothers.

3. A vasoconstrictor, such as epinephrine, can be given to a nursing mother. Although small amounts are excreted in breast milk, it will not harm the nursing child.

4. Mrs. Mendoza should be told the name of the local anesthetic and why she is receiving it. The dental hygienist should review potential adverse reactions that are associated with the local anesthetic. Mrs. Mendoza should be advised to let the dental hygienist or dentist know if she is feeling anxious, nervous, or if she is having heart palpitations. Most of these problems can be avoided by lowering the dose of the local anesthetic or switching to another local anesthetic.

  Lidocaine may cause sedation and Mrs. Mendoza should be advised of this. She should have someone drive her to and from the dental procedure, if possible. Mrs. Mendoza should also refrain from eating or drinking very hot or cold foods or drinks. The local anesthetic will make it difficult for Mrs. Mendoza to detect temperature changes and she may burn herself with hot food.

5. Adverse reactions include such central nervous effects as patient anxiety, apprehension, and nervousness. These can be minimized by having a calm staff member remain with the patient or by administering a lower dose of vasoconstrictor.

6. The two main systems affected by adverse reactions are the central nervous system (CNS) and the cardiovascular (CV) system. CNS adverse reactions include restlessness, tremors, and convulsions followed by CNS depression, respiratory and CV depression, and coma. Some patients may experience sedation with lidocaine. Cardiovascular adverse reactions include myocardial depression and cardiac arrest with peripheral vasodilation. Local adverse reactions may be a result of physical injury caused by injection technique or rate of administration.

7. Mrs. Mendoza should be told that it is all right for her to receive a local anesthetic even though she is nursing. Small amounts of drug may cross into breast milk and the child would then ingest the drug. The child may experience some sedation if the local anesthetic is lidocaine. The child may be sleepy and will just sleep off the effects of the lidocaine. Mrs. Mendoza could nurse the baby just prior to the procedure or immediately afterward and avoid nursing during peak lidocaine levels. Mrs. Mendoza may also want to express milk prior to the procedure and give this to the baby instead of nursing after the procedure.

CHAPTER 5

Case Study: Shalanda Riviera

1. The dental hygienist would ask Ms. Riviera what medications she may be taking (prescription and nonprescription), allergies to medications, and any medical problems such as heart disease, stomach problems, or asthma. The dental hygienist should also ask about family histories regarding health and medication. The dental hygienist should ask if there is any possibility that Ms. Riviera may be pregnant.

2. Since general anesthetics are inhaled, her cold could make it difficult for Ms. Riviera to inhale the anesthetic. The surgery should be scheduled after her cold has cleared up.

3. Any one of the volatile general anesthetics could be used. The choice of anesthetic would be dependent on the dentist and her comfort level with the anesthetic.

4. Halothane is a potent anesthetic with an MAC of 0.75 that is nonflammable, nonexplosive, and has a distinct fruity odor. It provides for smooth rapid induction of anesthesia with little laryngeal and bronchial spasm. Muscle relaxation is not complete and patients may require d-tubocurarine, a peripheral neuromuscular-blocking drug. Recovery is largely due to exhalation of the anesthetic from the lungs (80%).

    Halothane does cause respiratory depression and the dose must be carefully titrated to avoid respiratory depression. Halothane also causes cardiovascular depression and presents as bradycardia and hypotension, and can also cause arrhythmias. Other adverse reactions include uterine smooth muscle relaxation and depressed renal function.

    Enflurane is a colorless, nonflammable liquid with a sweet odor and an MAC of 1.68 that is lowered to 0.57 when combined with nitrous oxide. Its low

MAC allows for both rapid induction of and recovery from anesthesia. Skeletal muscle relaxation occurs to a greater extent with enflurane than halothane. Enflurane also causes respiratory depression, depression of myocardial contractility, and low blood pressure. Arrhythmias are less likely to occur with enflurane than with halothane. Adverse reactions include seizure activity, hypotension, and a transient decrease in kidney function.

Isoflurane is a potent agent with a pungent smell and is the most commonly used general anesthetic. Its low tissue solubility allows for rapid induction and recovery of anesthesia. Isoflurane's pungent smell may make it difficult for some patients to have a smooth induction period. This can be minimized by giving the patient an intravenous barbiturate as the induction to anesthesia. Isoflurane also produces respiratory depression, hypotension, and smooth muscle relaxation. It does not sensitize the heart to epinephrine and it does not produce seizure-like activity. The most serious adverse reaction is respiratory acidosis with deeper levels of anesthesia.

5. Ms. Riviera should be told the name of the drug and any possible adverse reactions. She should also be told that she will feel tired after the procedure and she should have someone drive her to and from her appointment.

6. An opioid analgesic may be necessary after the procedure. General anesthetics provide pain control during the procedure and are of no use once the medication has been stopped. An opioid analgesic may be of use for home pain control.

CHAPTER 6

Case Study: Kathleen Fitzpatrick

1. Mrs. Fitzpatrick requires an antibiotic prior to each dental appointment for prophylaxis against bacterial endocarditis.

2. Antibiotic prophylaxis is recommended for the following conditions: prosthetic heart valves, previous bacterial endocarditis, even in the absence of heart disease, history of bacterial endocarditis, congenital heart malformations, rheumatic heart disease, hypertrophic cardiomyopathy, and mitral valve prolapse with valvular regurgitation.

Many dental procedures can cause bacteremia and they include any dental procedure known to induce gingival or mucosal bleeding, including oral prophylaxis. Endocarditis prophylaxis is not indicated in dental procedures not likely to induce bleeding such as simple adjustments of orthodontic appliances or fillings above the gum line.

3. Amoxicillin is the drug of choice as long as Mrs. Fitzpatrick is not allergic to it. The dose is 3 grams 1 hour before the procedure and 1.5 grams 6 hours after the initial dose. If Mrs. Fitzpatrick were penicillin allergic then she could be prophylaxed with either erythromycin or clindamycin as follows:

Erythromycin stearate—1 gram 2 hours before the procedure, then 500 mg 6 hours after the initial dose

Clindamycin—300 mg 1 hour before the procedure, then 150 mg 6 hours after the initial dose

4. Mrs. Fitzpatrick should be told the name of the antibiotic, the strength of the antibiotic, and how to take it. The dental practitioner should also review potential adverse reactions or symptoms of allergic reactions with Mrs. Fitzpatrick and what to do should they occur.

5. The most common adverse reactions associated with amoxicillin are gastrointestinal and include gastrointestinal upset, nausea, vomiting, and diarrhea. There is also the possibility of allergic reaction. Mrs. Fitzpatrick should be told to try to take the amoxicillin on an empty stomach. She can take it with food or milk if it causes gastrointestinal upset. The dental practitioner should also tell Mrs. Fitzpatrick what she should do in case she experiences symptoms of an allergic reaction.

6. Mrs. Fitzpatrick could be noncompliant with her medication because of adverse reactions, because she did not understand the directions, or because she does not believe that the medication is necessary.

CHAPTER 7

Case Study: James Smith

1. Mr. Smith has an ulcer and NSAIDs or aspirin would aggravate his ulcer. Acetaminophen is not irritating to the stomach and is better suited for patients with ulcers.

2. Mr. Smith would probably benefit from two 650 mg tablets of acetaminophen every 4 to 6 hours for 1 to 2 days.

3. Acetaminophen has been associated with both nephrotoxicity and hepatotoxicity.

4. The doses required for these adverse reactions are constant and are usually taken over a long period of time. Long-term, chronic dosing could cause these adverse reactions. Those doses and duration used in dentistry are usual doses, yet short in duration, and should not present a significant problem in dentistry.

5. Mr. Smith can avoid acetaminophen toxicity by taking the medication as directed by his dentist or pharmacist. He should call his dentist if he continues to experience pain and not self-treat with higher doses of acetaminophen.

6. His risk would be further increased if he were taking aspirin or an NSAID in conjunction with the acetaminophen.

7. Acetaminophen possesses analgesic and antipyretic effects comparable to aspirin with no clinically significant antiinflammatory effects.

8. Acetaminophen is used to treat pain and fever and only poses antipyretic and analgesic effects. Aspirin, however, has antipyretic, analgesic, and antiinflammatory effects. Aspirin can be used to treat pain, fever, and inflammation.

9. The risk for developing hepatoxicity is further increased when combined with alcohol consumption. This could be avoided by not drinking alcoholic beverages while taking acetaminophen.

10. The dental hygienist should review all instructions that the dentist has given to Mr. Smith about acetaminophen and how to take it. The dental hygienist could also let Mr. Smith know that alcohol consumption could increase his

risk for hepatotoxicity and that Mr. Smith may want to avoid alcohol when taking acetaminophen.

CHAPTER 8

Case Study: Sam Smith

1. The main concern with this patient is that he is a substance abuser in search of medication to support his habit. The dentist and dental hygienist should examine the patient to determine the cause of his pain. Nonsteroidal antiinflammatory drugs should be the drugs of choice for his pain and this is all that Mr. Smith should be offered.
2. Other red flags associated with opioid addiction include patient (1) claims allergies to NSAIDs or lower-potency opioid analgesics; (2) calls with a request for an opioid analgesic just as the office is closing or after hours; (3) cancels the dental appointment but still requests the opioid analgesic even though he will be out of town "on business"; and (4) often changes dental providers because no one understands his "low pain threshold."
3. The addictive potential for opioid analgesics and other drugs is based on the schedules of the Controlled Substance Act of 1970. Drugs such as heroin and morphine have a higher potential for abuse than cough syrups that contain codeine.
4. Opioid addiction should not be a concern for patients (non–substance abusers) who may require an opioid analgesic to treat moderate to severe dental pain. The duration of opioid analgesic use is limited and not a long-term process. The concern arises for people with a history of substance abuse problems.
5. Hydrocodone is a weak opioid analgesic that produces fewer adverse reactions and has less potential for abuse than morphine. It is used for the relief of mild to moderate pain in patients who cannot tolerate NSAIDs or in whom NSAIDs are ineffective. It is effective in treating and/or managing dental pain.
6. This patient should return to his previous dentist for a complete follow-up examination. He should be prescribed an NSAID if he insists that he is in pain.

CHAPTER 9

Case Study: Leslie Fitzsimmons

1. Ms. Fitzsimmons appears to be having situational anxiety as a result of coming to the dentist's office.
2. Ms. Fitzsimmons could be scheduled for a morning appointment, the dental practitioner could talk with her and calmly reassure her, or the dental practitioner could provide Ms. Fitzsimmons with a set of headphones during the procedure. Ms. Fitzsimmons could listen to relaxation tapes or the tape of her choice to occupy herself during the procedure.
3. Benzodiazepines are used to treat anxiety because they have relatively fast onset of action and their duration of action is either short, intermediate, or long. These drugs are safe and effective in the treatment of anxiety.
4. The most common adverse reactions associated with benzodiazepines are drowsiness, sedation, blurred vision, ataxia, and psychomotor impairment.

Disorientation, confusion, aggressive behavior, and excitement can occur, especially in the elderly. There have been reports of benzodiazepines producing xerostomia, swollen tongue, increased salivation, and a metallic or bitter taste. Other adverse reactions include diplopia and nystagmus, and they can affect the gastrointestinal (GI) and genitourinary (GU) tracts.

5. Benzodiazepines are associated with amnesia. The memory loss is limited to events occurring after drug administration and most likely results from impaired consolidation processes that store information. Ms. Fitzsimmons should be counseled about the amnestic qualities of benzodiazepines. She should be instructed not to operate heavy machinery or equipment and Ms. Fitzsimmons should avoid any activity that requires thought or concentration. Lastly, she should have someone drive her to and from her appointment.

6. Since this is a limited one-time prescription for a benzodiazepine, Ms. Fitzsimmons should not be overly concerned about becoming addicted to benzodiazepines. Physiologic addiction usually occurs after an extended period of large doses of benzodiazepines.

7. Ms. Fitzsimmons should be told the name and dose of the medication and how she should take it. She should also be counseled about the additive CNS depressant effects with alcohol, opioid analgesics, and other CNS depressant medications. She should be counseled about the sedating and amnestic properties of benzodiazepines.

CHAPTER 10

Case Study: Destiny Savoy

1. The dental hygienist should be concerned about the fact that the water is not fluoridated.

2. A fluoride supplement may be necessary because the drinking water is not fluoridated. Any one of the oral fluoride preparations would be appropriate. The tablet preparation may be appropriate for Destiny because she is 2 years old and can probably chew the tablets.

3. Acute toxicity is due to the ingestion of lethal doses of fluoride and the patient can die if not treated immediately. Signs of acute toxicity include nausea, salivation, abdominal pain, vomiting, and diarrhea. Other symptoms include muscle hyperirritability or convulsions, sweating, thirst, followed by cardiovascular collapse, coma, and death. Patients require immediate, emergency care.

    Chronic toxicity is the result of long-term exposure to fluoride preparations. A fluoride ion concentration of more than 2 ppm in the drinking water can lead to fluorosis during the time of crown formation of the permanent teeth. It is characterized by whiter opaque lines, brown discoloration of the tooth surface, or enamel hypoplasia as the water concentration of fluoride increases.

    The dental hygienist should discuss the signs and symptoms of both acute and chronic fluoride toxicities with Ms. Savoy and how they can occur. Ms. Savoy should be instructed to call her dental practitioner should there be a change in the fluoride content of the drinking water. The combination of fluoride supplements and fluoridated water may increase the likelihood of fluoride toxicity. Ms. Savoy should carefully monitor the amount of fluoridated toothpaste that Destiny uses. Too much toothpaste can also lead to chronic fluoride toxicity.

4. The dental hygienist should be concerned about this because Destiny may decide to ingest a full tube of fluoridated toothpaste or ingest small amounts over a long period of time. Both could result in fluoride toxicity. Ms. Savoy should be instructed to place a very small amount (pea size) on Destiny's toothbrush and have Destiny rinse her mouth with water and spit this into the sink. However, the rinsing may be difficult because of Destiny's age.

5. Ms. Savoy may benefit from a fluoride supplement since she is also drinking from the same water supply as Destiny.

6. Ms. Savoy could be started on professionally applied topical fluoride preparations and follow this with home care. This would include a fluoridated dentrifice and a fluoridated mouth rinse. The dental practitioner may want to consider a 1.23% acidulated phosphate fluoride because it is administered at 6- or 12-month intervals. The dentrifice and mouth rinse should be approved by the American Dental Association's Council on Dental Therapeutics.

CHAPTER 11

Case Study: Paula Juaneza

1. Ms. Juaneza has scurvy (vitamin C deficiency).

2. Sources of vitamin C include citrus fruits, green peppers, tomatoes, strawberries, broccoli, raw cabbage, potatoes, and papaya.

3. Megadoses (greater than 1 gm/day) of vitamin C can precipitate oxalate stones in the urinary tract. Megadoses can also destroy vitamin B_{12}, reduce copper absorption, and increase plasma cholesterol.

4. Vitamin C has no significant pharmacologic actions though it has been used to prevent and treat the common cold.

5. Vitamin C is thought to play a major role in oxidation-reduction reactions and is essential for the normal synthesis and maintenance of collagen, which is necessary for wound healing.

6. Ms. Juaneza would probably benefit from a vitamin C supplement. Her family members should be instructed on the importance of eating fresh fruits and vegetables. They should also be encouraged to take Ms. Juaneza shopping once a week to purchase fruits and vegetables and to help Ms. Juaneza with her English lessons.

7. Estrogen-containing oral contraceptives, salicylates, and tetracycline antibiotics can cause a vitamin C deficiency.

CHAPTER 12

Case Study: Blake Blackstone

1. Ms. Blackstone has early-onset periodontitis that is further classified as localized juvenile periodontitis.

2. Localized juvenile periodontitis is characterized by minimal gingival inflammation with rapid and severe vertical bone loss, deep pocket formation,

and mobility and migration of incisors and first molars in patients under 20 years of age.

3. Refer to this section in the text for this answer. The student should compare signs and symptoms and age of onset.

4. Treatment consists of mechanical debridement with scaling and root planing in conjunction with antibiotic therapy.

5. Antibiotic therapy is indicated for patients who do not respond to debridement with scaling and root planing and good personal plaque control. It is also indicated when a bacterium has been identified.

6. Ms. Blackstone should be instructed on the importance of maintaining meticulous oral hygiene at home. She should brush and floss to maintain good plaque control.

CHAPTER 13

Case Study: Nina Papadopulos

1. High cholesterol is a result of excessive amounts of lipids in the body and is often caused by high-fat, high-cholesterol diets. Elevated plasma lipid levels above accepted normal values are a significant risk for developing coronary artery disease, stroke, and hypertension.

2. Nonpharmacologic methods of lowering cholesterol include following a low-fat, low-cholesterol diet, exercise, and weight loss.

3. Lovastatin is an HMG-CoA reductase inhibitor that works by interfering with the synthesis of cholesterol in the liver.

4. The adverse reactions associated with lovastatin include elevated transaminase levels, myopathy, dyspnea, flatulence, constipation, and headache.

5. Bile acid sequestrants bind with bile salts in the small intestine and the bound bile acids become insoluble. The bile salts are normally used to make new cholesterol and can no longer do this once they become insoluble. Adverse reactions include bloating, constipation, epigastric pain, flatulence, nausea, and altered taste.

   Niacin decreases triglycerides, total serum cholesterol, and LDL (low-density lipoprotein) cholesterol, and increases HDL (high-density lipoprotein) cholesterol. Niacin also causes flushing dry skin, itching, headache, and hepatotoxicity.

   Gemfibrozil (Lopid) lowers plasma triglycerides and very low-density lipoprotein (VLDL) cholesterol and can increase HDL cholesterol. Adverse reactions include gastrointestinal complaints.

   Probucol generally lowers total cholesterol and LDL cholesterol and it also lowers HDL cholesterol. Probucol may prolong the QT interval and is not used very often. Patients also complain of gastrointestinal adverse reactions.

   HMG Co-A reductase inhibitors lower cholesterol by interfering with its synthesis in the liver, and they also lower LDL cholesterol. Adverse reactions include elevated transaminase levels, myopathy, dyspnea, flatulence, constipation, and headache.

6. The bile acid sequestrants do not taste good and may leave the patient with a bad taste in his mouth. The dental hygienist can work with the patient by

encouraging him to find a liquid that makes the drug palatable and to practice good oral hygiene after every dose of the medication.

Chapter 14

Case Study: Linda Thompson

1. The annual incidence of PUD is 1% and the lifetime prevalence for duodenal ulcers is 10% for men and 5% for women. It is important because PUD is one of the leading causes of significant morbidity and mortality in the United States.
2. Omeprazole is a proton pump inhibitor that irreversibly binds the proton pump, resulting in 90% or greater reduction in gastric acid secretion over 24 hours. It is indicated for the treatment of active duodenal ulcers, erosive esophagitis and the control of symptomatic gastroesophageal reflux disease (GERD) that is poorly responsive to customary medical treatment.
3. Adverse reactions include abdominal pain and headache. Oral adverse reactions include esophageal candidiasis, mucosal atrophy of the tongue, and dry mouth.
4. The oral cavity of patients taking proton pump inhibitors should be carefully examined for the presence of candidiasis, mucosal atrophy, and dry mouth. Instruct all patients on methods to avoid or minimize dry mouth. They include chewing sugarless gum, sucking on tart, sour, sugarless candy, and drinking plenty of water. Patients should avoid all caffeine-containing beverages and fruit juices. Caffeine can exacerbate dry mouth and fruit juices can increase the likelihood of dental caries. Also, stress the importance of good oral hygiene and regular dental examinations.
5. NSAIDs are among the leading causes of drug-induced peptic ulcer disease.
6. Misoprostol is used to treat and prevent NSAID-induced PUD. This drug is a synthetic analogue of prostaglandin PGE_2, which stimulates gastric mucosal defenses, thereby decreasing gastric acid production.
7. Pepcid AC is the nonprescription version of Pepcid (famotidine) and is indicated for the treatment of heartburn. There are no significant dental concerns with famotidine.
8. Ms. Thompson should be reminded that Pepcid AC is a drug and should be added to her medication/health history. She should also be advised to see her physician if her GI symptoms continue.

Chapter 15

Case Study: Jamil Jones

1. Cromolyn sodium is an antiinflammatory agent that prevents mast cell mediator release. Cromolyn sodium prevents the influx of calcium ions into the mast cell thereby preventing cell rupture. It is used as maintenance therapy for mild to moderate asthma and is used as prophylactic therapy for irritant-induced asthma.
2. Adverse reactions include bronchospasm, wheezing, and cough. There have been reports of dizziness, headache, and nausea.

3. The patient should be counseled to rinse carefully after each use. The spinhaler and MDI can cause dry mouth and the powder from the spinhaler may leave a bitter aftertaste. Remind the patient about the importance of good oral hygiene.
4. The adverse reactions associated with albuterol include nervousness, tachycardia, insomnia, and the inhalers can cause dry mouth.
5. Because these agents can increase heart rate, it is a good idea to measure a patient's blood pressure and pulse prior to administering a local anesthetic with a vasoconstrictor or prior to a dental procedure. Patients may also experience dry mouth with the inhalers. The dental practitioner should counsel Mrs. Jones and Jamil about the importance of rinsing his mouth out after each use and to practice daily oral hygiene.
6. Spacer devices are available to help improve delivery of MDI medication. Spacers reduce hand-lung coordination requirements, decrease oropharyngeal deposition, and enhance pulmonary deposition of medication. They are indicated for anyone having difficulty with proper MDI technique, especially preschool-age children and the elderly. They are also recommended for patients receiving inhaled steroids. Spacers help to decrease the risk of developing oropharyngeal candidiasis and enhance efficacy even if the MDI technique is optimal.

CHAPTER 16

Case Study: Jan Smith

1. First-generation antihistamines block histamine receptors and they also block acetylcholine and serotonin receptors. They are used to treat the symptoms of allergies and colds and are also used as sleep aids and as antiemetics.
2. The pharmacologic effects of antihistamines are due to their ability to block histamine and other receptor sites. Histamine-blocking effects include decreased pruritus, decreased vascular permeability, decreased flushing, headache, and tachycardia. CNS effects include drowsiness, sedation, and confusion. Restlessness and excitement can occur in young children and the elderly. Anticholinergic effects include dry mouth (xerostomia), blurred vision, constipation, urinary retention, and tachycardia. These drugs are effective in treating motion sickness and nausea and vomiting and can be used as local anesthetics.
3. The most common CNS adverse reactions are sedation, drowsiness, and confusion. Excitability and restlessness can occur in the elderly and small children. Other CNS adverse reactions include tinnitus, uncoordination, and fatigue.

    Anticholinergic adverse reactions include dry mouth, blurred vision, constipation, urinary retention, and tachycardia. GI adverse reactions include anorexia, nausea, and vomiting.

    Toxicity can occur and is normally characterized by sedation in adults and excitability in small children. The most predominant signs and symptoms are anticholinergic. Cardiac arrest and death may occur.
4. Mrs. Smith should be told to use these medications as directed by her health-care provider or according to the directions on the package or package insert.

She should maintain good oral health care while taking antihistamines because of the dry mouth associated with them. She should also be careful if a CNS depressant drug is prescribed because of the potential for increased sedation.

5. Antihistamines can interact with other CNS depressant drugs, anticholinergic drugs, and antiemetics. They can also interact with NSAIDs and cause increased GI discomfort.

6. The dental hygienist should counsel the patient on the importance of good oral hygiene and how to treat or minimize the xerostomia associated with these drugs. Mrs. Smith should be instructed to drink plenty of water and stay away from juices and caffeinated beverages. Juices can lead to an increased risk of dental caries and caffeine can exacerbate xerostomia. Patients can also chew tart, sugarless gum or suck on tart, sugarless candy.

The dental practitioner should instruct the patient to use caution if an antianxiety drug or an opioid analgesic is prescribed. These drugs are sedating and can cause increased sedation and confusion in patients taking antihistamines. Patients should not drive and should use caution when operating heavy machinery or equipment or doing anything else that requires thought or concentration.

The patient should be careful if an NSAID is required to treat dental pain. There may be increased GI irritation. The patient should take her medication after meals or with milk.

CHAPTER 17

Case Study: Carter Edwards

1. Diabetes mellitus can either be caused by a failure of β cells to produce adequate insulin or by the poorly timed secretion of insulin from the pancreas. Insulin production may be partial or completely absent. Signs and symptoms of diabetes include hyperglycemia, glucosuria, ketosis, polyphagia, polydypsia, polyuria, and dry mouth. Patients present with weight loss and wasting despite increases in appetite and they are often weak.

2. Type I diabetes begins early in life when the pancreas does not secrete insulin. These patients require insulin therapy. It is thought that Type I diabetes is due to a virus or toxins that produce an autoimmune response or it may be due to β cell abnormalities.

Type II diabetes begins during adulthood (over age 40) and the pancreas secretes insulin that is ineffective. These patients can be treated with either diet, oral hypoglycemic drugs, a combination of both, or with insulin. Type II diabetes is due to decreased tissue sensitivity to insulin and/or a decreased response of β cells to insulin.

3. Dental Caries

Patients with uncontrolled diabetes may be at greater risk for developing dental caries. Carter and his parents should be made aware of this and Carter should be commended for maintaining adequate control of his sugars. This should reinforce Carter's continual control of his sugar levels. The dental practitioner should also stress the importance of good oral hygiene (brushing and flossing) and commend Carter on his efforts.

Periodontal Disease

Patients with diabetes may experience mild gingivitis, painful periodontitis, and increased tooth mobility due to the destruction of supporting alveolar bone. Carter should be instructed to report any oral changes to his parents, dental hygienist, and dentist.

4. Carter's dental appointments should be scheduled around meal times and involve as little stress as possible. This should also mean that Carter's sugars are within "normal" range and he should not experience an episode of hypoglycemia.
5. The juice is indicated for the treatment of hypoglycemia.
6. Insulins are either short acting, intermediate acting, long acting, or available as mixed preparations. These products differ in terms of peak effect and duration of action. Short-acting insulins have their peak effect early and have a short duration of action. Intermediate-acting insulins peak midway through a dosing interval and have a longer duration of action than short-acting drugs. Long-acting insulins have an onset of action of 4–6 hours and a duration of action of 36 hours. Mixed preparations are a combination of short- and intermediate-acting insulins and often mean less injections for the patient.

   Insulins also differ in their makeup. Older preparations were derived from either pork or beef pancreases. Many patients were allergic to the beef preparations and some were allergic to the pork preparations. This led to the development of "human" insulin that is derived from either the gene splicing of *Escherichia coli* through recombinant DNA or through the transpeptidation of pork insulin.
7. The most common adverse reaction associated with insulin is hypoglycemia, which can be caused by insulin overdose, failure to eat, or increased exercise or stress. Symptoms include sweating, tachycardia, weakness, nausea, headache, blurred vision, mental confusion, incoherence, and eventually coma, convulsions, and death. Other adverse reactions include lipodystrophy at the site of injection and allergic reactions to noninsulin contaminants.
8. Carter probably does not need an antibiotic. Diabetes does delay wound healing and may place Carter at a higher risk for infection. However, this was a simple oral examination and cleaning. Carter and his parents should be told to watch for any signs and symptoms of infection and call should any occur.

CHAPTER 18

Case Study: Susan Brown

1. AIDS is the end result of the retrovirus HIV when the symptoms of HIV infection become very severe.
2. Nucleoside analogues work by inhibiting HIV reverse transcriptase, the enzyme responsible for viral replication. The nucleoside analogue enters

the CD4 T-cell and is converted into an active triphosphate moiety by cellular enzymes, and viral replication is inhibited by (1) competition between the drug and the naturally occurring nucleoside triphosphate for binding to the active site of HIV reverse transcriptase and (2) termination of DNA synthesis.

3. The four nucleoside analogues include AZT (zidovudine), ddI, ddC, and 3TC. Currently, AZT is the only drug used as first-line monotherapy. Didanosine and zalcitabine are indicated for those patients who cannot tolerate or who are not responding to AZT monotherapy. 3TC is only indicated as first-line therapy in combination with AZT. The other two drugs can also be used in combination with AZT. Please see Table 18-1 for the adverse reactions of each of these drugs.

4. Acetaminophen and aspirin may potentiate the toxicity of zidovudine and concurrent administration should probably be avoided. Extreme caution should be used if either analgesic is necessary. All four antiretroviral drugs have GI adverse reactions that could be potentiated with the addition of aspirin, nonsteroidal antiinflammatory drugs, or opioid analgesics. Lorazepam has been reported to increase the toxicity of zidovudine. The aluminum and magnesium in didanosine tablets chelates with tetracycline, which makes the tetracycline less active.

5. Both didanosine and zalcitabine can cause oral ulcerations and dry mouth.

6. HIV infection is a concern of both dental personnel and the patient. HIV infection cannot be spread through casual contact and dental personnel can take precautions to prevent its spread during dental procedures. This can be accomplished by using universal precautions.

7. Please look at Table 18-2 for the answer to this question.

8. Drugs used to treat esophageal candidiasis include fluconazole, ketaconazole, and itraconazole.

CHAPTER 19

Case Study: Mary Jones

1. These medications cause dry mouth, altered sense of taste, sensitivity of teeth and gums, mucosal pain and ulceration, and gingival hemorrhage.

2. Provide Mrs. Jones with information on good oral hygiene, plaque control, and periodontal disease, and treat any existing infections. Mrs. Jones should maximize her oral health care including brushing, flossing, and keeping scheduled oral health appointments.

3. Please see Table 19-2.

4. White blood cells are formed in the bone marrow. If bone marrow suppression occurs then white blood cells are not formed and the patient cannot fight off infections.

5. GI adverse reactions can affect oral hygiene. Nausea and vomiting may make it difficult for a patient to brush and floss teeth. Vomiting changes the make up of the mouth and can increase the risk of caries. Patients should rinse with a dilution of baking soda after vomiting. Brushing their teeth will only cause more harm.

CHAPTER 20

Case Study: Sammy Jones

1. Carbamazepine is structurally related to tricyclic antidepressants and is used to treat generalized tonic-clonic seizures, temporal lobe epilepsy, and mixed seizures.
2. The major classes of adverse reactions associated with carbamazepine are hematologic, central nervous system, gastrointestinal, and oral.
3. Central nervous system adverse reactions are a concern when a CNS depressant drug is prescribed or used in a dental office. The patient runs the risk of being sedated, confused, or dizzy. Patients should be instructed of this and advised against driving, operating heavy machinery, or doing anything that requires thought or concentration.
4. The pediatric dose form of carbamazepine contains sugar.
5. Mrs. Jones and Sammy should be instructed on proper brushing and flossing techniques, especially after Sammy has chewed the tablet.
6. Carbamazepine can cause oral adverse reactions. Mrs. Jones should learn about the different ways to help Sammy treat dry mouth. She should also be told to call the dentist and Sammy's doctor should he develop glossitis or stomatitis.

CHAPER 21

Case Study: Suzanne Fernandez

1. Mrs. Fernandez was diagnosed with depression.
2. The signs and symptoms of depression include increased or decreased sleep, weight gain or loss, feelings of worthlessness, low energy levels, and a lack of interest in what used to please the patient. Depression is a common psychiatric illness that affects approximately 13 million Americans.
3. Fluoxetine works by selectively blocking the reuptake of serotonin.
4. Fluoxetine can be irritating to the gastrointestinal tract. This effect may be exacerbated by the addition of aspirin or nonsteroidal antiinflammatory drugs.
5. There have been reports of anticholinergic (dry mouth) adverse reactions with fluoxetine.
6. Mrs. Fernandez should be instructed to take any aspirin product or nonsteroidal antiinflammatory drug with food or milk when taking them in conjunction with fluoxetine. The dry mouth should be treated as discussed in the previous case.

CHAPER 22

Case Study: Kirsty Bellows

1. Ms Bellows is experiencing hypoglycemia. This can be caused by her blood sugar dropping well below normal levels, which can be a result of stress or of Ms. Bellows taking her medication and skipping meals.
2. The quickest way to treat this is to have Ms. Bellows ingest a sugar source. Examples include orange juice or cake frosting. Other sugar sources include oral glucose.

3. Ms Bellows should be instructed to eat and not skip meals.
4. Elevated blood sugar levels can lead to diabetic coma.
5. The signs and symptoms of diabetic coma include frequent urination, loss of appetite, nausea, vomiting, excessive thirst, and acetone breath. The patient may also have hypercapnia, warm dry skin, rapid pulse, and decrease in blood pressure.
6. This is treated with insulin in a hospital.
7. This can be prevented by the patient taking her medication as prescribed, maintaining a well-balanced diet, and reporting any changes to her physician.

CHAPTER 23

Case Study: Sam Raphael

1. Low doses of caffeine make people feel more alert, dissipate drowsiness or fatigue, and help us to think. Cardiovascular effects include increased heart rate and blood pressure. Caffeine can also irritate the stomach. High doses of caffeine can cause nervousness, mental confusion, irritability, muscle twitching, and insomnia.
2. Physical dependence can occur with as little as 2–3 cups of a caffeine beverage per day. Millions of Americans are mildly addicted to coffee (Seymour and Smith, 1987).
3. The signs and symptoms of caffeine withdrawal include lethargy, irritability, disorientation, working difficulty, constipation, and a general intense headache.
4. Mr. Raphael is probably suffering the effects of excessive doses of caffeine. This is manifested by nervousness, anxiousness, and his problems with insomnia.
5. A person's body weight, amount of alcohol consumed, time passed since the last drink, and tolerance to alcohol after years of continuous drinking all affect alcohol metabolism.
6. Alcohol is a central nervous system depressant that slows heart rate and respiration, decreases muscle coordination and energy, and dulls the senses. It initially acts as a stimulant because it lowers inhibitions.
7. The chronic, long-term effects include poor diet, which leads to protein deficiency and mineral- and water-soluble vitamin deficiencies. Physical effects include cirrhosis of the liver, gastritis, esophageal varices, arrhythmias, and hypertension. Chronic use can also increase the risk of mouth, pharynx, larynx, esophagus, and liver cancer.
8. Caffeine is not effective in treating acute alcohol intoxication. It only serves to make the drunk individual wide awake. Liquids (water), moderate exercise (walking in the fresh air), and sleep can help the person who is "hung over." Benzodiazepines may be required for individuals undergoing withdrawal after long-term consumption of alcohol.

CHAPTER 24

Case Study: Lynn Watson

1. The time to perform an elective procedure is after Mrs. Watson has had her baby. However, the second trimester would be an appropriate time to perform an elective procedure if it had to be done before the baby was born.

2. Many medications pass into breast milk and the baby could ingest the milk if he is nursed after the mother has taken the drug.

3. The plasma concentration of the drug, its lipid solubility, degree of ionization, and protein binding determine how much drug is absorbed into breast milk.

4. Though both local anesthetics and epinephrine are excreted in breast milk they can be given to a breast-feeding mother.

5. Mrs. Watson should nurse her child prior to the injection of the local anesthetic with the vasoconstrictor. She may also want to express breast milk prior to coming to the dental office and use that to feed the baby after the injection. She should be able to resume nursing a few hours after the procedure.

Glossary

Absorption: uptake of substances into or across tissues.

Acetaminophen: analgesic drug used to reduce pain and fever.

Acetylsalicylic Acid: chemical name for aspirin.

Achlorhydria: lack of hydrochloric acid in gastric secretions.

Addiction: often equated with physical dependence and can be defined as the compulsive use of a substance despite adverse consequence. (Seymour and Smith, 1987).

Additive: substance added to another substance to improve its ability to remain in solution.

Adrenal Gland: gland responsible for the release of cortisol into the body.

Adrenergic Agonists: Drugs that mimic the effects of the sympathetic nervous system.

Adverse Reaction: exaggerated effect of a drug on target and nontarget tissues and organs.

Afferent: conducting toward a center or specific site.

Agonist: drug which can stimulate or enhance a receptor site.

Agonist-Antagonist: drug with the ability to either stimulate or block a receptor site.

Agranulocytosis: marked decrease in the number of granulocytes. Characterized by flu-like symptoms.

AIDS: the end result of the retrovirus human immunodeficiency virus (HIV) when the symptoms of HIV infection become very severe.

Akathesia: inability to sit still.

Akinesia: absence or loss of the power of voluntary motion.

Albuminuria: presence of albumin in the urine.

Alkalosis: accumulation of base or loss of acid from the body.

Alkylating Drugs: drugs that bind with DNA and inhibit cell reproduction during the S phase of the cell reproductive cycle.

Allergy: non-predictable, non-dose related reaction of a drug that is an immunologic response of the body towards the drug.

Alopecia: hair loss.

Alveolar Osteitis: also known as "dry socket," caused by loss or necrosis of a blood clot which exposes bone in the tooth extraction socket.

Amblyopia: dimness of vision without detectable organic lesion of the eye.

Amide: any compound derived from ammonia by substitution of an acid radical for hydrogen, or by replacing the OH group with NH_2.

Amnestic: pathologic impairment of memory.

Analgesia: relief from pain.

Anaphylaxis: exaggerated reaction of an organism to a foreign substance to which it had been previously sensitized.

Androgen: a asynthetic hormone that stimulates male sex characteristics.

Anesthesia: the combination of reversible unconsciousness and the absence of response to painful stimuli.

Angina Pectoris: pain and discomfort in the chest caused by a lack of oxygen to the cardiac muscle and an imbalance between myocardial oxygen supply and demand.

Anorexia: diminished appetite; aversion to food.

Antacid: medications that counteract stomach acidity.

Antagonism: bactericidal rate for two drugs is less than that of either drug alone.

Antiandrogenic: having activity against male sexual characteristics.

Antibacterial: any substance that destroys or suppresses the growth or multiplication of bacteria.

Antibiotic: any drug that is produced by other microorganisms to kill or inhibit the growth or multiplication of bacteria.

Anticholinergic: substances with the ability to block cholinergic/muscarinic receptors.

Antifungal: any drug that destroys or suppresses the growth or multiplication of fungi.

Antihistamine: medication that counteracts the effects of histamine.

Antiinfective: any drug that acts against or destroys infections.

Antiinflammatory: ability to decrease inflammation.

Antimetabolite: drugs similar to the metabolites found in the body that cells use for normal growth and function.

Antimicrobial: any substance that inhibits the growth of or kills a microorganism.

Antipsychotics: class of medication used to treat schizophrenia.

Antipyretic: ability to reduce fever.

Antiretroviral: class of medications used to treat HIV.

Antitussive: medication that suppresses cough.

Antiviral: any drug that destroys or suppresses the growth or multiplication of viruses.

Anxiety: an unpleasant emotional state characterized by apprehension and nervousness.

Aplastic Anemia: pertaining to defective regeneration of red blood cells.

Arrhythmia: loss of rhythm; irregular or atypical heartbeat.

Arthralgia: pain in a joint

Asthma: exaggerated bronchoconstriction caused by a hyperresponsiveness of the airway that results in reversible airway obstruction.

Ataxia: inability to coordinate voluntary muscle movement.

Atrophy: wasting away.

Auditory: pertaining to the ear; a sense of hearing.

Autacoid: an organic substance that is produced in one part of the body and travels by blood to another part of the body where it produces its effect.

Autonomic Nervous System: nervous system responsible for controlling involuntary physiologic functions such as breathing, heart rate, blood pressure, and digestion.

Bactericidal: an antibiotic that kills bacteria.

Bacteriostatic: an antibiotic that suppresses the growth or multiplication of bacteria.

Barbiturates: class of medications used to treat anxiety, insomnia, and seizure disorders; also used as a general anesthetic.

Benign: overgrowth of new cells but the overgrowth is slower and localized to a specific area.

Benzodiazepines: class of medications used to treat anxiety, insomnia, seizure disorders, and as part of general anesthesia.

Beriberi: thiamine (Vitamin B_1) deficiency.

Beta Adrenergic Agonists: class of medications used to treat asthma.

Bioavailability: degree to which a drug becomes available to the target or nontarget organ after it is administered into the body.

Bradycardia: slow heartbeat.

Bronchospasm: bronchoconstriction (narrowing) of bronchi and bronchioles as a result of spasm of bronchial smooth muscle.

Buspirone: medication used in the treatment of generalized anxiety disorder.

Capillary: minute vessels that connect arterioles and venules.

Candidiasis: infection caused by the fungi *candida.*

Carbamazepine: medication used to treat seizure disorders.

Cardiac Glycoside: major group of drugs used to treat congestive heart failure.

Cardiovascular Disease: disorders that primarily affect the heart and blood vessels.

Catabolism: breakdown of complex substances.

Catatonia: state of stupor.

Catecholamine: any of the group of sympathomimetic amines.

CD4 count: catagorizes the stage of HIV infection.

Cheilosis: a condition characterized by simple redness at the angles of the mouth that can progress to fissures, erosions, ulcers, or crusting and may or may not be painful.

Chemotherapy: treatment of disease by chemical agents.

Chloral hydrate: nonbenzodiazepine/nonbarbiturate used to treat insomnia.

Cholesterol: lipid substance essential for the formation of cell membranes, nerve tissues, and lipoprotein.

Cholinergic Agonists: drugs that mimic the effects of the parasympathetic nervous system.

Chronic Obstructive Pulmonary Disease: irreversible airway obstruction with either chronic bronchitis or emphysema.

Clonazepam: medication used to treat seizure disorders.

Coagulation: formation of a blood clot.

Conscious Sedation: condition in which patient is capable of responding to sensory stimuli while sedated.

Constipation: decrease in frequency of fecal elimination.

Controlled Substance Act of 1970: legislation that set the current requirements for the writing of prescription drugs that have a potential for abuse such as narcotic analgesics, antianxiety drugs, and barbiturates. It also placed medications with a potential for abuse into any one of five schedules.

Corticosteroids: class of medications used to treat asthma and other inflammatory processes.

Cretinism: a condition combining dwarfism with mental retardation; usually associated with hypothyroidism in children.

Cyanosis: bluish discoloration of the skin and mucous membranes due to excessive concentration of reduced hemoglobin in the blood.

Dental Caries: destructive process of decalcification of tooth enamel leading to continued destruction and decavitation of the tooth.

Dentrifice: a preparation for cleaning and polishing teeth.

Depressant: drugs which slow heart rate and respiration, decrease muscle coordination and energy, and dull the senses.

Depression: a lowering or decrease in functional activity or mood.

Diabetes: common disease of the endocrine system which is caused by failure of the β cells to produce adequate insulin, or poorly timed secretion of insulin from the pancreas.

Diaphoresis: excessive perspiration.

Diarrhea: symptom of increased GI motility that can either be acute or chronic.

Diplopia: the perception of two images of a single object; double vision.

Dissociative Anesthesia: sedation in which the patient, does not respond to sensory stimuli and does not remember what happened during the procedure; breathing and cardiac functioning remain normal.

Dissolution: the process by which one substance is dissolved in another.

Distribution: spreading of absorbed drug throughout the body.

Drug: biologically active substance that can modify cellular function.

Drug Dependence: the need or compulsion to take a drug to prevent withdrawal symptoms or the downside of not taking the drug.

Drug/Substance Abuse: the continued use of a drug that is inconsistent with medical practice.

Dynorphin: polypeptide with analgesic properties found in brain tissue.

Dyscrasia: any abnormal or pathologic condition of the blood.

Dysgeusia: impairment of the sense of taste.

Dysphonia: hoarseness.

Dysphoria: a feeling of unpleasantness or discomfort.

Dysplasia: abnormal developing cells.

Dyspnea: labored or difficult breathing.

Dystonia: involuntary, irregular muscular movements of the trunk and extremities.

Edema: an accumulation of excessive amounts of fluid in cells, tissues, or serous cavities.

Efferent: leading away from a central or specific center.

Efficacy: how well something works.

Embolus: a plug, composed of a detached clot, mass of bacteria, or a foreign body that can block a blood vessel.

Emergency Medical Kit: kit that contains medications suitable to treat common office medical emergencies.

Emesis: the act of vomiting.

Endorphin: opioid-like polypeptide found in the brain and other body parts that binds to the same receptors as opioids.

Endothelium: layer of epithelial cells lining the cavities of the heart, blood, and lymph vessels, and the serous cavities of the body.

Enkephalin: either of 2 naturally occurring peptides which produce opioid-like effects.

Eosinophilia: the formation and accumulation of an abnormally large number of eosinophils in the blood.

Epigastric: upper and middle region of the abdomen.

Epiphysis: the end of a long bone.

Erythema Multiforme: a symptom characterized by macular papules, vesicles, and bullae.

Ester: compound formed from an alcohol and an acid by removing the water.

Estrogen: female sex hormone.

Ethosuximide: medication used to treat seizure disorders.

Euphoria: a feeling of well-being commonly exaggerated and not necessarily well founded.

Excretion: elimination of an active or inactive drug from the body.

Exfoliative Dermatitis: a condition in which layers of the skin fall off.

Expectorant: medication that promotes expectoration.

Fat Soluble: readily dissolved in or absorbed by fat.

Federal Regulatory Agencies: agencies involved in the production, marketing, advertising, labeling, and prescribing of medication.

Felbamate: medication used to treat seizure disorders.

Fibrin: an elastic filamentous protein derived from fibrinogen by the action of thrombin, which leads to the formation of a blood clot.

Fluoride: thirteenth most common element found in the earth's crust.

Fluoridation: addition of fluoride to public drinking water.

Fluorosis: mottled enamel during the time of crown formation of the permanent teeth.

Focal Seizures: seizures which begin in a local area in one hemisphere of the brain and are further classified as simple or complex.

Food and Drug Administration (FDA) Categories of Pregnancy: proposed categories of fetal risk to help health professionals determine whether or not a drug should be used in a pregnant or lactating woman.

Gastroenteritis: inflammation of the stomach and intestines.

Gastroesophageal Disease (GERD): multifactorial process that involves lower esophageal sphincter (LES) incompetence, abnormal esophageal clearance, delayed gastric emptying, and the irritating effects of gastric contents.

Gels: a topical (oral) fluoride preparation.

General Anesthetics: group of chemical substances that produce anesthesia.

General Seizure: seizures which are bilaterally symmetrical and do not have a local onset. The seizures are usually accompanied by a loss of consciousness and may or may not be accompanied by convulsive movements.

Generic Equivalence: this means that the generic drug produces similar concentrations in the blood and other tissues as the trade drug.

Generic Name: official name of the drug that is determined by the United States Adopted Names Council.

Gingivitis: inflammation of the gingiva.

Glossitis: inflammation of the tongue.

Gluconeogenesis: formation of glucose from sources other than carbohydrates.

Glucosuria: increased levels of glucose in the urine.

Glycogenolysis: the breakdown of glycogen to glucose.

Goiter: enlargement of the thyroid gland, causing a swelling in front of the neck.

Gynecomastia: excessive development of male mammary glands.

H_2-Receptor Antagonist: class of medication used in the treatment of peptic ulcer disease. These medications work by blocking Histamine$_2$ receptors.

Half-life: the time it takes for half the drug to be excreted from the body.

Hallucinogen: drugs that can act as either stimulants or depressants and that can distort one's perception of reality.

Helicobacter pylori: bacteria which is thought to play a role in the pathophysiology of peptic ulcer disease.

Hematoma: bruising.

Hemolytic: the breaking down of blood cells so that hemoglobin is separated from the red cell.

Hemostasis: interruption of blood flow through any vessel; arrest of bleeding by drugs (vasoconstrictor), coagulation, or surgery.

Hepatitis: inflammation of the liver.

Hirsutism: abnormal hairiness, especially facial hair in women.

Histamine: biogenic amine that is found in almost every part of the body.

HIV: Human Immunodeficiency Virus

Hormone: chemical substances produced in the body which have specific regulatory effects on the activity of specific cells.

Hydantoin: class of medications used to treat seizure disorders.

Hydrolysis: the cleavage of a compound by the addition of water.

Hydrophilic: property of absorbing water.

Hydrophobic: repelling water.

Hypercapnia: an excess of carbon dioxide in the blood.

Hyperglycemia: excessive levels of glucose in the blood.

Hyperinsulinism: excessive secretion of insulin; insulin shock.

Hyperpyrexia: excessively high body temperature.

Hyperreflexia: exaggeration of reflexes.

Hypertension: systolic blood pressure (SBP) of 140 mm Hg or greater and/or a diastolic blood pressure (DBP) of 90 mm Hg.

Hyperthermia: greatly increased body temperature.

Hypocalcemia: abnormally low levels of calcium in the blood.

Hypoglycemia: abnormally low levels of glucose in the blood.

Hypophosphatemia: abnormally low levels of phosphorous in the blood.

Hypoplasia: incomplete development of an organ or tissue.

Hypoprothrombinemia: deficiency of prothrombin in the blood.

Hypotension: low blood pressure.

Hypothalamus: the part of the central nervous system (CNS) that controls the functions of the autonomic nervous system, many somatic functions, and the pituitary gland.

Hypoxia: reduction of oxygen in body tissues below physiologic levels.

Induction: the process or act of producing anesthesia.

Infection: the invasion of the body by pathogenic organisms and the body's response to that organism.

Inhalation Anesthetic: substances which are gases at standard temperature and atmospheric pressure, and volatile liquids.

Insomnia: insufficient or nonrestorative sleep.

Intraarterial: within an artery.

Intraarticular: within a joint.

Intracardiac: within the heart.

Intracutaneous: within the substances of the skin.

Intraosseous: within the bone.

Intrasynovial: within the synovial fluid.

Intrathecal: within the subarachnoid space.

Ionization: dissociation of a substance in solution to ions.

Kappa Receptor: receptor site which is responsible for miosis, sedation, and analgesia.

Keratinization: the development or conversion into keratin.

Keratotmalacia: irritation and inflammation on the cornea.

Ketosis: a condition that is characterized by the enhanced production of ketone bodies.

Lamotrigine: medication used to treat seizure disorders.

Laryngospasm: spasmodic closure of the larynx.

Lethargy: condition of drowsiness or indifference.

Leukopenia: reduction in the number of leukocytes in the blood.

Leukoplakia: white, thickened patches on the mucous membranes of the cheeks, gums, or tongue that can fissure and become malignant.

Lipodystrophy: any disturbance of fat metabolism.

Lipophilic: any drug which has an affinity for fat.

Lipophobic: any drug which has an aversion to fat.

Lithium: medication used to treat mania.

Local Anesthetics: drugs that produce a loss of sensation in a localized area of the body.

Malignant: rapid new overgrowth of cells that spreads locally or throughout the body.

Mania: a condition characterized by changes in mood which can range from euphoria to depression or a combination of both.

Medicine: any drug or remedy that is used in the diagnosis or treatment of disease and maintenance of health

Metastasis: the condition in which abnormal cells have spread to distant sites throughout the body.

Metabolism: series of chemical alterations of a drug, in the body, by enzymes.

Methylxanthines: class of medications used to treat asthma and emphysema.

Microcytic: a condition in which the red blood cells are small in size.

Minimum Inhibitory Concentration (MIC): lowest concentration needed to inhibit viable growth of an organism after 18–24 hours of incubation.

Miosis: contraction of the pupil.

Miotic: drug that causes the pupil to contract.

Mitosis: method of indirect cell division in which two daughter cells receive identical complements of the number of chromosomes characteristic of the somatic cells of the species.

Monamine Oxidase Inhibitor: class of medication used to treat depression.

Mu Receptor: receptor site that is responsible for respiratory depression, euphoria, and analgesia.

Muscarinic Receptors: receptors located in the parasympathetic nervous system that are stimulated by acetylcholine.

Myalgia: muscular pain.

Mydriasis: dilation of the pupil.

Myxedema: refers to symptoms of adults with hypothyroidism.

Narcosis: stupor or drugged sleep.

Narcotic: drug that produces stupor or sleep.

Necrolysis: exfoliation of necrotic tissue.

Necrosis: death of individual cells or groups of cells or localized areas of tissue.

Neoplasia: overgrowth of cells; increased mitotic activity with the production of abnormal cells.

Nephrotoxicity: destructive or toxic to the kidney.

Neuralgia: pain along the nerves.

Neuronal Agonists: medications that affect the release of norepinephrine from presynaptic nerve endings. They also decrease adrenergic activity and influence α- and β-receptor activity.

Neutropenia: diminished number of neutrophils in the blood.

Nicotinic Receptors: receptors located in the somatic and parasympathetic nervous systems that are stimulated by acetylcholine.

Nitrous Oxide: colorless gas with little or no odor used as a general anesthetic.

Nonbarbiturate/nonbenzodiazepine: class of medications used to treat insomnia.

Nonsteroidal Antiinflammatory Drugs: drugs that reduce pain, inflammation, and fever by blocking prostaglandin synthesis.

Nystagmus: involuntary rapid movement of the eye; can be horizontal, vertical, rotatory or mixed.

Omnipotence: having unlimited power or authority, "all knowing".

Onycholysis: loosening or separation of the nail from its bed.

Oogenesis: the process of the formation of female ova or eggs.

Opioid: morphine-like compound that effects or binds to opiate receptors.

Opportunistic Infections: infections that are able to survive when the body is immunocompromised.

Oral Lesion: traumatic discontinuity of tissue in or around the mouth.

Orthostatic Hypotension: a drop in blood pressure when arising from a sitting position.

Osteoblast: bone formation.

Osteodystrophy: abnormal development of the bone.

Osteomalacia: softening of the bones; resulting from vitamin D deficiency.

Ototoxicity: having ill effects on balance and hearing.

Pain: unpleasant sensory and emotional experience resulting from actual or potential tissue damage.

***p*-aminobenzoic acid (PABA):**   metabolite of procaine.

Pancreas: the organ responsible for the production of insulin and glucagon secreted by islands of cells located throughout the pancreas called the islets of Langerhans.

Pancytopenia: abnormal depression of all elements of the blood.

Parasympathetic Nervous System: the actions of the parasympathetic nervous system are more discrete and generalized and are referred to as "vegetative" responses that dominate when the body is at rest.

Pellagra: niacin (Nicotinic Acid) deficiency.

Peptic Ulcer Disease (PUD): refers to a group of ulcerative disorders of the upper gastrointestinal tract that form in the presence of stomach acid and pepsin.

Periodontitis: inflammation of the periodontium.

Peristalsis: movement of contents through the gastrointestinal tract.

Pernicious Anemia: caused by inadequate absorption of vitamin B_{12}.

Pharmacology: the study of drugs and their effects on living organisms.

pH: the amount of acidity or alkalinity.

Photophobia: abnormal vision intolerance to light.

Physical Dependence: continued use of the drug in order to maintain certain body functions. Withdrawal can lead to physical signs and symptoms.

Pituitary Gland: small gland attached to the hypothalamus at the base of the brain often referred to as the "master" endocrine gland.

pKa: the pH at which half of a compound is in the unionized state and the other half is in the ionized state.

Polydipsia: frequent drinking due to extreme thirst.

Polyphagia: excessive eating.

Polyuria: frequent urination.

Porphyria: a disturbance of porphyrin metabolism characterized by recurrent attacks of abdominal pain, gastrointestinal and neurologic disturbances, with excessive amounts of aminolevulinic acid and porphobilinogen in the urine.

Postural Hypotension: *See* Orthostatic Hypotension

Potency: the dose of drug that is needed to produce the desired therapeutic effect.

Prescription: order for a specific medicine for a specific patient with appropriate directions as to how a patient is to use the medicine.

Progesterone: female sex hormone.

Prostatic Hypertrophy: enlargement of the prostate gland.

Proton Pump Inhibitor: class of medication used to treat peptic ulcer disease.

Psychological Dependence: continued use of the drug for pleasure or to prevent discomfort.

Pubescent: arriving at the age of puberty.

Recommended Dietary Allowance (RDA): recommended daily dietary guidelines for essential vitamins and minerals.

Resistance: occurs when organism growth is not killed or suppressed by antimicrobial drugs.

Reyes Syndrome: syndrome characterized by accute encephalopathy and fatty degeneration of the viscera following acute viral infection.

Rhinitis: inflammation of the nasal mucous membrane.

Rhinorrhea: free discharge of thin nasal mucous.

Rickets: vitamin D deficiency which is the result of the inadequate absorption of calcium and phosphate with decreased calcium in plasma.

Salicylate: salt of salicylic acid.

Salicylism: toxic blood levels of salicylates.

Schizophrenia: disease characterized by such positive symptoms as delusions, hallucinations, and changes in thought content, and/or negative symptoms such as low levels of emotional arousal, mental activity, and social drive.

Scurvy: condition caused by vitamin C deficiency.

Sedation: causing or promoting a calming effect or sleep.

Selective Serotonin Reuptake Inhibitors: class of medication used to treat depression.

Serotonin/Norepinephrine Reuptake Inhibitors: class of medication used to treat depression.

Side-Effect: predictable, dose-related effect of a drug that acts on nontarget organs.

Sigma Receptors: receptor site responsible for dysphoria, hallucinations, anxiety, respiratory and vasomotor stimulation.

Solutions: referring to liquid (oral) fluoride preparations.

Solubility: susceptibility of being dissolved.

Somatic Nervous System: nervous system responsible for voluntary physiologic functions that involve skeletal muscles.

Spectrum: the range of activity of a drug.

Spermatogenesis: the process of the formation of spermatozoa.

Stevens-Johnson Syndrome: a severe form of erythema multiforme characterized by bullae on the oral mucosa, pharynx, ano-genital region, and the conujunctiva.

Stimulant: drug that excites the cardiovascular or central nervous system.

Stomatitis: generalized inflammation of the oral mucosa.

Substance Abuse: continued use of a drug that is inconsistent with medical practice.

Sucralfate: medication used to treat peptic ulcer disease.

Superinfection: caused by the overgrowth of bacteria different from the causative infection.

Sympathetic Nervous System: the actions of the sympathetic nervous system are generalized and widespread and are often referred to as "flight or fright" responses. The sympathetic nervous system is more dominant in times of stress, increased activity, or emergency situations.

Syncope: fainting; sudden fall in blood pressure resulting in cerebral anoxia and subsequent loss of consciousness.

Synergism: the combination of two antimicrobials that is more bactericidal than either drug used alone.

Tachycardia: rapid heartbeat

Teratogenic: leading to the development of abnormal structures in an embryo, resulting in a severely deformed fetus.

Therapeutic Index: ratio of the median lethal dose (LD_{50}) to the median effective dose (ED_{50}).

Thrombin: an enzyme that converts fibrinogen to fibrin.

Thrombocytopenia: an abnormally small number of platelets circulating in the blood.

Thrombophlebitis: venous inflammation with thrombus formation.

Thromboplastin: a substance that is necessary for the conversion of prothrombin to thrombin.

Thyroid: organ responsible for maintaining normal functioning of almost all organ systems, regulating metabolism, and controlling energy expenditure.

Tinnitus: ringing in the ears.

Tolerance: increasing doses of drug to produce the same effect.

Trade Name: registered property of the company that developed the drug that is protected for seventeen years under the Federal Patent Law.

Tricyclic Antidepressants: class of medications used to treat depression.

Tuberculosis: disease caused by the acid-fast bacterium *Mycobacterium tuberculosis* that is highly communicable.

Urticaria: eruption of itching and localized edema; hives.

Valproate: medication used to treat seizure disorders and mania.

Vasoconstrictor: class of drug that causes blood vessels to constrict and thereby decreases blood flow to the site of injection.

Vertigo: dizziness.

Vestibular: pertaining to the part of the ear that helps to maintain balance.

Villi: small vascular protrusions that help to propel material through the membrane.

Vitamins: organic compounds that are necessary for the maintenance of normal metabolic functions but are not synthesized by the body.

Volatile Anesthetic: liquids that evaporate easily upon exposure to room temperature and are classified chemically as halogenated hydrocarbons.

Water Soluble: readily dissolved in or absorbed by water.

Withdrawal: occurrence of objective signs of physical distress when a person abruptly discontinues a drug.

Xerophthalmia: abnormal dryness and thickening of the conjunctiva and cornea.

Xerostomia: dry mouth.

Zolpidem: nonbenzodiazepine sedative-hypnotic that decreases sleep latency and the number of nocturnal awakenings, and increases sleep duration.

Index